APPLICATION OF MONOCLONAL ANTIBODIES IN TUMOR PATHOLOGY

DEVELOPMENTS IN ONCOLOGY

Recent volumes

M.P. Hacker, E.B. Double and I. Krakoff, eds., Platinum Coordination Complexes in Cancer Chemotherapy. ISBN 0-89838-619-5
M.J. van Zwieten, The Rat as Animal Model in Breast Cancer Research: A Histopathological Study of Radiation- and Hormone-Induced Rat Mammary Tumors. ISBN 0-89838-624-1
B. Löwenberg and A. Hagenbeek, eds., Minimal Residual Disease in Acute Leukemia. ISBN 0-89838-630-6
I. van der Waal and G.B. Snow, eds., Oral Oncology. ISBN 0-89838-631-4
B.W. Hancock and A.H. Ward, eds., Immunological Aspects of Cancer. ISBN 0-89838-664-0
K.V. Honn and B.F. Sloane, Hemostatic Mechanisms and Metastasis. ISBN 0-89838-667-5
K.R. Harrap, W. Davis and A.H. Calvert, eds., Cancer Chemotherapy and Selective Drug Development. ISBN 0-89838-673-X
C.J.H. van de Velde and P.H. Sugarbaker, eds., Liver Metastasis. ISBN 0-89838-648-5
D.J. Ruiter, K. Welvaart and S. Ferrone, eds., Cutaneous Melanoma and Precursor Lesions. ISBN 0-89838-689-6
S.B. Howell, ed., Intra-arterial and Intracavitary Cancer Chemotherapy. ISBN 0-89838-691-8
D.L. Kisner and J.F. Smyth, eds., Interferon Alpha-2: Pre-Clinical and Clinical Evaluation. ISBN 0-89838-701-9
P. Furmanski, J.C. Hager and M.A. Rich, eds., RNA Tumor Viruses, Oncogenes, Human Cancer and Aids: On the Frontiers of Understanding. ISBN 0-89838-703-5
J. Talmadge, I.J. Fidler and R.K. Oldham, Screening for Biological Response Modifiers: Methods and Rationale. ISBN 0-89838-712-4
J.C. Bottino, R.W. Opfell and F.M. Muggia, eds., Liver Cancer. ISBN 0-89838-713-2
P.K. Pattengale, R.J. Lukes and C.R. Taylor, Lymphoproliferative Diseases: Pathogenesis, Diagnosis, Therapy. ISBN 0-89838-725-6
F. Cavalli, G. Bonadonna and M. Rozencweig, eds., Malignant Lymphomas and Hodgkin's Disease: Experimental and Therapeutic Advances. ISBN 0-89838-727-2
L. Baker, F. Valeriote and V. Ratanatharathorn, eds., Biology and Therapy of Acute Leukemia. ISBN 0-89838-728-0
J. Russo, ed., Immunocytochemistry in Tumor Diagnosis. ISBN 0-89838-737-X
R.L. Ceriani, ed., Monoclonal Antibodies and Breast Cancer. ISBN 0-89838-739-6
D.E. Peterson, G.E. Elias and S.T. Sonis, eds., Head and Neck Management of the Cancer Patient. ISBN 0-89838-747-7
D.M. Green, Diagnosis and Management of Malignant Solid Tumors in Infants and Children. ISBN 0-89838-750-7
K.A. Foon and A.C. Morgan, Jr., eds., Monoclonal Antibody Therapy of Human Cancer. ISBN 0-89838-754-X
J.G. McVie, W. Bakker, Sj.Sc. Wagenaar and D. Carney, eds., Clinical and Experimental Pathology of Lung Cancer. ISBN 0-89838-764-7
K.V. Honn, W.E. Powers and B.F. Sloane, eds., Mechanisms of Cancer Metastasis. ISBN 0-89838-765-5
K. Lapis, L.A. Liotta and A.S. Rabson, eds., Biochemistry and Molecular Genetics of Cancer Metastasis. ISBN 0-89838-785-X
A.J. Mastromarino, ed., Biology and Treatment of Colorectal Cancer Metastasis. ISBN 0-89838-786-8
M.A. Rich, J.C. Hager and J. Taylor-Papadimitriou, eds., Breast Cancer: Origins, Detection and Treatment. ISBN 0-89838-792-2
D.G. Poplack, L. Massimo and P. Cornaglia-Ferraris, eds., The Role of Pharmacology in Pediatric Oncology. ISBN 0-89838-795-7
A. Hagenbeek and B. Löwenberg, eds., Minimal Residual Disease in Acute Leukemia 1986. ISBN 0-89838-799-X
F.M. Muggia and M. Rozencweig, eds., Clinical Evaluations of Anti-Tumor Therapy. ISBN 0-89838-803-1
F.A. Valeriote and L. Baker, eds., Biochemical Modulation of Anticancer Agents: Experimental and Clinical Approaches. ISBN 0-89838-827-9
B.A. Stoll, ed., Pointers to Cancer Prognosis. ISBN 0-89838-841-4
K.H. Hollmann and J.M. Verley, eds., New Frontiers in Mammary Pathology 1986. ISBN 0-89838-852-X
D.J. Ruiter, G.J. Fleuren and G.O. Warnaar, eds., Application of Monoclonal Antibodies in Tumor Pathology. ISBN 0-89838-853-8

Application of Monoclonal Antibodies in Tumor Pathology

edited by

Dirk J. Ruiter
Department of Pathology, University Medical Center
Nijmegen, The Netherlands

Gert Jan Fleuren & Sven O. Warnaar
Department of Pathology, University Medical Center
Leiden, The Netherlands

1987 SPRINGER-SCIENCE+BUSINESS MEDIA, B.V.

Library of Congress Cataloging in Publication Data

Application of monoclonal antibodies in tumor pathology.

(Developments in oncology)
"Based on a post-graduate Boerhaave course on "Application of monoclonal antibodies in cancer diagnosis," held in Jan. 1986 in Leiden, the Netherland"--Introd.
Includes index.
1. Cancer--Diagnosis--Congresses. 2. Antibodies, Monoclonal--Diagnostic use--Congresses. 3. Tumor antigens --Analysis--Congresses. 4. Immunodiagnosis--Congresses. 5. Immunohistochemistry--Congresses. I. Ruiter, Dirk J. II. Fleuren, Gert Jan. III. Warnaar, Sven O. IV. Series. [DNLM: 1. Antibodies, Monoclonal--congresses. 2. Antigen-Antibody Reactions--congresses. 3. Neoplasms--immunology--congresses. W1 DE998N / QZ 200 A652 1986]
RC270.3.M65A67 1987 616.99'407583 86-31071

ISBN 978-94-010-7981-5 ISBN 978-94-009-3299-9 (eBook)
DOI 10.1007/978-94-009-3299-9

Book Information

This publication is based upon a Boerhaave course organized by the Faculty of Medicine, University of Leiden, The Netherlands in cooperation with the Pathological Society of The Netherlands (NPAV) and the Comprehensive Cancer Centre West (IKW), The Netherlands.

PREFACE

The development of monoclonal antibodies to human tumor associated antigens has greatly facilitated the application of immunohistochemical techniques to analyze surgically removed tissues. During the last few years this approach has been utilized by a progressively increasing number of investigators to analyze malignant cells. Although monoclonal antibodies to tumor associated antigens have not become yet routine reagents in immunopathology, they have provided new information which could not be obtained with conventional antisera or histochemical procedures. The following are representative examples. Tumor associated antigens have been identified which display a restricted distribution in normal tissues and therefore may represent useful markers for radio-imaging and appropriate targets for immunotherapy. In spite of undetectable differences with conventional histopathological approaches heterogeneity has been found in the antigenic profile of tumor cells within a lesion, in autologous lesions removed from different anatomic sites from a given patient and in lesions removed from different patients. Phenotypes of tumor cells have been identified which correlate with the biology of tumor cells and with the clinical course of the disease.

From a practical view point the use of monoclonal antibodies in immunopathology has enhanced interactions between pathologists and immunologists, as exemplified by the present book. Such interactions have contributed to the application of basic research to clinical problems.

The chapter of this book discuss investigations performed with monoclonal antibodies to antigens expressed by various types of normal and malignant human cells. This information will provide an useful background to newcomers and is likely to stimulate additional studies by the experts in the field. The data resulting from such investigations will eventually determine the impact of monoclonal antibodies on the analysis of tumors by pathologists.

S. Ferrone.

CONTENTS

LIST OF MAJOR CONTRIBUTORS.

- J.W. Arends, M.D., Department of Pathology, State University Maastricht. Tongersestraat 53, 6213 GA Maastricht, The Netherlands.
- F.T. Bosman, M.D., Professor of Pathology, Department of Pathology, State University Maastricht, Tongersestraat 53, 6213 GA Maastricht, The Netherlands.
- J.J.M. van Dongen, M.D.,Department of Immunology, Erasmus University Rotterdam, P.O. Box 1738, 3000 DR Rotterdam, The Netherlands.
- J.R.J. Elbers, M.D., Department of Pathology, St. Antonius Hospital, J.V. Scorelstraat 2, 3583 CP Utrecht (Nieuwegein), The Netherlands.
- G.J. Fleuren, M.D., Department of Pathology, State University Leiden, Wassenaarseweg 62, 2300 RC Leiden.
- Ph.C. Hageman, Ph.D., Department of Immunology, Antoni van Leeuwenhoek Ziekenhuis, Plesmanlaan 121, 1066 CX Amsterdam, The Netherlands.
- S.C. Henzen-Logmans, M.D., Department of Pathology, Free University Amsterdam, De Boelelaan 1117, 1081 HV Amsterdam, The Netherlands.
- L. de Leij, Ph.D., Department of Clinical Immunology, State University Groningen, Oostersingel 59, 9713 EZ Groningen, The Netherlands.
- C.J.L.M. Meijer, M.D., Professor of Pathology, Department of Pathology, Free University Amsterdam, De Boelelaan 1117, 1081 HV Amsterdam, The Netherlands.
- H. Mullink, Ph.D., Department of Pathology, Free University Amsterdam, De Boelelaan 1117, 1081 HV Amsterdam, The Netherlands.
- M. Nap, M.D., Streeklaboratorium voor de Volksgezondheid Friesland, Jelsumerstraat 6, 8917 EN Leeuwarden, The Netherlands.
- A.C. Nieuwenhuijzen Kruseman, M.D., Department of Endocrinology, State University Leiden, Rijnsburgerweg 10, 2300 RC Leiden, The Netherlands.
- S. Poppema, M.D., Professor of Pathology, Department of Pathology, State University Groningen, Oostersingel 63, 9713 EZ Groningen, The Netherlands.
- F.C.S. Ramaekers, Ph.D., Department of Pathology, Catholic University Nijmegen, Geert Grooteplein Zuid 24, 6525 GA Nijmegen, The Netherlands.
- D.J. Ruiter, M.D., Professor of Pathology, Department of Pathology, State University Leiden, Wassenaarseweg 62, 2300 RC Leiden, The Netherlands.
- A. Thor, M.D., Laboratory of Tumor Immunology and Biology, National Cancer Institute of Health, Bethesda MD 20205, Maryland, USA.
- G.P. Vooys, M.D., Professor of Pathology, Department of Pathology, Catholic University Nijmegen, Geert Grooteplein Zuid 24, 6525 GA Nijmegen, The Netherlands.

- S.O. Warnaar, Ph.D., Department of Pathology, State University Leiden, Wassenaarseweg 62, 2300 RC Leiden, The Netherlands.

INTRODUCTION

The development of monoclonal antibody technology has resulted in major advances in the clinical and laboratory diagnosis of diseases, particularly in oncology. Although the diagnosis of tumors continues to be based on conventional histopathology, there is a growing demand for additional diagnostic information that can be provided by immunohistochemical techniques.

Following the development of monoclonal antibodies the field of diagnostic immunohistochemistry has expanded tremendously, as can be judged from the marked increase in scientific publications on this subject during the last five years.Many tumor-associated antigens have been identified by monoclonal antibodies. These antibodies are powerful tools in the study of tumor cell differentiation, tumor progression and tumor immunology. Immunohistochemical identification of these antigens in addition may provide important diagnostic and prognostic information, thereby enriching the repertoire of the anatomical pathologist.

Most of the early publications assert antibody specificity for a certain tumor cell type, but later studies on a large volume of normal and abnormal tissues have clearly indicated that monoclonal antibodies with absolute specificity for a particular tumor are exceptional. Although this lack of absolute specificity complicates the application of immunohistochemistry in tumor diagnosis it has been shown convincingly that some antibodies have great diagnostic power, provided they are used in a proper setting.

The large number of tumor-associated antigens, the various immunohistochemical procedures involved and the required knowledge on the proper diagnostic approach and rapid developments of the field are somewhat confusing for the practical anatomical pathologist.

Although excellent books and reviews have been written on tumor markers, immunohistochemistry and application of monoclonal antibodies in certain areas of organ pathology, to our knowledge a comprehensive volume on the application of monoclonal antibodies in tumor pathology has not been published yet. We felt that such a book could be helpful in guiding the practical anatomical pathologist.

This book is divided into three different sections: I. Basic and technical aspects (chapters 1-3), II. Monoclonal antibodies defining tumor-associated antigens, such as cytoskeletal proteins, oncofetal antigens and tumor-type associated antigens (Chapters 4-16) and III. Practical application in tumor diagnosis, containing an introductional review (chapter 17) and a series of case-reports (chapters 18-26). The chapters contain lists of references as a source for further reading. Because the source of the antibodies used should be at hand an appendix with data on antibodies used by authors of various chapters has been compilated. It is hoped that the contents of the book will appeal to the practical anatomical pathologist and to other medical

specialists involved in oncology, to residents in pathology and other specialisms and to researchers in the field.
Both the framework of this book and most contributions are based on a post-graduate Boerhaave course on "Application of monoclonal antibodies in cancer diagnosis" that was held in January 1986 in Leiden, The Netherlands. The positive responses of the participants of the course have stimulated us to produce this book. We would like to show our gratitude to all authors of this book for their excellent cooperation. In addition we would like to thank Dr. Soldano Ferrone for preparing a preface, and Mrs. I.A. Bruinenberg-Kruyff for her skilfull secretarial assistance.

Leiden, June 1986

D.J. Ruiter
G.J. Fleuren
S.O. Warnaar

I. BASIC AND TECHNICAL ASPECTS

1. SELECTION OF MONOCLONAL ANTIBODIES.

S.O. WARNAAR

1. INTRODUCTION

The discovery by Köhler and Milstein (1) of a way to immortalize individual antibody producing cells has greatly expanded the potential to produce antibodies suitable for specific purposes.

For diagnostic pathology only a limited number of antibodies are of interest, i.e. those antibodies that have a restricted tissue distribution and that therefore can be used to distinguish between cell types and differentiation stages.

A number of well known antigens are expressed only in certain differentiated cells. These antigens include hormones, immunoglobulins, prostate specific acid phosphatase, HLA related molecules, cytoskeletal proteins etc. Most of these well known antigens are constitutive, but some oncofetal antigens like CEA and AFP are associated preferentially with malignant cells.

Other antigens specific for certain cell types have been discovered by means of monoclonal antibodies and some of these were subsequently shown to be specific for hitherto unrecognized cell types, e.g. various cell types involved in the immune response.

2. GENERAL ASPECTS

Before starting the preparation of new monoclonal antibodies it is advisable to reflect on the properties desired of these antibodies and to choose or - if necessary - develop selection methods that promote the detection of antibodies of interest.

In developing antibodies against known antigens it should be realized that epitopes are frequently shared between proteins belonging to protein families. Unrelated or presumably unrelated proteins however may also share antigenic amino acid sequences or sugar moieties. This has consequences for the selection procedures for monoclonal antibodies to be used in histopathology. All antibodies developed against known antigens have to be extensively screened on tissue sections for unexpected staining reactions due to epitopes shared between antigens, in order to ensure that the antibodies have sufficient selectivity.

In addition to high selectivity a number of other characteristics can be desirable such as specificity for distinct differentiation stages of cells, specificity for certain tumors, high or low affinity, capacity to react in immuno blots or to precipitate antigens, reaction with cell membrane molecules, specific subclasses of immunoglobulins etc. Depending on the relative weight of any of these desirable properties and the availability of antigens, suitable selection protocols can be devised.

Here it is intended to provide an outline of various steps in the generation and selection of hybridoma clones and to discuss solutions to technical problems from data in the literature and the home laboratory. The emphasis will be to supplement more general reviews of the recent past (2,3). The discussion will be limited to procedures that can be performed in laboratories that do not have access to specialized equipment as cell sorters and high voltage electrofusion apparatuses.

3. IMMUNIZATION PROTOCOLS

Although in the literature an immense variation of immunization schemes can be found only few systematic data are available. Considering the wide variability of physico-chemical properties of antigens and the variable responses to these antigens, depending among others on genetic make up of the mouse, the phenomena of low and high zone tolerance and the declining reactivity of the immune system in older mice, it is advisable, when possible, to inject several mice with different immunization schedules. In all cases young mice from 3-8 weeks should be used. Although there is no unanimous opinion on the question of whether it is possible to obtain monoclonal antibodies from mice that do not have elevated antibody titers, most workers agree that highly immune mice are to be preferred. From the data of Stähli et al (ref 3 pg 26) it was suggested that successful fusions were the result of fusion of a myeloma cell with a B lymphoblast. Therefore immunization schedules are currently aiming at obtaining a high number of antigen specific B blasts. This is effected by giving boosters in the period immediately before fusion. Successful protocols are described in ref.3,4,5. In more complicated immunization schedules spleens of immunized mice are removed and spleen cells are transferred into recipient mice either directly or after in vitro immune stimulation with antigen. The recipient mice can then be further boosted with antigen injections (6). For most antigens such fairly complicated schemes should not be necessary.

Selection of mice: Most workers have used BALB/c mice. Apart from general considerations such as age and H-2 determined sensitivity or resistance of the mice to immunization it is possible by using mice with a so called Robertsonian translocation to reduce the workload in obtaining useful hybrids. In the usual selection system hybridomas between spleen donor and myeloma cells are selected for in medium with aminopterine. This medium will not permit the growth of the parent myeloma cells, due to a deficient hypoxanthin phosphoribosyl transferase enzyme(HPRT). The HPRT enzyme is located on the X chromosome, whereas the immunoglobulin heavy chain is located on chromosome 12 and light chain genes on chromosomes 6 and 16 respectively. Surviving hybridomas must contain an X chromosome from the spleen donor. Potentially useful hybridomas that loose the spleen X chromosome are incapable of further growth in aminopterine. Surviving

hybridomas that loose the chromosomes 6,16 or 12 bearing information for light or heavy chains of immunoglobulins will become non secretors. As the production of antibody by the hybridoma cells is considerable and does not contribute to the cell maintenance, non secretors tend to grow faster and to overwhelm the antibody producing cells in mixed cultures. These problems are partially relieved in fusions with spleens from RBF/Dn mice (obtainable from the Jackson Laboratory, Bar Harbor, Maine 04609) with FOX-NY cells. In the RBF/Dn mice the genes for the heavy chains of Ig are translocated to chromosome 8 and are genetically linked to the genes for adenosine-phosphoribosyltransferase (APRT). The Fox-NY cells (7) are deficient in APRT. Hybridomas that do not contain the heavy chain gene cannot grow in the APRT selective medium. This greatly reduces the problem of instability of hybridomas due to overgrowth of non secretors or loss of X chromosomes.
The RBF/Dn mice are slightly more difficult to handle and in our hands the fusion efficiency between RBF spleens and FOX-NY cells was somewhat reduced.

4. FUSION PROTOCOLS

For the fusion process a myeloma cell line and immune spleen cells are brought closely together after which membrane fusion and heterokaryon production can take place by applying special fusion agents such as poly ethylene glycol, Sendai virus or electro shocks. Several factors are important. In the first place the myeloma cell line. Several cell lines are available that do not themselves synthesize immunoglobulin chains. Cell lines most frequently used are SP2/0, X63/Ag8653 and NSO/U (8,9). These cell lines originate from Balb/c mice. For fusions with spleens from RBF/Dn mice the FOX-NY cells should be used as explained before. The myeloma cells should be in optimal conditions, that is in the logaritmic phase of cell growth. It is advisable to preestablish that the cell line used is free of mycoplasm and capable of growing when plated at one cell per well in a microtiter plate. It helps to use cells that have been passaged a few times in soft agar, to select a more robust clone. With proper myeloma cells and a good fusion protocol about $5\text{-}10 \times 10^3$ individual hybridoma cells will be obtained from one mouse spleen. In the following paragraphs details will be given on the protocol used in our laboratory. For other protocols which may vary slightly, the reader may consult ref.2.

4.1 Culture medium
RPMI 1640 buffered with HEPES and containing 10% fetal calf serum, supplemented with 2×10^6 units penicillin and 50mg streptomycin per liter. To obtain optimal growth of parent myeloma cells 2×10^{-5} M β mercaptoethanol is added.
For selecting hybridomas HAT is added: aminopterin at 0.17 mg/l and hypoxanthin and thymidin at respectively 13.6 mg/L and 3.8 mg/L.

4.2 Myeloma cells in logarithmic phase are washed twice in RPMI .

4.3 Spleen cells.

Remove the mouse spleen aseptically and gently press the spleen cells through a metal gauze. Wash the cells down with RPMI and centrifuge the cells 5 min at 200g. Resuspend the spleen cells in 25 ml of erylysis buffer containing 8.3 gr NH_4 Cl 1.0 gr $KHCO_3$ 0.037gr EDTA/liter. Incubate 5-10 min at 37C. Add 50 ml of cold RPMI and centrifuge 5 min at 200g. Wash the pellet twice by resuspending in cold RPMI followed by centrifuging.

4.4 Fusion.

Count SP2/0 and spleen cells. Add 4 x 10^7 SP2/0 cells to 1 x 10^8 spleen cells in RPMI. Centrifuge and remove all liquid as well as possible. Tap centrifuge tube to loosen cell pellet. Warm cells to 37C. Add 0.5 ml of PEG solution (50% PEG 1500 from (BDH). Gently shake cells in PEG solution. After 1 min add 0.5 ml RPMI of 37C. Keep shaking slowly. Then over a period of 10 min add 50 ml of warm RPMI medium. At this stage the actual fusion has been performed. It is important to use PEG batches of proven quality and to keep the time of contact of cells with PEG short.

The main variations on the scheme above are the following:

a) Total spleen cells can be used including erythrocytes. In our hands the treatment of spleen cells with erylysis buffer effectively removes erythrocytes without loss of viability of spleen cells. When the fused cells are to be plated in soft agar removal of erythrocytes is essential.

b) PEG with different molecular weight can be used and the concentration can be between 35-50%. Also the time the cells are kept in contact with PEG is sometimes increased up to 5-6 minutes.

c) The ratio of spleen cells to myeloma cells can be varied from about 10/1 to 2/1. Most likely all these variables have only modest effects as the main factors responsible for successful fusions most probably relate to the conditions of the myeloma cells, spleen cells and the use of high quality reagents and sera.

4.5 Plating of cells.

After the fusion reaction has been completed the cells can be plated out. In case ELISA or RIA is going to be used to assay for positive clones the cells should be plated in 300-400 wells of microtiter plates in 0.1 ml of RPMI + HAT and placed in a CO_2 box at 37C. Many laboratories use seeding on feeder layers. Mouse peritoneal macrophages can be used, seeded at 10^4 cells per microtiter well the day before the fusion is planned. In our hands the macrophages remove not only dying myeloma cells but will also damage growing hybridomas. Therefore we do not use feeder cells. Instead it is recommended to add 10% of culture medium from a 6 day mixed lymphocyte culture derived from spleen cells of Balb/C and C57/BL6 mice.

In case antigen is amply available or when whole cells have been used as immunizing agents it is recommended to plate the fused cells in soft agar. For this end prepare 20 5cm dishes with 10 ml of RPMI-HAT containing 10% fetal calf serum 0.5 μg/ml lipo- polysaccharide and 10 μg/ml of concanavalin A with a final agar concentration of 1% (bottom agar). After the agar has set the fused spleen-myeloma cells in 30 ml of complete RPMI-HAT medium at 37C are added to 4.5 ml of 5% agar to yield a final concentration of 0.6% agar. After swirling, 1.5 ml of this suspension is added to the dishes containing bottom agar. The dishes are placed at 4C for 15 min to allow the agar to set. It is convenient to use low temperature gelling agar as this eliminates chances of subjecting the fusion mix to temperature shock and also eliminates undue gelling before the cells have been plated into the dishes.

After the agar has set the dishes are incubated in a CO_2 box at 37C.

When the cells are incubating at 37C they should be left undisturbed for at least 5 days. Then cells in microtiter plates can be inspected for growth and an additional 0.1 ml of complete RPMI plus HAT are added. Ten days after plating both the cells growing in microtiter plates and those in agar dishes can be tested for useful hybridomas.

5. DETECTION OF MONOCLONAL ANTIBODIES OF INTEREST

5.1 Introduction

Before discussing various protocols in detail some general comments should be made. It is very important to realize that no single test exists for the detection of all clones that produce antibodies against the antigen used for immunization and tests that may be extremely sensitive for certain antibodies may not detect anything at all with other relevant antibodies. The binding of antibody to antigen is sensitive to alterations in pH and ionic strength, factors that may alter the conformations of antibody binding sites and of the determinants recognized. Also other factors may be important, such as detergents, fixatives and reagents that break S-S bonds. Last but not least the way the antigen is presented is important, e.g. bound to a solid substrate, to a conventional antibody or free floating in solution as is most often the case in RIA assays.

To the above considerations it can be added that antibodies that react quite specifically with certain antigens under one set of conditions may show unwanted side reactions under different conditions. From these accumulated data it is clear that the reaction conditions of the detection method used should resemble as closely as possible the conditions under which the antibodies are to be used eventually. All data on specificity and binding constants will only be reliable under constant assay conditions.

After these initial remarks we can now turn to the problem of identifying hybridoma clones of potential interest.

5.2 Requirements of detection tests

All detection tests for monoclonal antibody production should be sensitive and simple to perform and should be able to handle large numbers (2-400) of samples in 1-2 days.

The tests more of less fullfilling these requirements are successively: radio immune precipitation (RIP), immune radiometric assays (IRMA), enzyme linked immuno sorbent assays (ELISA) and various dot assays. More time consuming are immunoblot assays and immunohistochemistry. The last assay however is essential in developing antibodies for diagnostic purposes in histopathology. All assays mentioned above can only be carried out with hybridoma supernatants. When the cells have been initially plated in soft agar a number of filter tests are available as will be discussed later.

5.3 Freezing of cells

In case many hybridomas are detected it can be necessary to freeze away as many clones as possible. Several papers have described the freezing away of cells still in the originally wells of microtiter plates (ref.17-18). While certainly useful it appears that cell viability is adversely affected and therefore loss of secretors is possible.

5.4 Radioimmune precipitation tests (RIP).

An extensive literature exists on the RIP and the related RIA test. For use in testing hybridoma supernatants the main disadvantages are the necessity to radioactively label the antigen and the need to separate bound from unbound antigen effectively. This necessitates a centrifugation step and washing of the pellets. The final precipitates can either be visualized by autoradiography (not very sensitive for short illuminations) or can be counted in a γ or liquid scintillation counter.

When protein A containing staphylococcus aureus is used to precipitate immune complexes it is possible to loose IgG1 producing clones due to poor binding of this subclass to protein A.

A protocol for handling hybridoma supernatants with a RIP test is given in the literature (11). When labeled antigen is available a variant of a dotting technique can also be used. Crude culture supernatants are fixed to nitrocellulose by dotting and the nitrocellulose is then incubated with labeled antigen. The dots can be counted or autoradiographed.

IRMA tests can be used only when conventional antibodies to the antigens of interest are available or when previous work has already resulted in a monoclonal antibody. Therefore these tests in general are not applicable. A four step IRMA test has been devised to select monoclonal antibodies to allergens (12). In this assay the monoclonal antibodies are fixed to a plastic support by means of an anti mouse kappa antibody. After reaction with allergen a patient serum containing Ig E antibodies is added. Detection is with ^{125}J labeled anti IgE.

5.5 ELISA tests.

These tests are very well suited for developing monoclonal antibodies to defined antigens provided these antigens are available in sufficient amounts and purity. Antigen is fixed to wells in microtiter plates, either directly or linked through a conventional antibody. After reaction with monoclonal antibody an anti mouse antibody conjugated to enzyme is added and the reaction is visualized by development with appropriate substrates. Al Moudallal et al (13) have compared different ELISA procedures, of the direct binding and the "sandwich" type, for the detection of antibodies to tobacco mosaic virus (TMV). The enzyme label used was alkaline phosphatase. For this antigen and the 9 monoclonal anti-TMV antibodies tested no reaction was found in procedures in which antigen was directly coated to the plates. In contrast in sandwich methods where antigen was bound to the plates by means of a conventional anti TMV antibody, all 9 antibodies reacted with TMV. This clearly shows that even within a single type of assay the way the antigen is presented is of utmost importance. This is also illustrated by Vaida et al (14) who reported that 4/7 antibodies positive in direct ELISA against creatin kinase were negative in a competition type ELISA or in RIA. Also 16 antibodies positive in ELISA against lactate dehydrogenase (LDH) were negative with radiolabeled or native LDH in solution.

The enzymes that are used in ELISA are either horse radish peroxidase (HRPO), alkaline phosphatase or β galactosidase. Porstmann et al (15) have compared the relative sensitivities of these enzymes, both in colorimetric and fluorimetric assays, for the detection of α fetoprotein. It was shown in this system that HRPO using ABTS as substrate was 5-7 fold more sensitive than the other two enzymes. If O-phenylene diamine is used the sensitivity of HRPO ELISA's can be further increased. The advantage of using β galactosidase is mainly in the fact that mammalian cells do not contain β galactosidase activity. In ELISA's on crude cell extracts this can be an advantage.

Basic ELISA protocol for soluble antigens.

1. Coat wells in microtiter plate with 0.1μg of antigen in 100μl of 0.1 M $NaHCO_3$ pH 9.5, by incubating overnight at 4C. Alternatively let fluid evaporate at 37C. This will give better results for many antigens.
2. Saturate remaining binding sites in plate with 1% bovine serum albumin (BSA) in phosphate buffered saline containing 0.5% Triton X-100. Other blocking agents such as ovalbumin and gelatin can also be used. Incubate plates at least 2 hrs with blocking solution.
3. Incubate 2-24 hrs with hybridoma supernatant, wash 3 times with PBS.
4. Incubate 1 hr with anti-mouse Ig conjugated to enzyme, preferably horseradish peroxidase. This conjugated antiserum should be preabsorbed with the protein used for blocking. After the incubation wash 3 times with PBS.
5. Add substrate for 20 minutes.
   For HRPO this is 40 mg of orthophenylene diamine in 100 ml of 0.025 M phosphate-citrate buffer pH 5.0. Immediately before adding this substrate solution to the microtiter wells add 40 μl of 30% H_2O_2. Stop with 50 μl of 2N H_2SO_4. For alkaline phosphatase use as substrate a solution containing 1 mg/ml para-nitrophenylphosphate dissolved in 10% diethanolamine pH 9.8. Stop with 50 μl 3N NaOH.
   For β galactosidase use 1 mg/ml O-nitrophenyl β-D galactopyranoside dissolved in 0.1M sodium borate, 0.1M

NaCl and 10mm $MgCl_2$ pH 8.5. Stop reaction with 50µl 1M $Na_2 CO_3$.

6. Read reactions with a spectrofotometer at 492, 405 or 420 nm respectively. For screening monoclonal antibodies visual inspection suffices.

Variations on this basic ELISA scheme involve the use of antibody to bind the antigen to the plastic. Other variations include a more complicated detection system. After the binding of monoclonal antibody to the antigen add unlabeled rabbit-anti-mouse Ig, followed by goat-anti-rabbit Ig conjugated to enzyme or, alternatively a mouse antiperoxidase-peroxidase complex (PAP complex). These modifications can greatly influence the outcome of the ELISA test, see Al Moudallal et al (13).

When using ELISA as initial screening for monoclonal antibodies it is also necessary to establish that clones that give a positive signal do not react with the blocking protein used for saturating the binding sites of the plate. This is best done by repeating the ELISA in wells not containing the relevant antigen.

In case many antibodies are detected in the initial screen it is worthwile to find out which antibodies have highest affinity for the relevant antigen. To determine relative affinities exactly is laborious, therefore one can assume that antibody production of each clone is roughly similar and proceed to determine which of the antibodies can be diluted furthest still giving a positive signal (16).

For performing ELISA tests on whole cells the following modifications of the basic ELISA can be useful.

1. Polylysine coupling. Dissolve poly-L-lysine in phosphate buffered saline to 10 µg/ml. Add 100 µl to each well of a microtiter plate (96 wells). Incubate overnight at 4C and wash with PBS. Prepare the cells in PBS at a concentration of 10^5 cells/ml. Add 100 µl to each well. Incubate for 45 minutes. Wash in PBS and add 0.3% glutaraldehyde in PBS for 5 minutes. Wash the plate with PBS and block remaining glutaraldehyde binding sites with 1% BSA in PBS overnight. The plates are now ready for use. Continue with step 3 of the basic ELISA described above.
2. Glutaraldehyde coupling. Add 100µl of 0.5% glutaraldehyde to the wells of a microtiter plate. Incubate for 2 hrs at 37C. Wash with PBS. Add 10^4 cells in 100 µl of PBS per well. Centrifuge the plate at 200 g for 10 min. Incubate for an additional 30 min. at 37C. Wash with PBS and block remaining glutaraldehyde binding sites with 1% BSA in PBS as described above. Continue with step 3 of basic ELISA protocol.

5.6 Dot and blot assays

Nitrocellulose will bind proteins virtually irreversibly and advantage has been taken of this fact to develop simple dot assays for detection of monoclonal antibodies specific for certain antigens.

The procedure is as follows:

1. Spot 1 µl of antigen in PBS in the center of a 4 mm nitrocellulose disk. The amount of antigen spotted can be as low as 0.1 ng although quantities of 5-10 ng are recommended for initial screening purposes.
2. Block remaining binding sites on the nitrocellulose with 1% BSA, ovalbumin or gelatin for at least 2 hrs.
3. Put filter disks in wells of microtiter plates. Add 100 µl of culture supernatants from hybridomas. Incubate 2 hrs at 37C, rock gently.
4. Wash disks 3 times with 0.01 M Tris HCl pH 7.4 containing 1% Triton X-100, 0.5 % Sarcosyl NL30 and 0.02% SDS (washbuffer).
5. Incubate for 1 hr with rabbit-antimouse-Ig conjugated to HRPO. This conjugate has to be preabsorbed with blocking protein.
6. Wash 3 times with wash buffer.
7. Develop with 0.03% 3,3 diamino benzidine 0.01% H_2O_2 and 1 mM imidazole in 50mM Tris-HCl pH 7.4 for 2-10 minutes. Stop with 0.01 M β mercaptoethanol.

This assay is comparatively simple, the only drawback being the necessity to punch the nitrocellulose disks. Bennett and Yeoman (19) have modified the procedure in the following way: 1µl dots are made on a sheet of nitrocellulose paper so that each dot can be centered over a well of a microtiter plate. After blocking the binding sites on the nitrocellulose, the sheet is clamped over a microtiter plate containing the hybridoma supernatants to be tested. After clamping the plate is inverted to allow contact of hybridoma medium with the nitro cellulose sheet. After incubation a protocol similar to that given above starting from step 5 is followed. The main difficulty is in preventing leakage from one well to the next.

We have found that a small antigen, epithelial growth factor, with a molecular weight of 6000D was not bound to the nitrocellulose unless it was allowed to thoroughly dry at 60C for at least 2 hrs. McDougal et al (20) report that also Ig preparations dotted on nitrocellulose will bind better when allowed to dry.

Several modifications of the dot assays have been described. McDougal et al (20) described a variation permitting the determination of heavy and light chains of immunoglobulins without having to concentrate the culture supernatants.

Briefly, isotype specific antibodies are immobilized as dots on nitrocellulose paperstrips. After incubation with the hybridoma supernatants any reaction is visualized with an antimouse Ig antibody conjugated to HRPO by developing with diaminobenzidine and H_2O_2. This procedure permits the rapid selection of hybridomas of preferred isotypes in cases when many clones have been generated.

When labeled antigen is available a variant of a dotting technique can be used (2). Crude culture supernatants are fixed to nitrocellulose by dotting and the nitrocellulose is then incubated with labeled antigen. The dots can be counted or autoradiographed.

Towbin et al (22) have reviewed the blotting and dotting of antigens and the use in hybridoma technology. Obviously

these procedures are related, the main differences being that immunoblotting also reveals the molecular weight of the antigen in cases where this is unknown.
For antigens that are closely related, such as antigens belonging to protein families it is advantageous to screen each antibody against a battery of spots each containing one of the related antigens. Occasionally it is easier to prepare immunoblots of complicated antigen mixes than to purify individual antigens for spotting. It is entirely feasible to screen 0.2 ml samples of hybridoma supernatants on narrow strips of immunoblotted extracts. In our laboratory we have repeatedly screened several hundred hybridoma supernatants on immunoblots of cytokeratin preparations. These proteins constitute a family of about 20 closely related protein chains. The generation of chain specific anticytokeratin antibodies would have been impossible without an early immunoblotting step.
When performing immunoblots or dots it is necessary to realize that different blocking agents can cause varation in the immunologic detection of antigens. Spinola and Cannon (23) have compared bovine serum albumin, milk protein and Tween 20 as blocking agents in immunoblots of several conventional antibody-antigen combinations. No single blocking agent consistently permitted detection of all possible bands, although BSA and Tween 20 gave best results. NP40 seemed to be deleterious for certain antigen-antibody complexes. In our own laboratory we have found that monoclonal antibodies to cytokeratins may show different specificities when tested in Tris-HCl or in phosphate containing buffers.

Towbin et al (23) have also published a method to blot glyco and sphingo-lipids after separating these substances on thin layer plates. Glyco-and sphingolipids are antigens associated with cell membranes and many monoclonal antibodies obtained after immunization with whole cells recognize glyco- or sphingo-lipids.

5.7 Filter tests

When the original spleen-myeloma fusion mix has been plated in soft agar the clones producing antibodies of interest can be detected using a filter assay (25).
For soluble antigens the procedure is as follows:
Sterile antigen at 20-50μg/ml in PBS is incubated with gentle shaking with sterile nitrocellulose filters of 48 mm diameter. For each filter 50-100 μg of antigen is ample. We have occasionally used filters coated with 1 μg of antigen. After shaking overnight at 4C remaining binding sites on the filters are saturated by incubating with 10% bovine serum. Control filters without antigen or with a related antigen to which antibodies of interest should not bind are similarly prepared.
For screening against cells, filters are placed on a millipore suction funnel and $5x10^5$-$2x10^6$ cells in 10 ml of PBS are sucked through. The filters are then sterilized by UV irradiation for a period of 2x20 min at 60 cm with a 60W UV lamp and washed extensively in sterile water. The sterilized filters are then saturated with 10% bovine serum.

As soon as the colonies growing in agar have the appropriate size (about 50-100 cells per colony), excess liquid on the agar plates is removed and the plates are placed at 4C for 15 min to stiffen the agar. Pairs of filters are placed on top of the agar, the negative control filter in contact with the agar and the antigen containing filter on top of the first filter. Three small asymmetrically placed holes have to be punched in the antigen filter to help find the proper orientation of filter on the agar. With a fine needle the negative control filters are punched through the holes in the upper filter. With a pencil the positions of the holes are marked on the bottom side of the agar dishes. Incubate the dishes for 16 hrs at 37C in the CO_2 box. The antibodies that are shed in the agar by hybridoma clones will diffuse towards the filter and, depending on the specificities, will bind either to the antigen-containing filter, to both filters or to none of the filters respectively. Shorter incubations are possible. We have incubated dishes with single filters for periods as short as 3-4 hrs. This allows a second negative control filter to be included in the first screening assay.
After incubating the dishes at 37C they are replaced to 4C for 15 min to facilitate removal of the filters. The dishes and corresponding filters are numbered.
The filters are then incubated at room temperature with rabbit antimouse Ig-HRPO for 2 hrs and washed with washbuffer (see 5.6). The washed filters are then developed with diaminobenzidine, imidazole and H_2O_2 as described above for dots. Then the filters are sorted in pairs and the spots that are present on the antigen containing filter and not present on the negative control filter(s) are punched out with a 2 mm punch. Then the antigen containing filter with the punched out spots is positioned under the corresponding dish, care being taken to align the asymmetric orientation holes to their proper positions.
With an inverted microscope it is now possible to view the relevant clones through the punches in the filters. With drawn out Pasteur pipettes with a skewed end it is possible to pick the individual clones out of the agar. These clones are then put into wells of 96 well microtiter plates in 200 μl of HAT complete medium + 10% conditioned medium from the SP2/0 parent myeloma and 5-10% of mixed lymphocyte culture medium prepared as described before. After 4-7 days the supernatant medium in these wells is ready for further testing.
This filter procedure is extremely simple and attractive as it enables one to immediately pick individual clones of interest. Some additional comments may be helpful. When filters have been sterilized with UV light it is very important to wash extensively with pyrogen free H_2O as apparently some toxic substances are generated that are difficult to remove. If these substances have not been removed completely before the filters are layered over the colonies in the agar one will still find spots due to antibody binding to the filters but the viability of the clones will be poor. Normally we find that from 60-90% of

picked clones will grow well when put into liquid medium. With toxic filters growth may be zero. Also it is important always to use a negative control filter. Many clones will produce antibodies that will stick to virtually anything. The percentage of interesting clones - depending on the immune status of the animal used may be anything from 0.1-5%, therefore with only an antigen containing filter too many irrelevant clones will be picked.
The filter detection method can be modified to identify clones secreting specific subclasses of immunoglobulins by using subclass specific second antibodies conjugated to HRPO. A very useful modification is an adaptation that will detect all antibody secretors.
The procedure is as follows:
Incubate 48 mm filters with 50-100 μg of rabbit anti mouse Ig in PBS. Alternatively this amount of antibody may be sucked through the filter similar to the procedure described for coating filters with cells. After saturating remaining binding sites with 10% FCS the rabbit anti mouse Ig(RAM) filters are placed on top of the agar that contains the colonies to be screened. Antibodies secreted by the clones will diffuse to the filter and will be bound by the RAM. After 16 hrs incubation the filters are removed and incubated with RAM conjugated to HRPO for 2 hrs. Development is as usual with diaminobenzidine, imidazole and H_2O_2.
This modification is extremely useful for recloning hybridomas of interest as the intensity of the spots is related to the amount of antibody produced by the clones. With unstable clones with heavy overgrowth by non secretors this procedure will easily pick up any secretors remaining as it is possible to seed about 500-1000 cells per dish. With limiting dilution procedures in microtiter plates such clones are almost always lost. We have used a similar procedure to identify human antibody producing clones with the use of goat anti-human Ig coated filters as catchers. It is also possible to use a filter procedure to detect class switch variants by coating the filter with Ig subclass specific antibodies. This may again prove easier than the limiting dilution method of Spira et al.(26).

5.8 Screening on tissue sections

When antibodies against known antigens are to be used for diagnostic purposes on histological preparations they have to be extensively screened against a very wide panel of normal and abnormal tissues to establish that no unwanted cross reactions occur. Many antibodies in the literature were initially claimed to be very specific but fell through when tested on wider panels of tissue sections.
When antibodies are being developed against as yet unknown antigens specific for certain cell types or differentiation stages or specific for certain tumor types and it is intended to use these antibodies in immunohistochemical identification of celltype(s), it is advisable to screen the hybridoma supernatants at a very early stage on tissue sections.

It has been found that the way the tissues have been treated before making the thin sections is very important for the final outcome of the immunohistochemical staining reactions. For most purposes the best way of handling tissue specimen is to freeze them as rapidly as possible in isopentane with frozen CO_2 and to store the frozen tissue blocks at -70C. Sections of 4μm can then be cut and mounted on gelatin coated glass slides. After an acetone fixation of 5 minutes the tissue sections are ready for use. Some antibodies however will not react with frozen sections but will only react with tissues that have been fixed with formalin, Bouin or other fixatives. A heat treatment step such as occurs when fixed tissues are embedded in paraffin may also be necessary. Presumably the antigenic determinants recognized by these antibodies are hydrophobic determinants that are normally hidden and that become exposed when the surrounding proteins and or polysaccharides are subjected to denaturing agents. Of course a number of antibodies will react both with frozen sections and with formalin fixed and paraffin embedded material. These remarks may be illustrated by the results of a typical fusion experiment in which antibodies were generated from a spleen of a mouse immunized with renal carcinoma cells. Out of 126 clones that were picked from agar plates as described before and screened with filters coated with renal carcinoma cells or liver cells (negative control), 66 clones reacted with frozen sections only, 13 clones reacted with frozen sections and paraffin sections and 5 clones reacted with paraffin sections only.
For small antigens it may be necessary to use a strong fixative such as formalin or Bouin as otherwise the antigen will be washed out of the section during the immune incubations. This holds for example for polypeptide hormones and for other small molecules like epidermal growth factor.
Screening of hybridoma supernatants on tissue sections is a very powerful discriminating tool, as in most tissues various different cell types are present. This usually gives a good impression of whether an antibody will show undesired side reactions. Due to the multitude of antigenic determinants present it is not advisable to assay the tissue sections with supernatants that may contain antibodies from more than one hybridoma clone, such as usually is the case when fusion mixtures have been plated directly in microtiter wells. For testing on tissue sections antibodies can best be developed using the nitrocellulose filter techniques described before . The clones that eventually are picked from the agar can be grown in liquid medium. The supernatant medium of these cultures can be applied to the tissue sections of interest.
In addition to fixation the conditions during the incubation of the antibodies with the sections is also important. Some antibodies will only react at low ionic strength whereas other antibodies may be quite specific at elevated ionic strength and show considerable nonspecific cross reactions when tested at low ionic strength. Sternberger et al (27) have described antibodies that will react in Tris buffered solutions but not in phosphate buffers. The determinants

recognized in this case were phosphorylated sites on neuronal proteins. For these reasons it is necessary to adhere to the protocols for which it has been demonstrated that a given antibody gives specific results. The reliability of staining results on tissue sections is related to the efforts made by the developer to ascertain the specificity of the staining reaction. A brief outline of a protocol for use on tissue sections is given below.

5.8.1 Protocol for paraffin embedded sections

a. Deparaffinize the sections in xylol and a graded series of ethanol-H_2O.
b. Block endogenous peroxidase activity by incubating for 5 minutes in methanol + 1% H_2O_2. This step is optional.
c. Hydrate sections for 5 minutes in PBS.
d. Incubate for at least 1 hr with 10% normal rabbit serum diluted in PBS.

5.8.2 Protocol for frozen sections

a. Fix sections for 10 min in aceton.
b. Hydrate sections for 5 min in PBS.

5.8.3 Continuation of protocols 5.8.1 and 5.8.2

The following steps are the same for both paraffin embedded and frozen sections.

1. Wipe the glass slide surrounding the section. Add 50-100 μl of hybridoma supernatant. Incubate for 2 hrs in a humid chamber.
2. Wash sections 3x5 min with PBS and wipe sections.
3. Apply 50-100 μl of rabbit anti mouse conjugated to HRPO (RAM-HRPO). This antibody has to be preadsorbed with 10% normal human serum for at least one hour. The RAM-HRPO should be allowed to react with any mouse Ig on the sections for 1-2 hrs.
4. Wash 3x5 min with PBS.
5. Incubate for 10 min in 0.03% diaminobenzidine (DAB) in 0.05M Tris pH 7.4 + 0.01 % H_2O_2 or alternatively with 3 amino 9-ethylcarbazole (AEC): 40 mg AEC + 10 ml formamide in 200 ml of 0.1 M NaAc pH 5.0.
6. Counterstain nuclei for 2 min in hematoxylin. Dry sections stained with DAB in graded alcohol and finally in xylol. AEC stain will dissolve in alcohol. These sections should be directly mounted with a coverslip using Aqua mount (Gurr) as mounting fluid.

The following notes may be useful:

1) The blocking of endogenous peroxidase is necessary only in cases where inflammatory cells possessing peroxidase activity disturb the proper interpretation or quality of the staining reactions. Antigenic determinants not related to peroxidase may be harmed by this step, therefore for screening it is usually omitted.

2) If paraffin sections are not preincubated with normal rabbit serum the background staining is increased.

3) If insufficient staining is obtained with DAB the reaction may be significantly enhanced by adding 1mM imidazole(28).
To make sure that the protocol has been followed correctly it is advisable to include positive controls (antibodies that in previous experience gave good staining results) and negative controls, such as supernatant medium from myeloma cells not containing mouse antibodies or irrelevant mouse antibodies and a section that is not incubated with RAM-HRPO.

5.9 Screening on cultured cells
Screening hybridoma supernatants on cultured cells permits the detection of antibodies affecting functional tests such as cell lysis, cell adhesion, alteration of cell morphology, migration etc. This is a comparatively poorly developed field that merits further study. Vollmers et al (29) have described antibodies that affect growth and morphology of B16 melanoma cells. The antibodies were found to induce more normal behaviour of the cells and were capable of reducing the number of lungtumors when injected into mice preinjected with B16 melanoma cells.
Cheresh et al (30) described a monoclonal antibody that recognizes a di-sialoganglioside on melanoma cells. This ganglioside can serve as a target for monoclonal antibody mediated cytolysis.
Other groups have described antibodies interfering with cell-cell adhesion in various systems.

5.10 Antibodies to carbohydrate or glycolipid determinants
Often it is difficult to establish the nature of the antigen that is recognized by monoclonal antibodies, especially when immunoblotting does not indicate a specific band.
In these cases it may be useful to extract gangliosides and glycolipids with chloroform-methanol-H_2O (31). These substances can then be subjected to thin layer chromatography and blotting (24) or may be used in ELISA tests.
A simple method to evaluate whether a monoclonal antibody is reacting with a determinant that contains vicinal hydroxyl groups, often present in carbohydrates, is to treat the antigen with 0.5 mM of sodium periodate at pH 4.5 for 1 hr (32).

6. ASCITES PRODUCTION/STORAGE
Although antibodies derived from tissue culture are to be preferred for most purposes, and existing technology is capable of producing large quantities of such antibodies it may nevertheless be practicable to produce a quantity in ascites as the antibody titer can be 100-1000 fold higher in ascites than in tissue culture medium. Broders et al have investigated some parameters of antibody yield when produced in ascites (33).
They found that the optimal inoculum of hybridoma cells was between $6x10^6$ and $32x10^6$ cells and that the receiving mice should be pretreated with 0.5 ml of pristane 14 days before

being injected with hybridoma cells. The mice should preferably be between 6 and 10 weeks old.
Truitt et al (34) have described that human-human hybridomas can be grown in ascites in nude mice after having had a passage in nude mice as a subcutaneously growing tumor. Underwood and Bean (35) have demonstrated that monoclonal antibodies from tissue culture or ascites can show altered crossreactivities after physical treatments that can occur in normal storage or purification. Freezing and thawing, heating to 60°C for short periodes (as is done when traces of complement have to be removed), short exposures to pH 3 or 10 were all found to alter the qualities of certain antibodies. The passage of hybridoma cells in ascites was in itself found to alter the specificity of a number of antibodies, possibly due to somatic mutation at the antigen recognition site during growth in the mouse peritoneal cavity. The authors therefore stress the importance of documenting the methods of production, purification and storage of particular monoclonal antibodies.

7. PERSPECTIVES

The monoclonal antibody field has already seen tremendous progress in virtually all aspects from immunization and in vitro immunization techniques, large scale production and purification to applications. These include applications in histopathological diagnosis, identification of functions of cell types, monitoring of patient sera for various tumor related antigens, immuno scintigraphic detection of tumors and - to some extent - as therapeutic agents.
The promising aspects of these applications have been recognized by various commercial companies. This has resulted in the allocation of large sums of money for further development of practical applications. For the pathologist it can be expected that progressively better antibodies will become available to help in the identification of poorly differentiated tumors. As all antibodies have to be extensively screened for specificity on normal and abnormal human tissues, departments of pathology are eminently suited to play a role in the development of new diagnostic reagents both for use in immunohistology as well as for scintigraphy and therapy.
However, in view of the heterogeneity of tumors, it seems unrealistic to expect that for each tumortype specific antibodies will eventually be produced that will react with all tumor cells of a given tumor.

References

1. Köhler G, Milstein C: Continuous cultures of fused cells secreting antibody of predefined specificity. Nature 256: 495-497, 1975.
2 Campbell AM: Laboratory techniques in biochemistry and molecular biology: Monoclonal antibody technology eds. A.H. Burdon and P.H. van Knippenberg,Elsevier-Amsterdam-New York-Oxford. 1984.
3. Langone JL, Vanakis H van (Eds) Methods in Enzymology. Academic Press. New York, London, 92: 1983.
4. Cianfriglia M. et al: Simple immunization protocol for high frequency production of soluble antigen-specific hybridomas. Hybridoma 2: 451-457. 1983.
5. Samoszuk MK, Parker JW: High-frequency production of cell-surface antigen-specific hybridomas. Hybridoma 3: 293-295, 1984.
6. Siraganian RS et al: Methods of enhancing the frequency of antigen specific hybridomas. Eds. A.M. Campbell Elsevier-Amsterdam-New York-Oxford pp 17-25, 1984.
7. Taggart RT, Samloff IM: Stable antibody-producing murine hybridomas. Science 219: 1228-1230.1983.
8. Kearney JF et al: A new mouse myeloma cell line that has lost immunoglobulin expression but permits the construction of antibody-secreting hybrid cell lines. J. Immunol.123:1548-1550, 1979.
9. Shulman M et al: A better cell line for making hybridomas secreting specific antibodies. Nature 276:269-270, 1978.
10. Fazekas de St.Groth S, Scheidegger D: Production of monoclonal antibodies:strategy and tactics. J.Immunol.Meth.35: 1-21, 1980.
11. McKendall RR, Woo W: Microtiter radioimmuno precipitation assay of HSV-1 polypeptides with recovery and SDS-PAGE analysis of precipitated proteins:usefulness as screening test for large numbers of specimen including hybridoma supernates. J.Immunol.Methods 72: 461-469, 1984.
12. Ley V et al: A four step sandwich radioimmuno assay for direct selection of monoclonal antibodies to allergen molecules. J.Immunol.Methods 84: 265-270, 1985.
13. Moudallal al Z et al: Comparative sensitivity of different ELISA procedures for detecting monoclonal antibodies. J. Immunol.Methods 68: 35-43,1984.
14. Vaidya HC et al: Inadequacy of traditional ELISA for screening hybridoma supernatants for murine monoclonal antibodies. Hybridoma 4: 271-275, 1985.
15. Porstmann b et al: Which of the commonly used marker enzymes gives the best results in colorimetric and fluorimetric enzyme immunoessays:horse radish peroxidase, alkaline phosphatase or ßgalactosidase. J:Immunol.Methods 79: 27-37, 1985.

16. Heyningen V van et al: A simple method for ranking the affinities of monoclonal antibodies.
J.Immunol.Methods 63: 147-152, 1983.
17. Patel R, Brown JC: Hybridoma preservation at -70°C:a simple and economical procedure for the short-term storage and individual recovery of hybridomas.
J. Immunol.Methods 71: 211-215, 1984.
18. Ley L de et al: Cryopreservation of newly formed hybridomas.
J.Immunol.Methods 62: 69-72, 1983.
19. Bennet FC, Yeoman LC: An improved procedure for the dot immunobinding analysis of hybridoma supernatants.
J.Immunol.Methods 61: 201-207, 1983.
20. McDougal JS et al: Immunodot assay for determining the isotype and light chain type of murine monoclonal antibodies in unconcentrated hybridoma culture supernatants.
J.Immunol.Methods 63: 281-290, 1983.
21. Holmberg M et al: A rapid screening technique for monoclonal antibodies with specificity for protein antigens.
J.Immunol.Methods 61: 9-16, 1983.
22. Towbin H, Gordon J:Immunoblotting and dot immunobinding - current status and outlook.
J.Immunol.Methods 72: 313-340, 1984.
23 Spinola SM, Cannon JG: Different blocking agents cause variation in the immunologic detection of protein transferred to nitrocellulose membranes.
J.Immunol.Methods 81: 61-165, 1985.
24. Towbin H et al: Glycosphingo lipid-blotting: an immunological detection procedure after separation by thin layer chromotography.
J.Immunol.Methods 72: 471-479, 1984.
25. Sharon J et al: Detection of specific hybridoma clones by replica immunoadsorption of their secreted antibodies.
PNAS 76: 1420-1424, 1979.
26. Spira G et al: The identification of monoclonal class switch variants by sibselection and an ELISA assay.
J. Immunol.Methods 74: 307-315, 1984.
27. Sternberger LA et al: Neurotypy: regional individuality in rat brain detected by immunocytochemistry with monoclonal antibodies.
PNAS 79: 1326-1330,1982.
28. Straus W: Imidazole increases the sensitivity of the cytochemical reaction for peroxidase with diaminobenzidine at a neutral pH. .
J.Histochem.Cytochem. 30: 491-493, 1980.
29. Vollmers HPet al: Monoclonal antibodies NORM-1 and NORM-2 induce more normal behavior of tumor cells in vitro and reduce tumor growth in vivo.
Cell 40:547-557, 1985.
30. Cheresh DA et al: Disialoganglioside GD_3 on human melanoma serves as a relevant target antigen for monoclonal antibody-mediated tumor cytolysis.
PNAS 82: 5155-5159, 1985.

31. Tettamanti G et al: A new procedure for the extraction purification and fractionation of brain gangliosides. BBA 296: 160-170, 1974.
32. Wood MP et al: Detection of monoclonal antibodies specific for carbohydrate epitopes using periodate oxidation. J.Immunol.Methods 78: 143-153, 1985.
33. Brodeus BR et al: Parameters affecting ascites tumour formation in mice and monoclonal antibody production. J.Immunol.Methods 71: 265-272, 1984.
34. Truitt KE et al: Production of human monoclonal antibody in mouse ascites. Hybridoma 3: 195-199, 1984.
35. Underwood PA, Bean PA: The influence of methods of production purification and storage of monoclonal antibodies upon their observed specificities. J.Immunol.Methods 80: 189-197, 1985.

2. IMMUNOCYTOCHEMICAL TECHNIQUES.

F.T. BOSMAN

1. INTRODUCTION

Immunocytochemistry was born in 1941 when Coons and coworkers (1) succeeded in labeling an antibody with fluoresceine. For 25 years immunofluorescence was the only available immunocytochemical method and although direct or indirect immunofluorescence was used for a variety of applications, mainly in immunopathological studies, it was not widely accepted for routine histo- en cytodiagnostic purposes for two reasons. Firstly, morphological details of the tissues are difficult to appreciate in fluorescence microscopy. Secondly immunofluorescence preparations cannot be dehydrated and permanently mounted and are therefore difficult to store for prolonged periods of time.

The introduction of the horseradish peroxidase labeled antibody method by Nakane and Pierce in 1966 (2) was a major breakthrough. Enzyme labels result in coloured end-products which can be examined by regular transmission light microscopy and counterstaining of the preparation allows the recognition of morphological features as in ordinary light microscopy. Furthermore, the preparations can be permanently mounted and stored without any special requirements. The development of the unabeled antibody methods, of which the peroxidase-antiperoxidase (PAP) complex method introduced by Sternberger et al. (3) has gained enormous popularity, was a decisive step in the acceptation of immunocytochemistry as a routine procedure in diagnostic pathology.

At that point immunocytochemical methodology had reached a high level of reliability and it was more and more appreciated that one of the most important determinants of the final result of any immunocytochemical procedure was the quality of the first antibody. Conventional immunizations, especially with immunogens which were not absolutely pure, frequently yielded antibodies which cross-reacted with unwanted tissue components and therefore a wide variety of purification techniques, including immune-adsorption and affinity chromatography, was developed. Against this background the introduction of hybridoma technology by Kohler and Milstein (4), which allowed the production of monoclonal antibodies, was again a major breakthrough. Initial enthousiasm, concerning the superior properties of monoclonal antibodies, was tempered somewhat when it became clear that monoclonal antibodies also have some limitations (to which we will return later). Undoubtedly, however, the enormous impact of immunocytochemistry on diagnostic pathology has been especially caused by the availability of well characterized monoclonal antibodies against various tissue antigens, as will be discussed in the other chapters of this volume.

It is the purpose of this chapter to discuss some general aspects of the immunocytochemical methodology, especially in relation to its application in conjunction with monoclonal antibodies. Special attention will be paid to principles of immunohistochemical techniques, labels and detection systems, conditions for optimal immunocytochemistry and interpretation of the results.

2. PRINCIPLES OF IMMUNOCYTOCHEMISTRY

Immunocytochemistry belongs to the group of **affinity cytochemical** techniques, which includes in addition to immunocytochemistry lectin cytochemistry, enzyme-substrate cytochemistry and hybridocytochemistry or in situ hybridization. All these techniques rely on the ability of a molecular probe to interact with high specificity and affinity with a cell or tissue component. For immunocytochemistry the probe is an immunoglobulin, for lectin cytochemistry a lectin, for enzyme-substrate cytochemistry a substrate molecule which is specific for the enzyme under investigation and for hybridocytochemistry a single strand sequence of DNA. A molecular probe can be **directly** tagged with a label which can be visualized by some form of microscopy but more frequently an **indirect** procedure is used in which a labeled second probe is used to detect the specific first probe. Immunocytochemistry, therefore, relies on a combination of a. the unique interaction between a specific immunoglobulin molecule and its corresponding antigen and b. the availability of microscopically detectable labels.

For the localization of tissue-bound specific immunoglobulin molecules, various labels and detection systems are available. Initially, the only available labels were fluorochromes, of which fluoresceine isothiocyanate (FITC) remains the most popular although, especially in double staining techniques, tetra-rhodamine isothiocyanate (TRITC) is also regularly used. As mentioned before, fluorescent labels have some disadvantages, which has resulted in the almost exclusive use of enzyme labels for diagnostic immunohistochemistry. It should be emphasized here, however, that there are very few, if any, principle differences between fluorescence- and absorption immunocytochemical techniques and that what can be achieved at the light microscopical level with immunoenzyme cytochemistry can also be done by immunofluorescence. For practical reasons, we will mainly focus on absorption immunocytochemical techniques.

3. IMMUNOHISTOCHEMICAL TECHNIQUES

Many different systems for the detection of bound primary antibody molecules have been developed. These are schematically represented in fig. I-III. Some of these are applicable in combination with any label whereas others have been specifically designed for use with one particular label, as indicated in the legends.

Direct methods are simple because they are single step procedures. They are, however, relatively insensitive and antibody inefficient and are therefore not routinely used.

The indirect labeled antibody methods are much more versatile because one labeled second antibody can detect many different primary antibodies, provided they were all raised in the same species. Furthermore, indirect methods are more sensitive and much more antibody efficient, especially in combination with enzyme labels. The initial enzyme-antibody conjugation procedures, (2, 5) being rather inefficient and reducing the immunoreactivity of the conjugated antibody, did not yield optimal

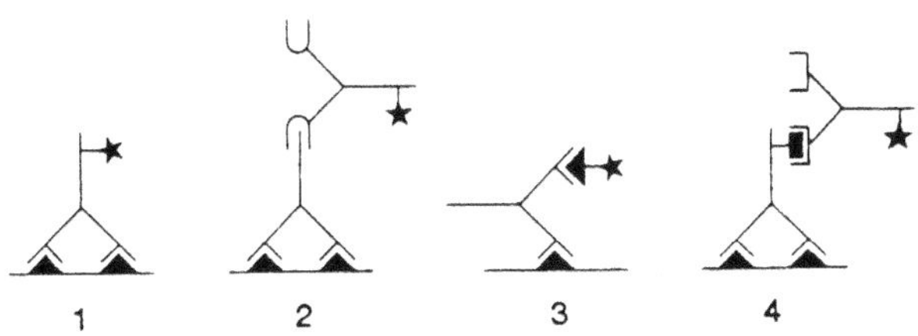

Fig. I 1. Direct labeled antibody method. 2. Indirect labeled antibody method. These two methods are suitable for almost any label. 3. Labeled antigen method, suitable for research purposes in combination with antigens and fluorochromes. 4. Hapten labeled antibody method. As hapten dinitrophenol (DNP) or biotin has been used. The method is suitable for most labels.
* label, antigen, hapten.

conjugates. The PAP complex method (fig. II 1), using immunologic linking of antibody and enzyme, and presumably resulting in more peroxidase molecules per molecule of bound first antibody, was claimed to be much more sensitive than the peroxidase labeled antibody method. Subsequent studies have shown, however, that when the presently available improved conjugation methods are used (6, 7) the indirect peroxidase labeled antibody method is almost as sensitive as the PAP method (8). Nevertheless the PAP complex method remains one of the most popular immunocytochemical techniques. With mouse monoclonal antibodies mouse PAP complexes have to be used. All available mouse PAP complexes are prepared with mouse monoclonal antiperoxidase antibodies (9).

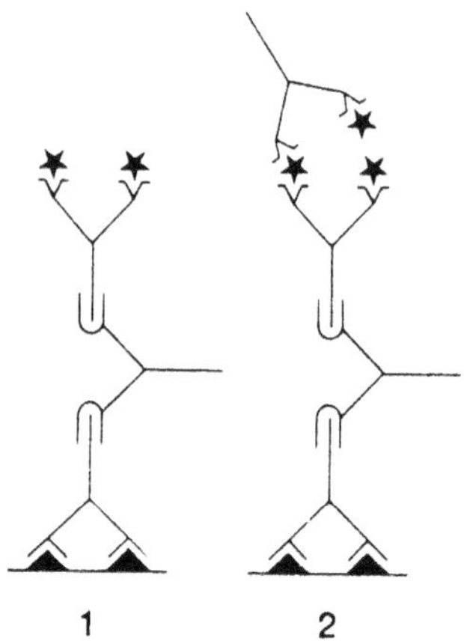

Fig. II.
1. Four step antibody-enzymebridge method which preceded the PAP technique. The primary antibody, linking second antibody, antiperoxidase antibody and peroxidase are sequentially applied. No longer in use. Was used only with enzyme labels.
2. Enzyme-antienzyme complex method. With peroxidase as label this three step technique, in which primary antibody, linking second antibody and enzyme-antibody complex are sequentially applied, is known as the PAP, with alkaline phosphatase as the APAAP method.
* = label, = antigen.

More recently developed detection systems use protein A or the avidin-biotin complex in the second step (Fig. III, 10, 11). Protein A reacts with the Fc fragment of IgG but not with all subclasses and not in all species and this method is therefore not very widely applied for light microscopical immunocytochemistry. In contrast, the avidin-biotin complex method has become fairly popular, especially in combination with monoclonal antibodies. Its main advantages are its versatility, the lack of background staining when used under appropriate conditions and its high sensitivity, due to the increased number of label molecules per bound molecule of first antibody (12, 13).

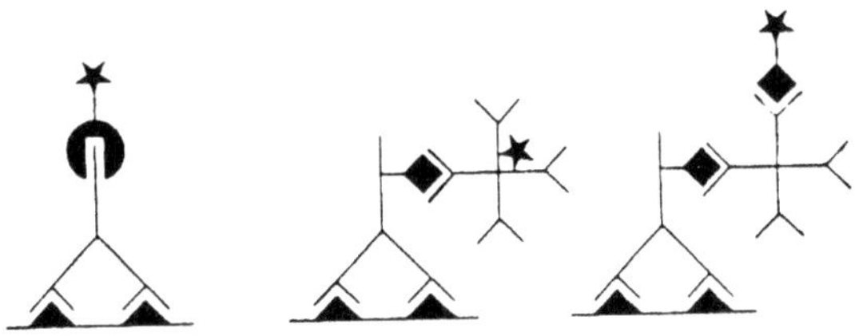

Fig. III

1. Protein A method. This technique is especially popular for colloidal gold label but can be used with any label. Not very suitable for monoclonal antibodies.
2. Avidin labeled avidin-biotin method. This method relies on the binding of an avidin-labeled conjugate with a biotinylated antibody. This technique is not widely used.
3. Avidin-biotin complex (ABC) method. Biotinylated labels (almost exclusively enzymes) are complexed with avidin. The complex then reacts with the biotinylated first antibody.

= protein A, * = label, = antigen, = biotin.

Numerous attempts have been made to increase the sensitivity of immunoperoxidase procedures by increasing the intensity of the enzyme-staining reaction. The addition of Co and Ni salts to the DAB substrate solution (14,15), indeed increases the staining intensity and furthermore alters the color of the reaction product, which may be useful for double staining procedures. Imidazole also intensifies the staining intensity of diaminobenzidine (DAB) (15). In a recent study De Jong et al (17) demonstrated that for visualization of peroxidase the sensitivity of these procedures is indeed significantly better than that of DAB alone. Silver intensification methods, applied after completion of the DAB reaction, have also been developed (18). All these methods undoubtedly increase the specific staining intensity but often also increase the amount of background staining.

Although DAB is still probably the most widely used chromogen for peroxidase several alternatives are available. Amino-ethylcarbazole (AEC) results in a red reaction product, which many users have found preferable in combination with monoclonal antibodies on frozen sections. The efficiency of the reaction equals that of DAB (19). The only disadvantage of AEC is the solubility of the reaction product in ethanol and xylene. Chloronaphthol (CN) results in a darkblue reaction product which is also soluble in alcohol and xylene (20). Furthermore the efficiency of the reaction is distinctly lower than that of DAB or AEC. CN has therefore been used mainly for double staining purposes in combination with DAB.

Various alternative enzymes have been applied for enzyme- immunocytochemical purposes. Alkaline phosphatase (AP) has been extensively tested (21, 22) and AP labeled antibodies as well as AP-anti-AP (APAAP) complexes are now commercially available. For this enzyme various chromogens with different colors are available. Fast red and Fast blue have become popular for use as AP chromogens (17) but their reaction products are soluble in ethanol and xylene. Bromo-4-chloro-3-indolyl phosphate (BCIP) results in a blue reaction product which is not soluble in organic solvents (23) and its reaction is at least as efficient as that of Fast blue and Fast red. For these reasons BCIP appears to be the best choice for visualization of AP (17). The main advantage of AP is that in most tissues endogenous enzyme levels are much lower than those for endogenous peroxidases, which alleviates the need for blocking procedures and may result in a better contrast. The sensitivity of AP immunocytochemistry appears to equal that of peroxidase procedures (17). A disadvantage is the higher cost of the reagents. Other enzymes that have been tested for enzyme-immuno-cytochemical purposes are glucose oxidase (24) and β-galactosidase (25). For reasons of lower efficiency and higher cost these labels are not recommendable for routine use. Overall, peroxidase remains the best with AP as a good second choice.

A fairly recent development is the use of colloidal gold labels for light microscopical immunocytochemistry which was first described by Faulk and Taylor in 1971 (26). The simplicity of the procedures for the preparation of colloidal gold and for the labeling of proteins (27), the high sensitivity and the resolution of the method, and the possibility to perform double labeling studies by using gold particles of different sizes (28) have rapidly given gold labels a leading position in immunoelectronmicroscopy. Gu et al. (29) discovered that under appropriate conditions gold labeled antibody deposits are visible by light microscopy. Subsequently Holgate et al. (30) developed a procedure to visualize gold particles by use of a silver reaction. Springall et al. (31) adapted this technique for use on routinely prepared tissue sections and demonstrated that it allows the use of higher primary antibody dilutions than more conventional immunocytochemical procedures, results in high contrast staining even in tissues with very low antigen concentrations, which might not be detected by conventional methods, and is useful in double staining procedures. The commercial availability of gold labeled antibodies as well as of silver staining kits may contribute to the growing popularity of this method.

4. ESSENTIAL CONDITIONS FOR IMMUNOCYTOCHEMISTRY USING MONOCLONAL ANTIBODIES.

In terms of essential technical requirements there are no differences between immunocytochemistry with polyclonal or with monoclonal antibodies. The primary antibodies should be of well established specificity, a suitable detection system should be available and the tissue specimen should be adequately processed. Each of these factors will be considered in more detail.

a. Antibody specificity. Monoclonal antibodies (MA) are by definition specific for a single antigenic determinant or epitope but not infrequently the distribution of the epitope is insufficiently known. This is rarely a problem when MA prepared against a defined antigen are used but many MA which are applied for the histopathological diagnosis of tumors were raised against undefined cell or tissue elements and often the precise nature of the corresponding antigen is not or only partly known. Consequently, the specificity of such antibodies is primarily defined by tissue binding characteristics. In this situation the reliability of specificity claims is exclusively determined by the thoroughness of mapping on various tissues of the immunoreactivity pattern of the MA. Numerous examples can be given of MA which were initially claimed to be tumor, organ- or celltype specific but on extensive testing were shown to be less "specific" and occasionally even fairly ubiquitous. Furthermore, such MA, even when specific for a unique epitope, may on occasion be found to show unexpected patterns of immunoreactivity. A striking example of such an occasion is the reactivity of the natural killer cell specific Leu-7 MA with small cell lung cancer cells (32). Such findings indicate that testing of MA for application in tumor diagnosis can never be too exhaustive and call for caution in the blind application of MA immunocytochemistry for the histopathological diagnosis of tumors.

It has become increasingly clear that the reactivity of MA should be analyzed in test-systems which correspond with the intended application. There are many examples of MA which reacted well in (solid or fluid phase) immunoassays but showed no reactivity on tissue sections and vice versa. In the preparation of MA, however, solid phase enzyme immunoassays remain for practical reasons one of the most important test systems.

The antigen spot test is a simple and reliable test system which can be used to determine antibody specificity (e.g. for antibodies against peptide hormones), the immunoglobulin class of a MA or the sensitivity of a detection system (8, 32). For the identification of the tissue antigen reacting with the MA, immunoblotting (34) has appeared to be a very powerful technique. In this technique a tissue extract is subjected to some form of separation procedure, usually sodium dodecyl sulphate polyacrylamide gel-electrophoresis, which separates proteins by molecular weight. The separated proteins in the gel are subsequently transferred to nitrocellulose sheets and reacted with the monoclonal antibody. In this way combined information concerning immunoreactivity as well as physicochemical characteristics of the reactant can be obtained.

b. Adequacy of tissue processing procedures

There is a widespread belief that MA can almost exclusively be used on very mildly fixed frozen sections or cytological preparations. This is not true. Clearly many available MA against cell surface determinants of differentation will only detect these determinants in the native (undenatured) form but that is an antigen- and not an antibody-related characteristic. It is important to emphasize here that for each antigen, and for MA even each epitope, the optimal preservation procedure will have to be established. The alternative approach is to select for MA that recognize epitopes which are stable under standard conditions of tissue processing. Unfortunately not all antigens contain such epitopes. For a fairly wide variety of antigens, however, MA exist which will detect the antigen after formalin fixation and paraffin embedding. For other MA mildly fixed (acetone or ethanol) cryostat sections or cytological preparations will remain the only suitable material. Therefore unfixed specimens of tumor tissue should always be kept adequately stored (at -70 °C). It will be clear that for MA adequate negative and positive tissue controls are as essential as for conventional polyclonal antibodies. It is important that control tissues were processed according to the same protocol as the tissue under investigation.

c. Suitability of the detection system.

For each application of a MA in an immunocytochemical test the optimal detection system will have to be selected. The various determinants of the detection system are listed in table I.

Table I. Determinants of the detection system

1.	reagent related	a.	choice of linking system (fig. I-III)
		b.	choice of label- fluorochrome - enzyme choice) of chromogen) - colloidal gold
2.	instrument related	a.	static microscopy
		b.	flow cytometry

The linking systems have already been discussed. The sensitivity of all systems is primarily determined by the quality of the applied reagents. If optimal reagents are used the ABC technique may be slightly better than the PAP technique, which in turn might be slightly better than the indirect antibody labeled technique. These differences will, however, not exceed a factor 2 to 3. It is therefore preferable to use one technique, gain experience with it and gradually improve on it.

The various labels have also been reviewed. Although in principle similar results can be obtained with fluorochromes and enzyme labels there is a clear preference for fluorochrome labeling when the antigen of interest is membrane bound and will be studied on cell suspensions. Also for the double labeling of two antigens on the same cell a combination of two fluorochromes (FITC and TRITC) is preferable. For the detection of antigens in tissue sections there is a clear preference for enzyme labels. As has been pointed out already, under optimal conditions the efficiency of the most frequently used labels (peroxidase and alkaline phosphatase) is equal. The experience with the immunogold-silver method is still too limited to fully substantiate the claims of its superior sensitivity. Nevertheless, this technique evidently has promising characteristics.

For quantitative evaluation of antigen expression on individual cells, both in terms of the number of immunoreactive cells as well as the amount of antigen per cell, flow-cytometry has gained wide acceptance (35). An important development in this area is the availability of new fluorochromes such as phycoerythrin, with high quantum efficiency and emission spectra which make them especially suitable for flow-cytometrical use (36).

5. INTERPRETATION OF STAINING RESULTS

Specific aspects of the interpretation of immunoreactivity patterns for various antigens will be discussed in the following chapters. Here we will only reemphasize some general rules. These are summarized in the following questions.

a. Were the applied techniques valid and the controls adequate?

The amount of background should be sufficiently low to enable the distinction between positive and negative. Postive control tissue should be positive with an acceptable staining intensity. Negative control tissue should be negative. The tissue specimen should have been adequately processed, including the control tissues. It should be reminded that only under very strict conditions the staining intensity can be regarded as a measure for the amount of antigen.

b. Is the distribution of the antigen known in sufficient detail?

As was pointed out before, the specificity of MA induced against unidentified cell- or tissue antigens relies entirely on the thoroughness of the tissue testing procedures. The potential user should ascertain that the MA is suitable for the intended use and has been sufficiently characterized.

c. Are markers of differentiation of normal cells also valid as markers of differentiation of neoplastic cells?
Marker-based classification relies on the assumption that neoplastic cells at least usually but hopefully always differentiate along the same lines as their normal counterparts and that markers of differentiation of normal cells will retain their differentiational specificity in neoplastic cells. This assumption leads to conclusions such as "neuroendocrine cells contain neuron specific enolase (NSE) and therefore NSE positive tumors are of neuroendocrine origin" or "myogenous (smooth and cross-striated muscle) cells contain desmin and therefore desmin positive tumors are of myogenous origin". Unfortunately, NSE has occasionally been found in non-neuroendocrine tumors (37) and, along the same line, it has been recognized that although neoplastic cells usually retain the intermediate filament protein characteristic of their normal ancestors unexpected patterns of intermediate filament expression do occur (38). Many case reports illustrate the potential for aberrant differentiational behaviour of neoplastic cells and call for cautious interpretation of marker patterns in the classification of tumors.

6. CONCLUSIONS AND FUTURE PROSPECTS

It is clear that marker immunocytochemistry using monoclonal as well as polyclonal antibodies is revolutionizing diagnostic pathology. This is an important development for two reasons. Firstly, the practising pathologist is provided with a vast array of new tools which will assist in the solving of diagnostic problems. Secondly, marker studies reestablish an essential connection between fundamental pathobiology and diagnostic pathology. It is equally clear, however, that the reliability of marker immunocytochemistry depends on three simple rules. The applied techniques should be appropriate, the primary antibodies should be adequately characterized and the interpretation should be careful, keeping in mind that "tumors break rules".

What will the future bring? Firstly, it can be expected that many new MA will be developed which will further improve the diagnostic accuracy of histo- en cytopathology. Especially promising in this respect are MA specific for the gene products of oncogenes and MA which will reliably detect antigens in routinely processed tissue specimens. Secondly, and maybe even more important, standardization in the use of MA reagents for immunomorphological tissue typing will be established. An important prerequisite for tumor classification is consensus. If there is no consensus it will be impossible to compare clinico-pathological studies or to develop uniform treatment protocols. If a majority of the laboratories continues to use their own highly interesting and very powerful panel of monoclonal antibodies uniformity will remain a distant dream and consensus will never be reached.

REFERENCES

1. Coons AH, Creech HJ, Jones RN. Immunological properties of an antibody containing a fluorescent group. Proc.Soc. Exp.Biol.Med. 1941, 47, 200-202.

2. Nakane PK, Pierce GB Jr. Enzyme-labeled antibodies: preparation and application for the localization of antigens. J. Histochem.Cytochem. 1966, 14, 929.

3. Sternberger LA, Hardy Ph Jr., Cuculis JJ, Meyer HG. The unlabeled antibody-enzyme method of immunohistochemistry. Preparation and properties of soluble antigen-antibody complex (horseradish anti-horseradish peroxidase) and its use in the identification of spirochetes. J. Histochem.Cytochem. 1975, 23, 208-215.

4. Kohler G, Milstein C. Continuous cultures of fused cells secreting antibodies of predefined specificity. Nature 1975, 256, 495-497.

5. Avrameas S. Indirect immunoenzyme techniques for the intracellular detection of antigens. Immunochemistry 1969, 6, 825-831.

6. Wilson JB, Nakane PK. Recent developments in the peroxidase method of conjugating horseradish peroxidase (HRPO) to antibodies. In: W. Knapp, K Holubar, G Wick (Eds.) Immunofluorescence and related staining techniques. Elsevier Amsterdam, 1978,215-224.

7. Avrameas S. Enzyme markers: their linkage with proteins and use in immuno-histochemistry. Histochem. J. 1972, 4, 321-330.

8. Bosman FT, Cramer-Knijnenburg G, van Bergen Henegouw J. Efficiency and sensitivity of indirect immunoperoxidase methods. Histochemistry 1983, 77, 185-194.

9. Naritoku WY, Taylor CR. A comparative study of the use of monoclonal antibodies using three different immunohistochemical methods: an evaluation of monoclonal and polyclonal antibodies against human prostatic acid phosphatase. J. Histochem. Cytochem. 1981, 130, 253-260.

10. Romans EL, Romano M. Staphylococcus protein A bound to colloidal gold: a useful reagent to label antigen-antibody sites in electron microscopy. Immunochemistry 1977, 14, 711-715.

11. Roth J, Bendayan M, Orci L. Ultrastructural localization of intracellular antigen by the use of the protein-A gold complex. J. Histochem.Cytochem. 1978, 26, 1074-1081.

12. Guesdon JL, Ternynck T, Avrameas S. The use of avidin-biotin interaction in immunoenzymatic techniques. J. Histochem. Cytochem. 1979, 27, 1131-1139.

13. Hsu S-M, Raine L, Fanger H. Use of avidin-biotin-peroxidase complex (ABC) in immunoperoxidase techniques. J. Histochem.Cytochem. 1981, 29, 577-580.

14. Hsu S-M, Soban E. Color modification of diaminobenzidine (DAB) precipitation by metallic ions and its application for double immunohistochemistry. J. Histochem.Cytochem. 1982, 30, 1079-1082.

15. Adams JC. Heavy metal intensification of DAB-based HRP reaction product. J. Histochem.Cytochem. 1981, 29, 775.

16. Straus W. Imidazole increases the sensitivity of the cytochemical reaction for peroxidase with diaminobenzidine at neutral pH. J. Histochem.Cytochem. 1982, 30, 491-493.

17. De Jong ASH, Van Kessel- van Valk M, Raap AK. Sensitivity of various visualization methods for peroxidase and alkaline phosphatase activity in immunoenzyme histochemistry. Histochem.J. 1985, 17, 1119-1130.

18. Gallyas F, Görcs T, Merckenthaler I. High-grade intensification of the end-product of the diaminobenzidine reaction for peroxidase histochemistry. J. Histochem.Cytochem. 1982, 30, 183-184.

19. Graham RC, Lindholm U, Karnovsky M. Cytochemical demonstration of peroxidase activity with 3-amino-9-ethyl-carbazole. J. Histochem.Cytochem. 1965, 13, 150-152.

20. Nakane PK. Simultaneous localization of multiple tissue antigens using the peroxidase labeled antibody method: a study in pituitary glands of the rat. J. Histochem.Cytochem. 1968, 16, 557-560.

21. Mason DY, Sammons RE. Alkaline phosphatase and peroxidase for double immunoenzymatic labeling of cellular constituents. J. Clin.Pathol. 1978, 31, 454-462.

22. Malik NJ, Daymon ME. Improved double immunoenzyme labeling using alkaline phosphatase and horseradish peroxidase. J. Clin. Pathol. 1982, 35, 1092-1094.

23. McGradey J. A tetrazolium method for non-specific alkaline phosphatase. Histochimie 1970, 23, 180-184.

24. Masseyeff HR, Maiolini R. A sandwich method of enzyme immunoassay. Applications to rat and human α-fetoprotein. J. Immunol.Methods 1975, 8, 223-234.

25. Bondi A, Chieregatti G, Eusebi V, Fulcheri E, Bussolatti G. The use of beta-galactosidase as a tracer in immunocytochemistry. Histochemistry 1982, 76, 153-158.

26. Faulk WP, Taylor GM. An immunocolloid method for the electron microscope. Immunochemistry 1971, 8, 1081-1083.

27. De Mey J. Colloidal gold probes in immunocytochemistry. In: Immunocytochemistry (JM Polak, S van Noorden, Eds.). Wright, Bristol. 1983, pp. 82-112.

28. Geuze H, Slot J, van der Ley P, Schutter R, Griffith J. Use of colloidal gold particles in double labeling immuno-electron microscopy of ultrathin frozen tissue sections. J. Cell Biol. 1981, 89, 653-655.

29. Gu J, De Mey J, Moermans M, Polak JM. Sequential use of the PAP and immunogold staining methods for the light microscopical double staining of tissue antigens. Reg. Peptides, 1985, 15, 365-374.

30. Holgate CS, Jackson P, Cowen CN, Bird CC. Immunogold-silver staining: new method of immunostaining with enhanced sensitivity. J. Histochem.Cytochem. 1983, 31, 938-944.

31. Springall DR, Hacker GW, Grimelius L, Polak JM. The potential of the immunogold-silver staining method for paraffin sections. Histochemistry 1984, 81, 603-608.

32. Bunn PA Jr, Linnoila L, Minna JD, Carney D, Gazdar AF. Small cell lung cancer, endocrine cells of the fetal bronchus and other neuroendocrine cells express the leu-7 antigenic determinant present on natural killer cells. Blood 1985, 65, 764-768.

33. Herbrink P, van Bussel F, Warnaar SO. The antigen spot test (AST): a highly sensitive assay for the detection of antibodies. J. Immunol. Meth. 1982, 48, 293-298.

34. Towbin H, Staehelin T, Gordon J. Electrophoretic transfer of proteins from polyacrylamide gels into nitrocellulose sheets: procedure and some applications. Proc.Natl.Acad.Sci. USA 1979, 76, 4350-4354.

35. Thornthwaite JT, Seckinger D, Sugarbaker EV, Rosenthal PK, Vazquez DA. Dual immunofluorescent analysis of human peripheral blood lymphocytes. Am.J.Clin.Pathol. 1984, 82, 48-56.

36. Oi VT, Galzer AN, Stryer L. Fluorescent phycobilinoprotein conjugates for analysis of cells and molecules. J. Cell Biol. 1982, 93, 981-986.

37. Schmechel DE. Gamma subunit of the glycolytic enzyme enolase: non-specific or neuronspecific. Lab. Invest. 1985, 52, 239-247.

38. Gould VE. Histogenesis and differentiation. A reevaluation of these concepts as criteria for the classification of tumors. Human Pathol. (in press).

3. DOUBLE IMMUNOENZYME STAINING METHODS WITH SPECIAL REFERENCE TO MONOCLONAL ANTIBODIES.

H. MULLINK, D.M. BOORSMA, S.C. HENZEN-LOGMANS, C.J.L.M.MEIJER

INTRODUCTION

Immunohistochemical methods have been developed to evaluate the distribution patterns of different antigens (e.g. each characteristic for a certain cell type) simultaneously in tissue sections. These methods have relevance, especially for research in (tumor) cell biology. The demonstration of co-expression of cytoskeletal proteins in a single cell or the presence of different hormones in adjacent cells are good examples of such application. In the past double immunofluorescence techniques have been most widely used for this purpose. Double immunoenzyme staining however, is in many cases more attractive than double immunofluorescence because the preparations are permanent and the evaluation of the staining in relation to morphology is simple. Although several methods for double immunoenzyme staining have been published, their execution often remains problematic, especially when monoclonal antibodies (MoAb's) are used. In this chapter we will review some of these methods and pay special attention to their practical applicability. Moreover, a method for double staining with MoAb's will be described. For the common immunocytochemical techniques, the reader is referred to chapter 2.
Two main methods using one or two enzymes respectively, can be distinguished. If one enzyme is used the contrasting colours are obtained by using different chromogens. The immunostaining for the first antigen has to be finished before starting the incubations for the second antigen: a sequential method. If two different enzyme labels are used, the incubations for both antigens can be performed either simultaneously or sequentially.

ENZYMES

One of the conditions to be fullfilled in immunocytochemical double staining is a clear contrast between the colours obtained. When both antigens are expected to be present on the same structure, a mixed intermediate staining clearly distinguishable from the primary colours should be obtained. Although the number of enzymes which are in use for immunocytochemical purposes is restricted these requirements can be met. Enzymes which are commonly used are: horseradish peroxidase (HRP), alkaline phosphatase (AP) (usually derived from calf intestine) and glucose oxidase.
If, in a sequential assay, HRP has to be used twice, there are a number of possibilities. The most suitable chromogens are: diaminobenzidine (DAB) (brown), 4-chloronaphtol (4CN) (blue-grey) and 3-amino-9-ethylcarbazole (AEC) which gives a bright-red reaction product. The combination DAB with 4CN was the first to be used (1), although the contrast is not really optimal and an intermediate colour is not easily distinguished. AEC with 4CN

gives a better contrast, but for other reasons the use of DAB in double HRP stainings is preferable (see below). With the combination DAB-AEC the contrast is often insufficient. Sometimes it is possible to use metallic ions in combination with DAB in a sequential method. The very-dark-blue reaction product of DAB-cobalt, for instance, can be used in combination with normal DAB or AEC staining (2).
The use of 2 different enzymes, e.g. HRP and AP, makes it possible to use a number of different colour combinations. As AP can be revealed with several blue and red reaction products, by means of different diazo reagents its use in combination with HRP is ideal. In our experience, DAB or AEC in combination with the blue reaction product of AP obtained with naphtol AS-MX phosphate and Fast Blue BB gives optimal results (3,4). When this AP reaction product is combined with AEC in cells containing both antigens, a distinct violet mixed colour is obtained, contrasting well with both primary colours (4,5).
Good results can also be obtained with the combination HRP (DAB or AEC) with glucose oxidase which gives a bluish-purple reaction product (6). As glucose oxidase is not found in mammals it might be an alternative to HRP or AP in tissue with much endogenous activity of the latter enzymes.
Although in paraffin sections endogenous peroxidase can be blocked sufficiently by methanol-H_2O_2 (7) and endogenous AP activity is destroyed, their presence may lead to problems in frozen sections. In this case the commonly used peroxidase-inactivating methods are often harmful to the antigenicity of the tissue components under investigation. Tissue AP activity in frozen sections may be blocked sufficiently by levamisole in the substrate reaction mixture (8). However intestinal AP is not inhibited by levamisole and therefore one may encounter difficulties with AP as marker enzyme in the study of antigens in intestinal tissue.
The double use of AP only in a sequential method has been described (9). As AP can be revealed with different red and blue colours, good combinations may be obained. There is however a risk of the primary applied enzyme coreacting in the second enzyme reaction, giving rise to spurious mixed staining.

INCUBATION METHODS

The main problem in double immunoenzyme staining is how to prevent cross-reactions.
The antibodies and the conjugates intended for the demonstration of one antigen should in no way react with the second antigen and its antibody layers. This means that high demands are made upon all antibodies with respect to specificity and purity. Since in multistep techniques the secondary antibodies are always anti Ig, care should be taken that no interspecies reactions can occur. For this reason the number of different antibody layers should be restricted as much as possible.
As indicated above, sequential and simultaneous incubation methods can be distinguished. The sequential method is the oldest and was introduced by Nakane (1). It is based on two indirect immunostainings both usually performed with HRP as marker enzyme and with antibodies derived from the same species. Therefore the antibodies and the enzyme used in the first staining have to be removed before the second incubation

sequence can be started. The coloured reaction product is retained in the section.
This removal can be performed by acid elution (1) electrophoresis (10) or permanganate oxidation (11). The decomposition of the antibody complexes is not always complete however and traces of the first antibody sandwich are often retained (11). Furthermore the possibility exists that this treatment is harmful to other antigens, especially when frozen sections are used.
Another approach came from Sternberger and Joseph (12) who reported that the DAB reaction product of HRP would block both antigenic sites on the primary antibody as well as the enzyme activity. Thus an elution step could be omitted without risk of spurious double labelling. However, recent studies by Valnes and Brandtzaeg (13) and our group have shown that this blocking does not occur under all reaction circumstances. We found that better blocking is obtained by the use of an indirect avidin-biotin-peroxidase method for the first antigen. In this way the antigenic sites of the first sequence are often effectively blocked, probably by means of steric hindrance through the avidin-biotin-enzyme complexes.
The need to remove or to block the immunoreagents of the first sequence can be avoided by using unrelated primary antibodies and to use developing antibodies labelled with different enzymes in the two sequences (6). In this way it is also possible to perform the incubation steps simultaneously (3). Now the different primary antibodies, and enzyme-linked secondary antibodies, respectively are mixed and the sections are incubated with these mixtures in sequence. Subsequently the respective enzyme reactions are performed separately. An absolute prerequisite for these two- or multi-step techniques is that both antigen-antibody layers are unrelated.
When the two antigens to be demonstrated are localized very near to each other, e.g. on the same cell membrane, simultaneous methods are preferable. In these cases sequential methods carry the risk of masking the second antigen by the immunoreagents applied in the first sequence. In a simultaneous method both primary antibodies can compete for their respective sites.
With two different enzymes, the following simultaneous methods can be distinguished.

1. Double-direct.

The most simple and rapid method (4): Two enzyme-linked primary antibodies, e.g. rabbit antikappa-HRP plus rabbit antilambda-AP are incubated together. In this case antibodies can even be derived from the same species, e.g. two monoclonal antibodies, and the risk of cross reactivity is minimal. However, the method is very inefficient and most antibodies are not commercially available as enzyme-conjugates, at least not with AP. When antibody-enzyme conjugates with high affinity are available, this method is preferred.

2. Double-indirect.

When two primary antibodies from different species are used and species-specific enzyme-linked anti-immunoglobulin antibodies are available, this method is suitable. All 4 antibodies should be raised in different species. For examle, (1) rabbit anti kappa + mouse anti lambda; (2) swine anti rabbit Ig-HRP + horse anti mouse Ig-AP.

3. Combination Direct-Indirect.

This method is often usable. E.g. (1) rabbit anti kappa - HRP + mouse anti lambda; (2) goat anti mouse Ig - AP.

4. Double - three stage method.

This method, which was originally described by Mason and Sammonds (3), can be used to demonstrate antigens present in low amounts. These are detected by simultaneous treatment of the sections with the classical peroxidase antiperoxidase (PAP) procedure for one antigen and the comparable APAAP (AP anti AP) method for the second one. In this method the risk for cross reactivity is considerable because six different immunoglobulins are used. E.g.: rabbit anti kappa + mouse anti lambda; (2) swine anti rabbit IgG + goat anti mouse IgG; (3) rabbit anti HRP-HRP (PAP) + Mouse anti AP-AP (APAAP).

5. Combinations

of direct or indirect with 3-stage methods are possible, provided both detection systems are unrelated.

6. Labelled antigen method

This highly specific 2-step method was introduced by Falini et al (14). Application of a mixture of two primary antibodies - which can be raised in the same animal species - is followed by incubation with the enzyme-labelled antigens. The applicability of the method is restricted by the often limited availability of purified antigens for coupling with the marker enzymes. For this reason the method is less suitable for routine use in the detection of changing pairs of antigens.

7. Biotin-Avidin Methods

Several immunoenzyme staining methods have been described which make use of the extremely high affinity between biotin and avidin, using biotin-labelled primary or secondary antibodies. Subsequently enzyme-labelled avidin or avidin-biotin-enzyme complexes (ABC) are used in the next step (15,16).

The combined use of two avidin-biotin methods is not suitable in simultaneous double-labelling, but they may be used in combination with other methods (18), e.g. hapten-antihapten sandwich techniques (17), APAAP methods, or enzyme-labelled primary antibody methods (19).

If simultaneous methods are not possible, it is often recommendable to use an ABC-HRP method in the visualization of the first antigen in a sequential assay (20). The sequential use of two ABC-HRP methods has also been described (21).

8. Hapten anti hapten and hapten sandwich methods

Although several immunocytochemical methods have been described which make use of haptenated antibodies (22-26), surprisingly few reports exist concerning their actual use in double-labelling studies. This is remarkable because hapten-labelling methods are often developed and recommended for this purpose (19,27,28).

Two types of methods can be distinguished:

a. Hapten anti-hapten methods, analogous to the conventional indirect assay. A mixture of two primary antibodies, which may be derived from the same animal species, are linked with different hapten groups (e.g. arsanilate (26), dinitrophenyl (DNP), (22,29), glutamate (26) or oxazolone (29). In the second step enzyme-linked anti-hapten antibodies are used. The method has been used by Wallace and Wofsy (23), but with fluorochrome in stead of enzyme labels.
b. Hapten sandwich procedures. Incubation with primary haptenated antibodies is followed by unlabelled anti-hapten

antibody and then haptenated PAP or APAAP complex (25). Both anti hapten antibodies should be non-crossreacting.
The main disadvantage of these methods is that it is not easy to obtain pure haptenated antibodies, while the enzyme-linked anti-hapten antibodies are not available commercially. Hapten techniques may also be combined well with other methods to obtain double-stained sections (5,17,29).

DOUBLE IMMUNOENZYME STAINING USING MONOCLONAL ANTIBODIES

As the overwhelming majority of monoclonal antibodies (MoAb's) is of the same (mouse) origin, their use in double-labelling studies offers particular problems. It is not possible to use simultaneous two- or multi-step procedures because the secondary antibodies generally do not distinguish between the two primary MoAb's. If the antigens however are expected to be localized on the same structure, it is recommendable to use simultaneous methods in order to give both antibodies a fair chance to occupy their antigenic sites. For this reason only pairs of MoAb's should be used, which have been linked directly to different groups: enzymes, haptens or biotin.

a. If possible the double direct method should be used. Good results, including intermediate staining, were obtained by incubation with a mixture of two MoAb's conjugated with HRP and AP, respectively (4). However, the efficiency is relatively low while conjugation of the antibodies requires a certain experience and also substantial amounts of the MoAb's.
b. When the MoAb's to be used are of different classes or subclasses (e.g. Mouse IgM, IgG1, or IgG2a), class- or subclass-specific developing antibodies may be used in double sandwich techniques. There is a risk, however, that the anti-subclass antibodies are not truly specific and are only low-titered (27). Tidman (30) used this method succesfully in double immunofluorescence studies, and van Rooyen and Kors (5) used a combination of HRP-conjugated anti subclass antibody with AP-labelled hapten in the detection of subclass and specificity of antibodies present in the tissue.
c. As indicated above, double hapten-antihapten or hapten sandwich techniques theoretically offer great possibilities, but their practical use is hampered by the limited availability of the immunoreagents. In certain cases the quick haptenation procedure we developed for small amounts of MoAb's with dinitrofluorobenzene (DNFB) or oxalone may be used (29). Good results have been obtained with the combined use of mouse monoclonal anti human IgM-DNP and biotinylated anti-T-helper monoclonal antibody with subsequent incubation of guinea pig anti-DNP-HRP and avidin-AP conjugate.
A variation of these simultaneous methods was described by Boorsma et al (19). They visualized pairs of cell-surface antigens in the same section with mixtures of (a) MoAb1-HRP with MoAb2-biotin, followed by (b) avidin-AP. With this method the simultaneous presence of cell-surface antigens, e.g. specific for pan T and T suppressor lymphocytes, were demonstrated by the formation of a mixed intermediate staining.

Sequential methods

In many instances, however, these simultaneous techniques cannot be used because direct conjugates of the MoAb's are not available or difficult to prepare. Moreover, the quantities of MoAb's that may be obtained commercially are often extremely small, too small anyhow to allow chemical modification. Taking into account that labelled and purified antigens are hardly available either, only sequential techniques are left.

Of these sequential methods one might select the original method of Nakane (1) or other methods as mentioned above, which may include elution of the primary and developing antibodies applied in the first sequence. In our experience, however, with MoAb's directed against cell-surface antigens, the second and third antibodies (like PAP complexes) are easily removed, but the primary, MoAb's, are often much more persistent. In these cases the elution procedure is of no help, and gives an even better exposure of the first MoAb to the developing antibodies of the second sequence, causing spurious double staining.

In order to solve this problem, we explored several combinations of incubation methods in sequential double-stainings with two MoAb's. In our experience the best method which could be applied most generally, was the combination of an indirect biotin-avidin complex method with DAB-HRP staining (although AEC can often be used also) with subsequent application of the APAAP method for the second antigen. Good results were obtained with several pairs of MoAb's, e.g. specific for cell-surface antigens of lymphocytes: Leu 1 or Leu 4 with Leu 12 or Leu 14 (T and B lymphocytes, resp.); Leu 2a with Leu 3a (T suppressor/cytotoxic and T helper/inducer, resp.); Leu 2a or Leu 3a with anti HLA-DR, etc. We were also able to visualize vimentin and cytokeratin simultaneously within the same cell using MoAb's (20,31). The bulky tree of antibodies with ABC, covered with the DAB polymer, efficiently masks the primary MoAb applied, preventing cross-reactions in the second sequence.

As the second antigen might be masked a little when present on the same cell, it is necessary to use an amplification step in the second sequence. For this, the APAAP method, with monoclonal antiAP, is ideal. It combines high sensitivity with exposure of AP, which can be demonstrated with high contrast and intensity, e.g. with the combination of naphtol AS-MX phosphate and Fast Blue BB (3,27). The full method is described below.

But also this method should be carried out critically. When both antigens to be stained are localized very near to each other or one of both is only present with few determinants whereas the other has many antigenic sites, problems may arise. In order to get the right balance between the two stainings, preliminary experiments should be performed to determine the optimal dilutions of the antibodies, which may be different from those in single stainings. Also the best sequence of applying them has to be determined. For example, when trying to stain T lymphocytes of the suppressor/cytotoxic and helper phenotype using this method, one will notice that the assay is only reliable when the T suppressor /cytotoxic (T8) cells are reacted first (with the ABC-HRP-DAB method) and subsequently the T helper (T4) cells (with the APAAP method).

SELECTION OF THE BEST TECHNIQUE

As can be concluded from the above, the method to be selected is predominantly dependent on the antibodies available. Generally it is recommendable to use a technique with simultaneous incubation steps and with different enzyme labels, e.g. peroxidase and alkaline phosphatase.

a. If enzyme-conjugates are available of one or both primary antibodies, it is advantageous to use them, for example in double direct or combined direct-indirect assays.
b. As at present anti-IgG antibodies of several animal species specificity can be obtained as HRP, AP as well as glucose oxidase conjugates, the double indirect technique is usually possible if both primary antibodies are also from different species. In the same way a combined PAP-APAAP technique has to be considered.
c. When one of both antigens is weakly staining, it is often possible to enhance its staining intensity by means of PAP, APAAP or avidin-biotin. Often several incubation steps can be performed simultaneously in combination with a direct or indirect method.
d. Only when the primary antibodies have the same species specificity (like most MoAb's) and are not available as conjugate with enzyme, hapten or biotin, a sequential technique should be considered.

CLOSING REMARKS

Double immunoenzyme staining of 2 antigens in tissue sections is not just a combination of two conventional single staining methods. Even higher demands are made upon the immunoreagents concerning their specificity and purity than in single immunostainings. If possible the detection systems for both antigens should be unrelated.

But which technique whatsoever has been chosen, it is always necessary to perform some preliminary experiments in order to determine if it works anyway, the proper dilutions of the immunoreagents and to make sure that no spurious mixed staining does occur. Also a careful comparison with both single stainings should be made. Sufficient control sections have to be included: deletion of one single step of antibody should result in a staining not different from the corresponding single staining.

When a sequential technique has to be used, it should be determined which antibody may be used best in the first and which one in the second sequence.

APPENDIX

Double immunoenzym staining of two unlabelled monoclonal antibodies

Pretreatment and preincubation of the sections should be the same as in the individual single stainings.
Subsequently the following incubations are performed:

1. MoAb 1; 60 min.
2. anti Mouse Ig-biotin* (e.g.Horse anti Mouse Ig-biotin,Vector, 1:250) 30 min.
3. Preformed Avidin-biotin-HRP complex*; 60 min.
4. Develop HRP staining **
5. MoAb 2; 60 min.
6. anti Mouse Ig (e.g.Rabbit anti Mouse Ig (DAKO) 1:25 or 1:50) 30 min.
7. monoclonal APAAP (e.g. DAKO, 1:50); 30 min.
8. Develop AP staining ***; 20-40 min.
9. Mount the wet sections directly with Kaiser's glycerin-gelatin or any other aequous mounting medium.

Between all steps thoroughly washing with Tris-buffered saline (TBS) /or phosphate-buffered saline (PBS) is necessary. Antibodies and conjugates are diluted in TBS or PBS.

* Avidin and biotin immunoreagents may be obtained from the Vectastain kit (Vector) and prepared according the directions indicated.

** Diaminobenzidine (0.5 mg/ml) plus 0.03% H_2O_2 and 0.07% imidazole in Tris-HCl buffer, pH 7.6. Stain for 5-10 min. Often 3-amino-9-ethylcarbazole (AEC) may be used as well: dissolve 4 mg AEC in 0.25 ml dimethylformamide (DMF) in a glass tube. Add to this solution 10 ml 0.05 M sodium acetate buffer, pH 4.9, and add 200 ul 1% H_2O_2. Filter this solution onto the slide. Incubate 10-15 min.

*** Dissolve 10 mg naphtol AS-MX phosphate in 0.2 ml DMF. Add 40 ml 0.2 M Tris-HCl buffer, pH 8.5. Immediately before use, dissolve 40 mg Fast Blue BB salt in this buffer and add 10 mg levamisole. After filtration, the solution may dripped directly onto the slide or the slides may be incubated vertically within a Coplin jar. Incubate for 20-40 min. Wash with buffer and tap water respectively.

REFERENCES:

1. Nakane PK: Simultaneous localisation of multiple tissue antigens using the peroxidase-labelled antibody method. J. Histochem. Cytochem. 16: 557-560, 1968.

2. Hsu SM, Soban E: Color Modification of diaminobenzidine precipitation by Metallic Ions and its application for double immunohistochemistry. J. Histochem. Cytochem. 30: 1079-1082, 1982.

3 Mason DY, Sammons R: Alkaline phosphatase and peroxidase for double immunoenzymatic labelling of cellular constituents. J. Clin. Pathol. 31: 454-460, 1978.

4. Boorsma DM: Direct immunoenzyme double staining applicable for monoclonal antibodies. Histochemistry 80: 103-106, 1984.

5. Van Rooyen N, Kors N: Double immunocytochemical staining in the study of the antibody-producing cells in vivo. J. Histochem. Cytochem. 33: 175-178, 1985.

6. Campbell GT, Bhatnagar AS: Simultaneous visualization by light microscopy of two pituitary hormones. J. Histochem. Cytochem. 24: 448-452, 1976.

7. Streefkerk JG: Inhibition of erythrocyte pseudoperoxidase activity by treatment with hydrogen peroxide following methanol. J. Histochem. Cytochem. 20: 829-831, 1972.

8. Borgers M: The cytochemical application of new potent inhibitors of alkaline phosphatase. J.Histochem. Cytochem.21: 812-824, 1973.

9. Feller AC, Parwaresch MR, Wacker HH, Radzun HJ, Lennert K. Combined immunohistochemical staining for surface IgD and T-lymphocyte subsets with monoclonal antibodies. Histochem. J. 15: 557-562.

10. Van de Sande F, Dierickx K: Immunocytochemical demonstration of separate vasotocinergic and mesotocinergic neurons in the amphibian hypothalamic magnocellular system. Cell Tissue Res. 175, 284-289, 1976.

11. Tramu G, Pillez A, Leonardelli J: An efficient method of antibody elution for the succesful simultaneous localization of two antigens. J. Histochem. Cytochem. 26: 322-324, 1978.

12. Sternberger LA, Joseph FA: The unlabelled antibody method. Contrasting color staining of paired pituitary hormones without antibody removal. J.Histochem. Cytochem. 27, 1424-1429, 1979.

13. Valnes K, Brandtzaeg P: Comparison of paired immunofluorescence and paired immunoenzyme staining based on primary antisera from the same species. J.Histochem. Cytochem. 30, 518-524, 1982.

14. Falini B, De Solas I, Halverson C, Parker JW, Taylor CR: Double labelled-antigen method for demonstration of intracellular antigens in paraffin-embedded tissues. J. Histochem. Cytochem. 30: 21-26, 1982.

15. Guesdon JL, Ternynck T, Avrameas S: The use of avidin-biotin interaction in immunoenzymatic techniques. J. Histochem. Cytochem. 27: 1131-1139, 1979.

16. Hsu SM, Raine L, Fanger H: Use of avidin-biotin peroxidase complex (ABC) in immunoperoxidase techniques. J. Histochem. Cytochem. 29: 577-580, 1981.

17. Caligaris-Cappio F, Gobbi M, Bofill M, Janossy G: Infrequent normal B lymphocytes express features of B-chronic lymphocyte leukemia. J. Exp. Med. 155, 623-628, 1982.

18. Klareskog L, Forsum U, Wigren A, Wigzell H: Relationship between HLA-DR-expressing cells and T lymphocytes of different subsets in rheumatoid synovial tissue. Scand. J. Immunol. 15: 501-507, 1982.

19. Boorsma DM, Van Bommel J, Van der Raay-Helmer EMH: Simultaneous double staining using two different enzymes linked directly to monoclonal antibodies or with biotin-avidin. J. Microscopy 1986, in press.

20. Mullink H, Henzen-Logmans SC, Alons-van Kordelaar JJM, Tadema TM, Meijer CJLM: Simultaneous immunoenzyme staining of vimentin and cytokeratins with monoclonal antibodies as an aid in the differential diagnosis: malignant mesothelioma - pulmonary adenocarcinoma. Virchows Arch B (Cell Path) in press, 1986.

21. Butterworth BH, Khong TY, Loke YW, Robertson WB: Human cytotrophoblast populations studied by monoclonal antibodies using single and double biotin-avidin-peroxidase immunocytochemistry. J. Histochem. Cytochem. 33:977-983,1985.

22. Farr AG, Nakane PK: Use of anti-hapten immunohistochemistry and immunoassay. J. Histochem. Cytochem. 29: 891, 1981.

23. Wallace EF, Wofsy L: Hapten Sandwich Labelling IV. Improved procedures and non-cross reacting hapten reagents for double-labelling cell surface antigens. J. Immunol. Meth. 25: 283-289, 1979.

24. Hewlins MJE, Weeks I, Jasani B: Non-deleterious dinitrophenyl hapten labelling of antibody protein. J. Immunol. Meth. 70: 111-118, 1984.

25. Jasani B, Wynford Thomas D, Williams E: Use of monoclonal antihapten antibodies for immunolocalisation of tissue antigens. J. Clin. Pathol. 34: 1000-1002, 1981.

26. Cammisuli S: Hapten-modified antibodies specific for cell-surface antigens as a tool in cellular immunology, in Lefkovits I, Pernis B (eds): Immunol. Meth. New York Acad. Press, Vol. 2, pp 139-162, 1981.

27. Mason DY, Abdulaziz Z, Falini B, Stein H: Double immunoenzymatic labelling. Polak JM, Van Noorden S: Immunocytochemistry. London Wright PSG, pp 113-128, 1983.

28. Falini B, Taylor CR: New developments in immunoperoxidase techniques and their application. Arch. Path. Lab. Med. 107: 105-117, 1983.

29. Mullink H, Scheper RJS, Boorsma DM, Klein JC, Oostendorp R: A rapid and simple hapten conjugation method of monoclonal antibodies and its application in immunohistochemical double staining procedures. To be published.

30. Tidman N, Janossy G, Bodger M, Granger S, Kung PC, Goldstein G: Delineation of human thymocyte differentiation pathways utilising double staining techniques with monoclonal antibodies. Clin. Exp. Immunol. 45: 457-467, 1981.

31. Henzen-Logmans SC, Mullink H, Ramaekers FCS, Meijer CJLM: Cytokeratin patterns and co-expression of cytokeratin and vimentin in epithelial cells of normal and pathologic thyroid glands. Pathol. Res. Pract. 180: 276, 1985.

II. TUMOR ASSOCIATED ANTIGENS

4. MONOCLONAL ANTIBODIES TO ONCOFETAL ANTIGENS.

M. NAP

1. INTRODUCTION

Oncofetal antigens can be defined as antigens that are expressed during intrauterine life, diminish strongly or disappear after birth and reappear in situations of repair or neoplastic growth in those organs where they appeared during gestation in the fetus (1). It should be emphasized that in this situation a normal fetal antigen is reexpressed not only in neoplastic cells of the adult, but also in cells involved in regenerative processes.
The position of oncofetal antigens can be looked at from different view points.
One is the observation that tumor cells morphologically resemble embryonic or immature cells and thereby may recapitulate a fetal type composition of their cell products and antigenicity (2).
Another point is the observation that immunization with fetal tissue could elicit an immune response to tumor antigens in the experimental model (3). However, not all tumor antigens are oncofetal and not all fetal antigens are expressed by tumor cells. Immunization with fetal material does not always result in production of antibodies the same as immunizations using tumor material and not all antibodies directed against tumor antigens are reactive with fetal antigens. Despite morphological and functional resemblances also differences between tumor cells and fetal cells exist. Fetal cells do proliferate but in general do not infiltrate whereas tumor cells proliferate and often infiltrate. One has to be well informed about the distribution of antigens, in normal adult tissues and during development before an antigen can be regarded as an oncofetal antigen.

2. ONCOFETAL ANTIGENS AND MONOCLONAL ANTIBODIES

The contribution of monoclonal antibodies to the field of oncofetal antigens probably is mainly in the more precise identification of oncofetal epitopes and altered expression of epitopes on the same molecules in the fetus and adult.
In various types of tumors oncofetal antigens have been described, of which alpha fetoprotein (AFP) (4) and carcinoembryonic antigen (CEA) (5) probably are the ones that we know most of. Perhaps AFP and CEA together with several other antigens illustrate best how careful preparation of antigens and antibodies, and documentation of antigen distribution contribute to the insight in their possible function and utility in cancer diagnosis and monitoring.
Although antigens with oncofetal properties are reported mostly in association with epithelial tumors, also in malignant tumors from the haematopoetic system, in melanomas and neurogenic tumors, antigens have been described

associated with a specific period during maturation of the normal counterpart (3).
As Sell pointed out so nicely in his book "Cancer Markers", that although oncodevelopmental antigens are important in diagnosis and prognosis of cancer; "they did not originate for the convenience of the physician or scientist but must play an important role in the normal developing embryo or in adult proliferating tissue" (6). This attitude is of importance to improve our knowledge about these antigens and their relation to cancer and immediately implicates that our studies should not be focussed to much on the neoplastic cell but also on regenerative situations in the normal adult and on cells in the developing individual.

2.1. Alpha fetoprotein

AFP, initially described by Abelev (4), appeared to be a protein that could be isolated from the amniotic fluid, and demonstrated in yolk sac epithelium, fetal hepatocytes and primary hepatocellular carcinoma. Chapters dealing with AFP in "Cancer Markers" edited by Sell and in "Fetal antigens in cancer" of the 96th Ciba Foundation Symposium summarize much of the information available on AFP (7).
In situations of congenital malformations of the neural tube elevated levels of AFP can be found in the maternal serum and also errors of metabolism in the liver can be associated with increased plasma concentrations of AFP in the newborn. Increased levels of AFP in plasma after birth are associated with liver cell proliferation either of regenerative nature or in liver cell neoplasia. However, also tumors with yolk sac differentiation produce AFP and sometimes AFP production can be found in carcinoma of the intestine (8), which, like the liver, has its relation with the yolk sac by its endodermal origin. Because AFP and albumin show many similarities in chemical composition but differ markedly in distribution between fetal and adult tissues, AFP has been considered to be a precursor of albumin (7). Some suggestions have been put forward about its function one of which is supported by experimental data (9, 10, 11).
Its role in the developing liver was once thought to be in the orientation of hepatocytes (7) and its production by the yolk sac epithelium was brought in connection with a possible immunological function in keeping the fetus from rejection by the mother's immune system (3). Indeed for this immunological function supportive evidence has been obtained (9,10,11). AFP was found to have a stimulatory effect on T-suppressor cells and administration of AFP in an animal model could prevent an allergic encephalitis (12).
AFP corresponds to the definition of an oncofetal antigen as outlined in the beginning and a functional aspect has been demonstrated. Whether or not AFP has a similar function in cancer and regeneration is uncertain at the moment. Up till now polyclonal antisera and monoclonal antibodies to AFP have shown similar specificities for the antigen (Uriel, pers. communication). The advantage of monoclonal antibodies here is a general one, namely that large quantities of constant specificity can be produced (13).

2.2. Mucus associated antigen M_1

Whereas AFP is truly an oncofetal antigen in the liver and yolk sac, other antigens can be of oncofetal nature at one localization and belong to the normal products of adult tissue at another place.

The group of M_1 antigens is an example of this phenomenon. M_1 antigens, mucus associated antigens, have been extensively studied by Bara and co-workers (14, 15, 16, 17) whereas Higgins et al. (18) have reported on similar antigens which occur in the normal adult gastric foveolar mucus cells, in mucinous ovarian cysts, in the adult endocervical gland epithelium and in the goblet cells of the fetal colon, but not in the normal adult colonic epithelium (14).

The name M_1 was given by Bara based on reaction patterns in tissue sections using antisera to mucus cyst fluid. Staining reactions in the foveolar gastric epithelium only was called M_1 reactivity. Antiserum that stained mucus neck cells, subesophageal glands, cardiac and pyloric glands and the Golgi apparatus of the intestinal absorptive cells, represented M_2 reactivity. Antiserum reactive with the goblet cells of small and large intestine represented M_3 reactivity.

M_1 belongs to a group of highly sialilated fucomucins all reactive with the polyclonal antiserum. The initial results concerning the M_1 antigens were obtained using polyclonal antisera which needed extensive absorptions to red blood cells, normal human serum components and other normal tissue components. These results have now been confirmed by studies with monoclonal antibodies. At present five monoclonal antibodies have been produced all recognizing different epitopes on the protein moiety of the M_1 molecule.

Because M_1 reactivity could not be observed in normal adult colonic mucosa, but was present in fetal colonic goblet cells its possible role in neoplastic disorders of the colon was studied both in the rat model (19) and in man (16). Expression of M_1 antigens in the rat colonic mucosa was found early in the process of experimental carcinogenesis, i.e. two weeks after administration of the carcinogen (19). In the human situation M_1 expression can be found in adenomatous polyps and in the mucosa adjacent to carcinomas. A tendency for increased M_1 expression with increase in size of the adenoma and loss of M_1 positivity together with loss of goblet cells in dysplasia has been reported (14). In carcinomas M_1 expression was found to be relatively low (14).

In a recently completed study (20) on colorectal adenomas we have compared the staining patterns of four monoclonal anti-M_1 antibodies with the results of flow cytometric DNA profile measurements obtained on the same adenomas in a previous study (21).

Our results were compatible with those published before by Bara on M_1 distribution in colorectal adenomas. There was no correlation between the classical goblet cell staining by M_1 antibodies and DNA ploidy data. One of the monoclonals, however, in addition to goblet cell staining showed a predominant cytoplasmic staining. The staining pattern of antibody 1-13 M_1 showed a strong correlation ($p<0.001$) with aneuploid DNA profiles. These observations illustrate that different epitopes on an oncofetal antigen like M_1 may have different biological implications. However, cross reactivity with an unknown determinant cannot be excluded. The cytoplasmic staining pattern obtained with antibody 1-13 M_1 has not been observed before, using polyclonal antisera to M_1. This may be explained by assuming that antibodies to the epitope recognized by antibody 1-13 M_1 comprise a minor part of the polyclonal antiserum to M_1 and cannot display their reactivity due to steric hindrance or competition. Separate incubation of the different moabs may eliminate this inhibitory effect.

Studies performed on the distribution of M_1 using both polyclonal and monoclonal antibodies have dealt mostly with neoplastic and fetal colonic epithelium and with normal adult colonic mucosa (14-17). However, another aspect of the oncofetal character of M_1, its expression in regenerative epithelium of the adult colonic mucosa has not obtained much attention. Both histochemical and immunohistochemical studies have shown altered mucin composition in the colon mucosa involved in inflammatory disease (22, 23). Using the same panel of monoclonal anti-M_1 antibodies we have studied cases of ulcerative colitis, Crohn's colitis, acute self limiting colitis, schistosomiasis, diverticular disease and other mucosal disorders of the colon. It appeared that staining of goblet cells for M_1 could be found in all inflammatory conditions and also in reactive changes without active inflammation (Maes et al., manuscript in preparation).

Nutritional factors and changes of the bacterial flora in the colon have been reported to play a role in the etiology of colorectal cancer. The objective registration of epithelial damage in the colon mucosa due to these factors might contribute to the understanding of the possible relation between chronic irritation and the development of neoplasia. Immunohistochemistry using anti-M_1 antibodies may provide tools for registration of these changes.

The knowledge obtained by this method might be useful as a tool in preventive medicine, i.e. in the identification of individuals at risk for colorectal cancer.

2.3. Pancreatic oncofetal antigens

The pancreas has been the subject of many studies concerning detection and management of malignant tumors arising mainly from its exocrine component (24 -30).

Because of its difficult accessability both for diagnostic and therapeutic approaches many investigations have been executed in order to identify an antigen, produced by neoplastic or preneoplastic lesions and secreted into the blood stream which could indicate tumor activity. However, not all antigens studied in this respect appear to be of oncofetal nature, which does not necessarily mean that they are less important in the diagnosis and monitoring of cancer of the pancreas.

Of the antigens related to pancreatic adenocarcinoma the GICA (24) and Dupan 2 (25) are most clearly of non-oncofetal nature but represent normal antigens of the digestive tract (31) which are expressed in increased amounts also in pancreatic adenocarcinoma. This applies also to pancreatic oncofetal antigen (POA), described by Homma et al. (26) which can be demonstrated both in fetal and adult pancreatic ductal epithelium and in tumors.
An antigen with the same name but different molecular weight was described earlier by Banwo (27) using polyclonal antisera. The results obtained by them and later by others (28) showed that increased POA reactivity in the serum of patients with carcinoma was not restricted to carcinoma of the pancreas but could be found in 20 - 36% of cancers from the lung, head and neck region and bile ducts as well as in 27% of benign liver disorders. These observations illustrate the wrongly applied terminology. One should exercise caution in labeling an antigen as oncofetal too early in the characterization studies and await extensive immunohistological testing of normal tissues and non-neoplastic conditions.
It is currently not known if the pancreatic antigens described by the group of Escribano (29, 30) are of oncofetal nature. Using a polyclonal antiserum many oncofetal characteristics have been demonstrated that now have to be confirmed by monoclonal antibodies. Immunoblotting experiments using a polyclonal antiserum demonstrated five different bands in a fetal pancreatic extract which are absent in extract from adult pancreas. Antigen reactivity can be found in acinic cells of the developing fetal pancreas leaving the ductal elements unstained. During intrauterine maturation maximal staining of acinar cells is observed around the fifth month, declining thereafter. In the adult pancreas no positive staining is found. In a large number of fetal and adult non-pancreatic tissues and carcinomas of the colon, stomach, liver and biliary tree, lungs, salivary glands, kidney, ureter, urinary bladder and prostate no reactivity was found using the polyclonal antiserum . The majority of pancreatic tumors, however, focally express the antigen. Interestingly the preexisting acinar cells surrounding the tumor show a strong cytoplasmic staining. This phenomenon was also observed in pancreatic acinar tissue surrounding a metastatic melanoma. In samples of pancreatitis individual acinar cells were positive. Apparently the increased expression of this antigen is also associated with reactive changes of acinar pancreatic cells. A recently developed monoclonal antibody reactive with two bands in immunoblotting of compatible molecular weight as demonstrated by the polyclonal antiserum reacted strongly with fetal acinar cells but also with some acinar cells in the normal adult pancreas. No reactivity was seen in normal duct epithelium but in hyperplastic altered epithelium of pancreatic ducts some reactivity was seen.
The results still are preliminar but it seems worthwhile to proceed and prepare monoclonal antibodies recognizing

different epitopes on the antigens identified by the polyclonal antiserum in order to establish the oncofetal character. Such antibodies may become useful in the diagnosis and management of pancreatic adenocarcinoma.

2.4. Carcino Embryonic Antigen

An antigen which is also associated with cancer of the pancreas and with many other carcinomas of intestinal and non-intestinal origin is the carcinoembryonic antigen (CEA) described by Gold and Freedman (5). CEA probably is one of the tumor associated antigens that has been subjected to much critizism but nevertheless remains an antigen valuable as a marker of many different tumors during follow-up after treatment (32 - 45).
Although CEA is not an oncofetal antigen and therefore perhaps should not be discussed in this chapter, its historical relation with them and the fact that by demonstration of the absence of an oncofetal nature of this antigen it becomes more useful in differential diagnosis, justifies its presence here.
The main problem concerning the interpretation of immunohistochemical and immunochemical data on CEA has been the influence of cross reactive antibodies to CEA and related antigens such as NCA, NCA$_2$ and BGP$_I$ (46). With the introduction of monoclonal antibodies to CEA it was hoped to overcome the laborous absorption procedure necessary to render polyclonal sera monospecific for CEA. However, it appeared that most antibodies produced by hybridoma technique, although reactive with CEA, also reacted with epitopes that were present on both CEA and other antigens (47, 48).
This observation confirmed the mechanism of the cross reactions and proved that the cross reactions obtained with polyclonal antisera were not due to impurities of the antigen preparation used for immunization. In figure 1 a schematic proposition is given to illustrate this mechanism.

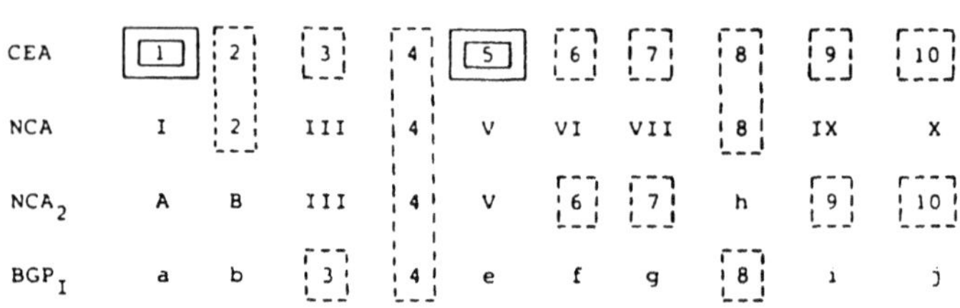

Fig.1 Schematic illustration if the possible mechanism of cross reactions between CEA and related antigens.

In this figure CEA and its main cross reacting antigens NCA, NCA_2 and BGP_I have been given 10 theoretical epitopes represented by different symbols. Those epitopes that CEA has in common with one or more of the other antigens retain the symbol of the corresponding epitope on the CEA molecule. It is evident that immunization with pure CEA always results in a mixture of crossreactive antibodies and monospecific antibodies constituting the antiserum. Absorption with NCA, NCA_2 and BGP_I removes the crossreactive antibodies resulting in a monospecific antiserum (46). Monoclonal antibodies to one of the common epitopes on CEA, NCA, NCA_2 or BGP_I will also show cross reactivity but because of their monoclonal nature absorptions cannot remove their crossreactivity.
Only a limited number of publications on monoclonal anti-CEA antibodies provide convincing evidence with respect to monospecificity (49,50,51). The difficulty to find monospecific anti-CEA antibodies may be reflected in the scarcity of epitopes specific for CEA illustrated in fig. 1. Knowledge of the reactivity of both monospecific and cross reactive antibodies seems helpful in understanding the possible different positions taken by CEA during development and in the adult with or without carcinoma. Using monospecific polyclonal and monoclonal antibodies to CEA recognizing exclusively the 180 kd glycoprotein of a perchloricacid extract from colonic adenocarcinoma, we have studied the organ distribution of CEA in over 90 embryo's, fetusses and in the normal adult. It appeared that CEA could be demonstrated exclusively in certain segments of the digestive tube (52). CEA could be demonstrated starting from early fetal life throughout the intra uterine period and also in adult tissues at the tongue, esophagogastric junction, gastric antrum and pyloric region and the entire colon and appendix. Organs outside this tube such as liver, pancreas, kidney, ureter, urinary bladder, lungs, thyroid, salivary glands, breast, skin and spleen, were consistently negative for CEA. These observations made it possible to arrange a large group of carcinomas into three different classes according to their CEA production in relation to the development and normal adult situation of the tissue of origin.
Tumors could belong to expected positives: colon, stomach, esophagus, small intestine, or expected negatives; kidney, liver, prostate, thyroid (papillary and follicular) and the third category, a group of tumors that unexpectedly produce CEA: lung, breast, pancreas, urinary bladder and the medullary thyroid carcinoma.
In the first category CEA immunohistochemistry can be of help to decide if serial CEA serum samples will be useful for follow-up or, if the tumor is CEA negative, other markers should be looked for (53).
CEA immunohistochemistry can also be of help in the case of differential diagnostic problems about the origin of metastatic tumors. A CEA positive tumor at the anatomical site of expected CEA negativity most likely is of metastatic origin.
In carcinomas of the third category the relation between CEA production by the tumor and the corresponding normal

developing or adult organ is absent. However, it is this category in which CEA positivity seems to be closely related with malignancy (50), as an ectopic production by neoplastic cells, possibly due to inappropriate DNA expression. This ectopic CEA production is especially valuable in the diagnosis of tumors with a high degree of CEA positivity, such as pancreatic adenocarcinomas and medullary carcinoma of the thyroid. CEA possitivity may be of help to discriminate carcinoma from reactive changes. These possible benefits from CEA immunohistochemistry clearly show the impact of commercially available pure and specific reagents.
In addition the cross reaction between CEA and another antigen has been shown to be of diagnostic importance. Cross reactivity with BGP_1 results in bile canalicular staining of normal liver tissue (46). This type of staining in the absence of true CEA reactivity was seen in approximately 80% of primary hepatocellular carcinomas and never in tumors from non-hepatic origin, thus being highly diagnostic for the hepatocellular origin of a tumor (54). Unfamiliarity with this phenomenon may result in misinterpretation of the CEA reactivity in primary liver cancer (45) and the loss of potential use of anti-CEA antibodies in differential diagnostic problems.

3. CONCLUSIONS

I have tried to illustrate different aspects of antigens generally referred to as oncofetal antigens i.e. (table 1) the existence of truly oncofetal antigens like AFP, the possibility that antigens can be oncofetal in one organ but belong to the normal structure of another organ (M_1), the confusion which can occur if an antigen is introduced as an oncofetal antigen without sufficient proof (pancreas, CEA) and how the unraveling of the different characteristics of antibodies to an antigen can result in better understanding of their possible usefulness in diagnostic pathology (CEA and related antigens).

Table I
Oncofetal antigens of epithelial cells classified by their distribution in fetal, and adult organs and in regeneration and neoplasia, as demonstrated by immunohistochemistry.

Antigen	Class*	fetal organs	normal adult	regeneration	(from related tissue) related neoplasia	(from different germ layer) unrelated neoplasia
1 AFP	I	liver, yolksac	not detectable	liver	hepatoma yolksac tumor intestinal tumors	breast, ovarian epithelial tumors
2 M_1	II	colon, stomach endocervix	stomach, endocervix	colon stomach endocervix	adenomatous polyps of colon, endocer vical tumors, mucinous ovarian tumors, gastric tumors	unknown
3 GICA (CA 19-9)	III	colon, stomach pancreatic ducts	colon, stomach pancreatic ducts, endocervix	unknown	colon, stomach pancreatis/adeno-carcinoma endocervix	unknown
4 $Dupan_2$	III	pancreatic ducts	pancreatic ducts	unknown	pancreatic adenocarcinoma	
5 P.O.A.	III	pancreatic	pancreatic	unknown	pancreatic adenocarcinoma salivary gland tumors	
6 F.P.A.	I	pancreatic acinar cells	not detectable	pancreatic acinar cells	pancreatic adenocarcinomas	none
7 C.E.A.	III	tongue, stomach colon	tongue, stomach colon	as adult	intestinal neoplasms	breast, thyroid lung, pancreas urinary bladder

* Antigen class
I = truely oncofetal at one or more places
II = oncofetal at some, normal antigens at other places
III = not oncofetal due to constant presence at the same localization

REFERENCES

1. Uriel J., Retro-differentiation and fetal patterns of gene expression in cancer. Adv. Cancer Res. 1979; 29: 127-174.
2. Chism S.E., Oncofetal transplantation antigens. In: Sell S. ed. Cancer Markers. Humana Press 1980, pp. 115-132.
3. Coggin J.H. Jr., Embryonic antigens in malignancy and pregnancy: common denominators in immune regulation. In: Fetal antigens and cancer. CIBA Foundation, Symposium 96. Egeret D. and Whelan J., eds., Pitman 1983, pag. 28-54.
4. Abelev G.J., α-Foetoprotein in ontogenesis and its association with malignant tumors. Adv. Cancer Res. 1971; 14: 295-358.
5. Gold Ph. and Freedman S.O., Specific carcinoembryonic antigens of the human digestive system. J. Exp. Med. 1965; 121: 467-479.
6. Sell S., In Cancer Markers, Sell S. ed., Humana Press 1980, preface pag. VII.
7. Sell S., α-Fetoprotein. In: Cancer Markers, Sell S. ed., Humana Press 1980, pag. 249-293.
8. Leader M., Jass J.R., Increased α-fetoprotein concentration in association with ileal adenocarcinoma complicating Crohn's disease. J. Clin. Pathol. 1984; 37: 293-297.
9. Gershwin M.E., Castles J.J., Ahmed A., Makishima R., The influence of α-fetoprotein on Moloney sarcoma virus oncogenesis: evidence for generation of antigen nonspecific suppressor T cells. J. Immunol. 1978; 121: 2292-2298.
10. Murgita R.A. and Wigzell H., Regulation of immune functions in the fetus and newborn. Prog. Allergy 1981; 29: 54-133.
11. Gershwin M.E., Castles J.J. and Makishima R., Accelerated plasmacytoma formation in mice treated with alpha-fetoprotein. J. Nat. Cancer Instit. 1980; 64: 145-149.
12. Abramsky O., Brenner T., Mizrachi R. and Soffer D., Alpha-fetoprotein suppresses experimental allergic encephalomyelitis. J. Neuroimmunol. 1982; 2: 1-7.
13. Köhler G. and Milstein C., Continuous cultures of fused cells secreting antibodies of predefined specificity. Nature 1975; 256: 495-497.
14. Bara J., Burtin P., Mucus associated gastro-intestinal antigens in transitional mucosa adjacent to human colonic adenocarcinomas: their "fetal type" association. Eur. J. Cancer 1980; 16: 1303-1310.
15. Bara J., Loisillier F. and Burtin P., Antigens of gastric and intestinal mucus cells in human colonic tumors. Brit. J. Cancer 1980; 41: 209-221.
16. Bara J., Languille O., Gendron M.C., Daher N., Martin E. and Burtin P., Immunohistological study of precancerous mucus modification in human distal colonic polyps. Cancer Res. 1983; 43: 3885-3891.

17. Bara J., Malarewicz A., Loisillier F. and Burtin P., Antigens common to human ovarian mucinous cyst fluid and gastric mucosa. Brit. J. Cancer 1977; 36: 49-56.
18. Higgins P.J., Friedman E., Lipkin M., Hertz L., Attiyeh F. Stonehill E.H., Expression of gastric associated antigens by human premalignant and malignant colonic epithelial cells. Oncology 1983; 40: 26-30.
19. Deceaens C., Bara J., Rosa B, Daher N., Burtin P., Early oncofetal antigenic modifications during rat carcinogenesis. Cancer Res. 1983; 43: 355-362.
20. Ingh van den H.F., Bara J., Cornelisse C.J., Nap M., Aneuploidy and expression of gastric-aassociated mucus antigens M_1 and CEA in colorectal adenomas. Accepted for publication in Am.J.Clin.Path.
21. Ingh van den H.F., Griffioen G., Cornelisse C.J., Flow cytometric detection of aneuploidy in colorectal adenomas. Cancer Res. 1985; 45: 3392-3397.
22. Philipe M.I., Branfoot A.C., Abnormal patterns of mucus secretion in apparently normal mucosa of large intestine with carcinoma. Cancer 1974; 34: 282-290.
23. Biasco G., Lipkin M., Minarini A., Higgins P., Miglioli M., Barbara L., Proliferative antigenic properties of rectal cells in patients with chronic ulcerative colitis. Cancer Res. 1984; 44: 5450-5454.
24. Magnani J.L., Steplewski Z., Koprowski H., Ginsburg V., Identification of the gastro-intestinal and pancreatic cancer associated antigen detected by monoclonal antibody 19-9 in the sera of patients as a mucin. Cancer Res. 1984; 43: 5489-5492.
25. Lan M.S., Finn O.J., Fernsten P.H.D. Metzgar R.S., Isolation and properties of a human pancreatic adenocarcinoma associated antigen DU-PAN-2. Cancer Res. 1985; 45: 3005-3010.
26. Homma T., Ogushi H., Kawa S., A pancreatic oncofetal antigen: its partial purification and clinical application. Gastroenterology Jpn. 1983; 18: 487-491.
27. Banwo O., Versey J. and Hobbs J.R., New oncofetal antigen for human pancreas. Lancet 1974; 1: 643-645.
28. Gelder F.B., Reese C.J., Moosa A.R., Hall T. and Hunter R., Purification, partial characterization and clinical evaluation of pancreatic oncofetal antigen. Cancer Res. 1978; 38: 313-324.
29. Benedi V.J., Escribano M.J., Zuinghedau J. and Burtin P., fetal pancreatic antigens in the Serian golden hamster and their relationship to development and carcinogenesis. Cancer Res. 1984; 44: 1135-1141.
30. Escribano M.J., Cordier J., Nap M., Kate ten F.J.W., Burtin P., Antigens of differentiation in fetal human pancreas and their reexpression in cancer. Int. J. cancer, in press.
31. Bara J., Herrero Zabaleta E., Mollicone R., Nap M., Burtin P., Distribution of GICA in Normal Gastrointestinal and Endocervical Mucosae and in Mucinous Ovarian Cysts, using antibody NS 19-9. Am. J. Clin. Path 1986; 85: 152-159,

32. O'Brien M.J., Zamcheck N., Burke B., Kirkham S.E., Saravis C.A., Gottlieb L.S., Immunocytochemical localization of carcinoembryonic antigen in benign and malignant colorectal tissues. Am. J. Clin. Pathol. 1981; 75: 283-290.
33. Franchimont P., Zangerle P.F., Hendrick J.C., Renter A., Colin C., Simultaneous assays of cancer associated antigens in benign and malignant breast disease. Cancer 1977; 39: 2806-2812.
34. Kuhajda F.P., Offutt L.E., Mendelsohn G., The distribution of carcinoembryonic antigen in breast carcinoma. Cancer 1983; 52: 1257-1264.
35. Nap M., Fleuren G.J., Immunohistochemical demonstration of carcinoembryonic antigen in lung cancer, its localization in relation to tumor type and differentiation. Protides of the biological fluids. Peters H. (ed.), 31: 333-335 (1983).
36. Vincent R.G., Chu T.M., Lane W.W., The value of carcinoembryonic antigen in patients with carcinoma of the lung. Cancer 1979; 44: 685-691.
37. Shevchuk M.M., Fenoglio C.M., Richart R.M., Carcinoembryonic antigen localization in benign and malignant transitional epithelium. Cancer 1981; 47: 899-905.
38. Moore T.L., Kupchik H.Z., Marcon N., Zamcheck N., Carcinoembryonic antigen assay in cancer of the colon and pancreas and other digestive tract disorders. Am. J. Dig. Dis. 1971; 16: 1-7.
39. Rapp W., Wurster K., The CEA positive cancer and non-cancer cells of the stomach. Diagnostic and histogenetic significance. In: Carcinoembryonic Proteins, Vol. II, Lehman F.G. (ed.), Elsevier, North-Holland Biomedical Press 1979, pp 29-37.
40. Burtin P., Calmettes C., Fondaneche M.C., CEA and non-specific cross reacting antigen (NCA) in medullary carcinomas of the thyroid. Int. J. Cancer 1979; 23: 741-745.
41. Heald J., Buckley C.H., Fox H., An immunohistochemical study of distribution of carcinoembryonic antigen in epithelial tumors of the ovary. J. Clin. Pathol. 1979; 32 (no 9): 918-926.
42. Charpin C., Bhan A.K., Zurawski Jr. V.R., Scully R.E., Carcinoembryonic antigen (CEA) and carbohydrate determinant 19-9 (CA 19-9). Localization in 121 primary and metastatic tumors: an immunohistochemical study with the use of monoclonal antibodies. Int. J. Gynecol. Pathol. 1982; 1: 231-245.
43. Van Nagell J.R. and Goldenberg D.M., Carcinoembryonic antigen staining of endometrial and endocervical carcinomas. Lancet 1980; 213.
44. Caselitz T.J., Seifert G., Immunohistochemical detection of carcinoembryonic antigen (CEA) in parotid gland carcinomas. Virchows Arch. (PA) 1981; 394: 49-60.

45. Roncalli M., Borzio M., De Biagi G., Servida E., Cantaboni A., Sironi M., Taccagni G.L., Liver cell dysplasia and hepatocellular carcinoma: a histological and immunohistochemical study. Histopathol. 1985; 9: 209-221.
46. Nap M., Hoor ten K.A., Fleuren G.J., Cross reactivity with normal antigens in commercial antisera used for immunohistology; their need for tissue controls and absorptions. Am. J. Clin. Pathol. 1983; 79: 25-31.
47. Neumaier M., Fenger U., Wagener C., Monoclonal antibodies for carcinoembryonic antigen (CEA) as a model system: identification of two novel CEA-related antigens in meconium and colorectal carcinoma tissue by Western blots and differential immuno affinity chromatography. J. Immunol. 1985; 135: 3604-3609.
48. Hedin A., Hammerström S., Larsson A., Specificities and binding properties of eight monoclonal antibodies against Carcinoembryonic Antigen (CEA). Mol. Immunol. 1982; 19: 1641-1648.
49. Bosslet K., Lüben G., Schwarz A., Hundt E., Harthus H.P., Seiler F.R., Muhrer C., Klöppel G., Kayser K., Sedlacek H.H., Immunohistochemical localization and molecular characteristics of three monoclonal antibody defined epitopes detectable on Carcinoembryonic Antigen (CEA). Int. J. Cancer 1985; 36: 75-84.
50. Nap M., Keuning H., Burtin P., Oosterhuis J.W., Fleuren G.J., CEA and NCA in benign and malignant breast tumors. Am. J. Clin. Pathol. 1984; 82: 526-534.
51. Nap M., letter: Carcinoembryonic Antigen (CEA) and cross reacting antibodies. Arch. Pathol. Lab. Med. 1985; 109: 482.
52. Nap M., Møllgård K., Burtin P., Fleuren G.J., What is oncodevelopmental about Carcinoembryonic Antigen (CEA)? Tumor Biology 1985; 6: 329.
53. Midiri G., Amanti C., Benedetti M., Kampisi C., Santeusanio G., Castagna G., Peronace L., Di Tondo U., Di Paola M., Pascal R.R., CEA tissue staining in colorectal cancer patients. A way to improve their usefulness of serial serum CEA evaluation. Cancer 1985; 55: 5624-5629.
54. Koelma I.A., Nap M., Huitema S., Krom R.A.F., Houthoff H.J., Hepatocellular Carcinoma, Adenoma and Focal Nodular hyperplasia. A compararive histooathologic study with immunohistochemical parameters. Arch. Path. Lab. Med., 1986 in press.

5. CYTOSKELETAL PROTEINS AS MARKERS IN SURGICAL PATHOLOGY.

F.C.S.RAMAEKERS, A.HUIJSMANS, G.SCHAART, O.MOESKER, G.P.VOOIJS

1. INTRODUCTION

Within the cytoskeleton of the cell three different types of filaments can be distinguished on basis of their ultrastructural appearance and biochemical composition. Next to microfilaments and microtubules, filaments measuring 8-11 nm in diameter are commonly seen in mammalian cells. These so-called intermediate-sized filaments, which often constitute a considerable part of the intracellular matrix (Figure 1), are extremely insoluble and show a protein composition which is completely different from that of microfilaments and microtubules. Biochemical and immuno(cyto)chemical studies have demonstrated that five different types of intermediate filament proteins (IFP) can be distinguished in mammalian

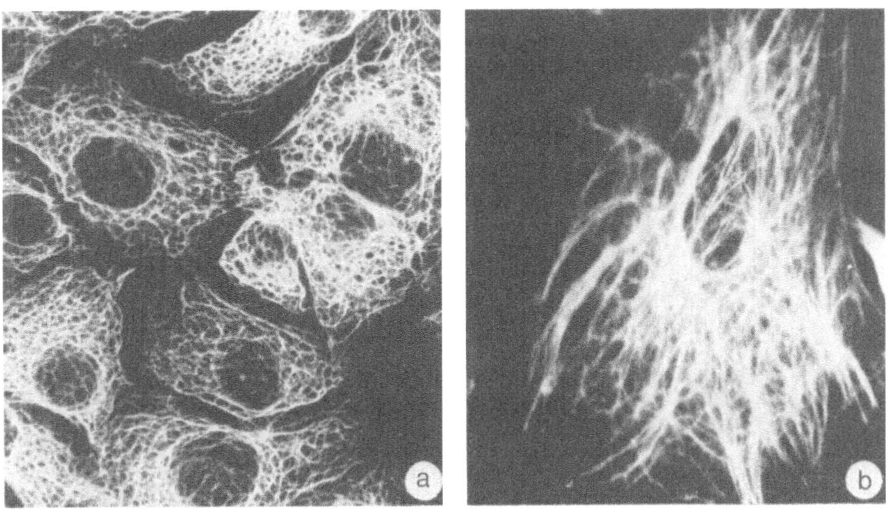

FIGURE 1. Cytokeratin intermediate filament organization as detected by the indirect immunofluorescence technique with specific cytokeratin antibodies in a) cultured human hepatocellular carcinoma cells (RGE 53, a monoclonal antibody to cytokeratin 18) and b) guinea pig hepatocellular carcinoma cell in culture (rabbit antiserum to human skin keratins).

cells (1). These include the cytokeratins, vimentin, desmin, glial fibrillary acidic protein (GFAP) and the neurofilament protein triplet. This chapter will concentrate on the use of (monoclonal) antibodies to these IFP in diagnostic histopathology.

2. TISSUE-SPECIFIC DISTRIBUTION OF IFP

The different types of IFP are distributed in a tissue-specific manner, and from Table 1 it may be obvious that the subdivision made between tissues on basis of their IFP content corresponds strikingly well with the major tissue classification based on histologic principles.
Monoclonal and polyclonal antibodies to the different types of IFP have been prepared by several groups working in the field (1-5) and many of them are commercially available now. Normally the polyclonal antibodies are raised in rabbits, sheep or goat by injection of highly purified intermediate filament proteins (see for example reference 5). As an example, Figure 2 illustrates the purity of a desmin preparation from chicken gizzard. This muscle-specific IFP was injected into rabbits and the resulting antiserum absorbed on skin keratins to remove cross-reactivity with epithelial tissues. Immunoblotting assays show that this rabbit antiserum reacts only with desmin (Figure 2f).

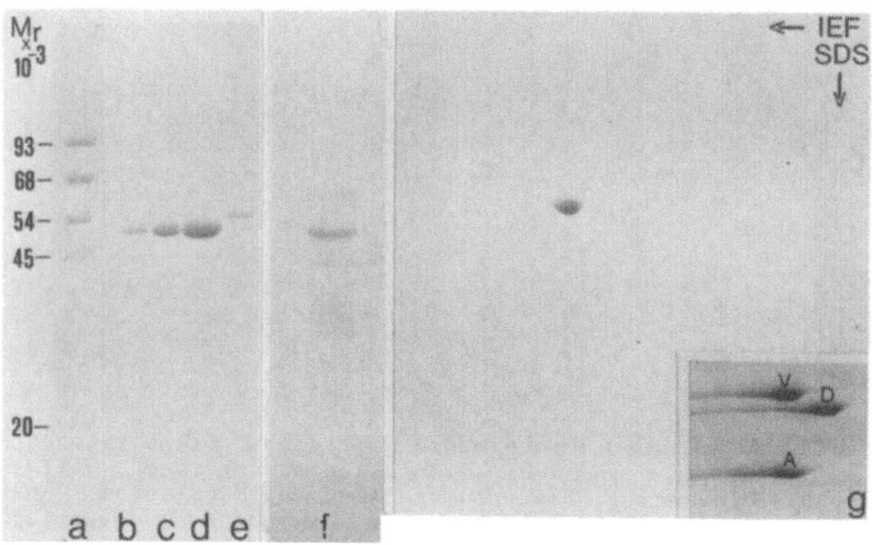

FIGURE 2. Gel electrophoretic analysis of a desmin preparation isolated from chicken gizzard muscle tissue and used for immunisation of rabbits. a) Marker proteins. b-d) The desmin preparation. e) Purified vimentin from bovine lens as reference. g) Two-dimensional gel showing purity of the desmin preparation and the mobility of desmin (D) relative to vimentin (V) and actin (A) (insert). f) Immunoblot of the rabbit antidesmin serum on human muscle proteins.

For the preparation of monoclonal antibodies to IFP it is not necessary to inject mice with highly purified protein preparations. In many instances total cytoskeletal fractions (which also contain nuclear and some membrane proteins) of specific cell types have been used for immunisation. Normally, such antibodies are tested for specificity by immunofluorescence- and immunoblotting assays. Figure 3 shows the reaction pattern of several monoclonal IFP antibodies on immunoblots of cytoskeletal preparations from diverse sources.

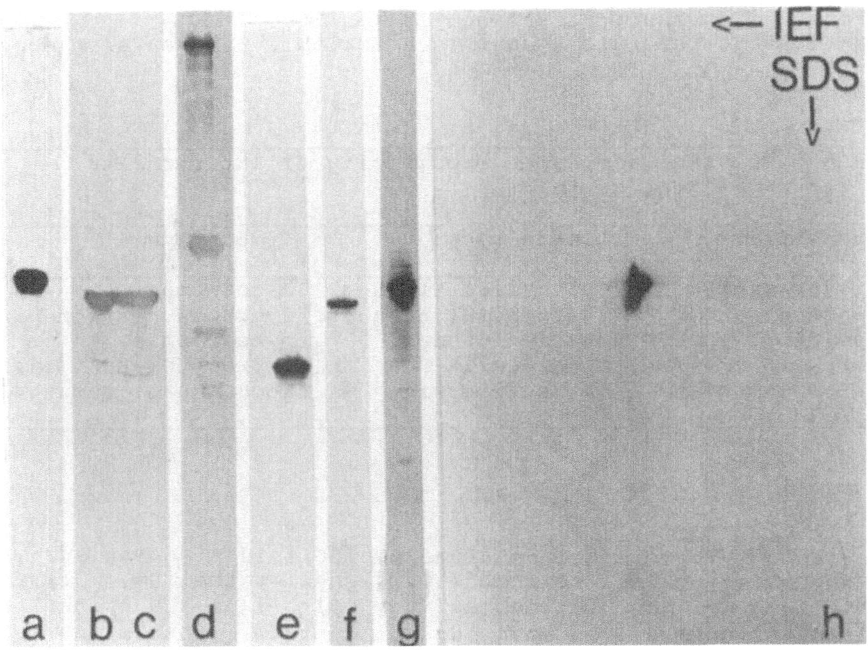

FIGURE 3. Immunoblotting of several monoclonal IFP antibodies showing their specificity.
a) A monoclonal antibody to vimentin (RV 201) tested on proteins present in a cytoskeletal preparation from bovine lens.
b,c) A monoclonal antibody to desmin (RD 301) blotted on a cytoskeletal preparation from BHK cells (b) and from a human leiomyosarcoma (c).
d) A monoclonal antibody to neurofilaments (MNF, obtained from Euro-Diagnostics BV, Apeldoorn) mainly reactive with the 200 kDa and to a lesser extent with the 68 kDa neurofilament protein in a preparation from bovine brain.
e) The monoclonal antibody RGE 53, specific for cytokeratin 18, and tested on a cytoskeletal preparation from cultured bovine hepatocytes.
f) A monoclonal antibody specific for cytokeratin 7 (RCK 105) tested on a cytoskeletal preparation from HeLa cells.
g,h) The monoclonal antibody RKSE 60, specific for cytokeratin 10, tested on a one-dimensional (g) and a two-dimensional immunoblot containing human skin keratins.

Most of the antibodies described sofar could be shown to react in a tissue specific manner (Figure 4), meaning that in general antibodies to cytokeratin react only with epithelial tissues, antibodies to desmin only with muscle tissues, GFAP antibodies react only with glial cells and neurofilament antibodies react with neural cells. Antibodies to vimentin normally react only with cells and tissues of mesenchymal origin, but for this type of IFP some exceptions are known (see below). The different types of normal tissues denoted in Table 1 can thus be distinguished by immunocytochemical methods, using specific antibodies to IFP.
Exceptions to the rule as outlined in Table 1 have also been

TABLE 1. Tissue- and tumor specificity of intermediate filament proteins

Type of IFP	Tissue type	Tumor type
cytokeratins	epithelial tissues	carcinomas
vimentin	mesenchymal tissues	lymphoma, sarcoma
desmin	muscle tissues	myosarcomas
GFAP	glial cells	astrocytomas
neurofilaments	nerve tissues	some neural tumors

described. These include some epithelioid tissues, such as the seminiferous epithelium (6), lens epithelium, pigment epithelium in the retina, ciliary epithelium and epithelial cells covering the iris which do not contain cytokeratins but posses vimentin IFP (7). Mesothelial cells have been shown to co-express cytokeratins and vimentin (8), a phenomenon also seen in some other types of epithelial cells (9). Some types of neurons are completely devoid of intermediate filaments (10), while some types of vascular smooth muscle cells contain either vimentin alone or vimentin as well as desmin (11).

Furthermore, it should be kept in mind that certain tissue types in developing embryos may contain IFP different from those present in their adult counterparts. For example myoblasts contain vimentin instead of desmin (12) and neonatal glial cells may contain vimentin in addition to GFAP (13). Some types of kidney epithelial cells transiently express vimentin during embryogenesis (14). Finally, cells brought into tissue culture commonly express vimentin next to their cell type specific IFP (15).

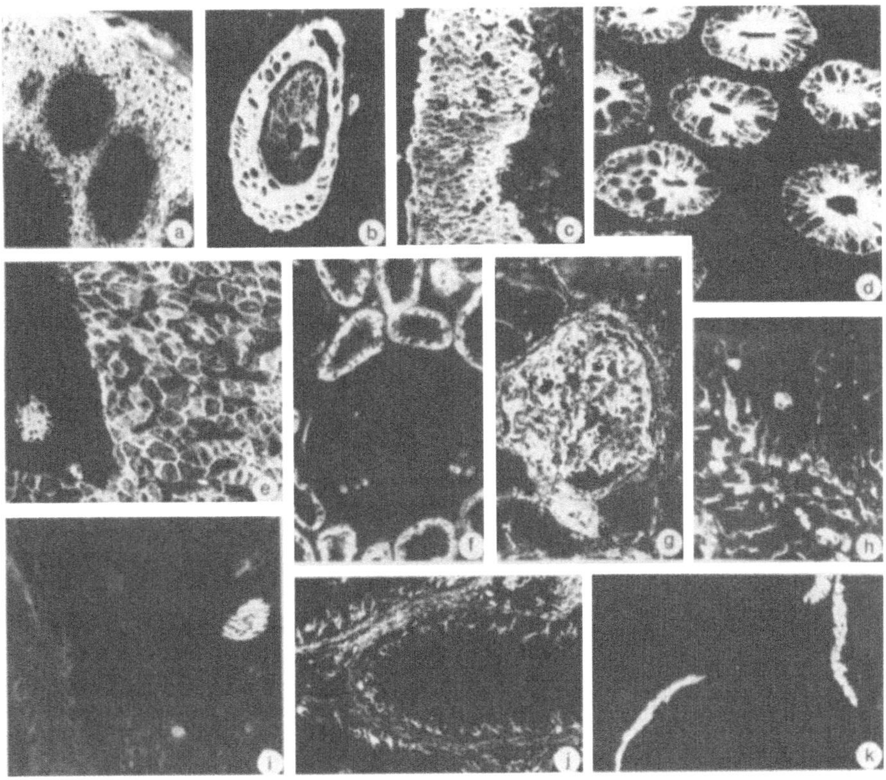

FIGURE 4. Tissue-specific distribution of intermediate filament proteins as shown in the indirect immunofluorescence technique on frozen sections of human tissues. Cytokeratins occur only in epithelial tissues such as the epidermis (a), and epidermal adnexes such as hair root sheats (b), transitional epithelium of the urinary bladder (c), colon epithelium (d), hepatocytes and bile duct epithelium (e), and kidney tubules (f). Some of the epithelioid tissues, such as the seminiferous epithelium, do not contain cytokeratins, but instead express vimentin (j). Furthermore, vimentin is expressed in many cell types of mesenchymal origin, such as fibroblasts and Langerhans' cells in the skin (h), some smooth muscle cells, endothelial cells and glomerular components (g). Neurofilaments occur only in nerve cells (i), while desmin is specific for smooth muscle cells, such as those surrounding the sebaceous glands of the skin (k).

3. ANTIBODIES TO IFP IN TUMOR HISTOPATHOLOGY

Antibodies to IFP have been tested extensively for use in tissue characterization in the past few years and from the data obtained in these studies it is obvious that IFP can be used as powerful markers in tumor typing (Table 1 and for reviews see 2,3,5). Most important, it has been shown that generally tumor cells retain their original IFP, with the exception of a few types of neoplasms (16). Therefore, carcinomas can be stained with antibodies to cytokeratins, while mesenchymal tumors such as lymphomas (17), most soft tissue sarcomas (18), melanomas (19), seminomas (20) and Schwannomas are negative for cytokeratins, but positive for vimentin.

Tumors derived from striated- or smooth muscle tissues, i.e. rhabdo- and leiomyosarcomas can be differentiated from other soft tissue tumors because of their reactivity with desmin antibodies (21-23). Astrocytomas are strongly positive for GFAP, while ganglioneuroblastomas, and part of the neuroblastomas are positive with neurofilament antisera. However, also some neuroendocrine tumors such as pheochromocytomas (24), pulmonary carcinoids (25), oat cell carcinomas (26), Merkel cell tumors (27) and pancreatic islet tumors (28), have been described to contain neurofilament proteins, often in addition to cytokeratins.

For some examples of reactivity patterns of several tumor-types see Figures 5 and 6.

Table 2 summarizes some typical examples of cases of differential diagnoses where routine histology may fail to give conclusive results and where application of intermediate filament immunohistochemistry may be of help.

Since treatment protocols for these tumors differ, an accurate diagnosis is imperative for optimal therapy.

In the differentiation between an anaplastic carcinoma (Figure 5) and a lymphoma (Figure 6) in the case of a lymph node biopsy, antibodies directed against cytokeratins and vimentin can be very helpful (17). When routine staining procedures do not permit a diagnosis in case of a lymph node metastasis, a positive reaction for cytokeratin clearly points to a carcinoma, whereas a positive reaction for vimentin (without a positive reaction for cytokeratin) is suggestive for a lymphoma.

Routine histological diagnosis of small-round-cell tumors of childhood (including lymphomas, neuroblastomas, Ewing's sarcomas, nephroblastomas and embryonal rhabdomyosarcomas) is often difficult or impossible due to the lack of differentiation of the tumor cells. The use of antibodies directed against IFP, however, can help considerably in establishing the diagnosis. Table 2 also contains the reaction patterns of the various types of childhood tumors with IFP antibodies. In the case of spindle cell tumors, antibodies to cytokeratin, vimentin and desmin can be helpful in diagnosis. Table 2 summarizes cases of spindle cell tumors, such as malignant fibrous histiocytoma (MFH), spindle cell type mesothelioma and leiomyosarcoma. MFH is only positive for vimentin and does not react with antibodies to

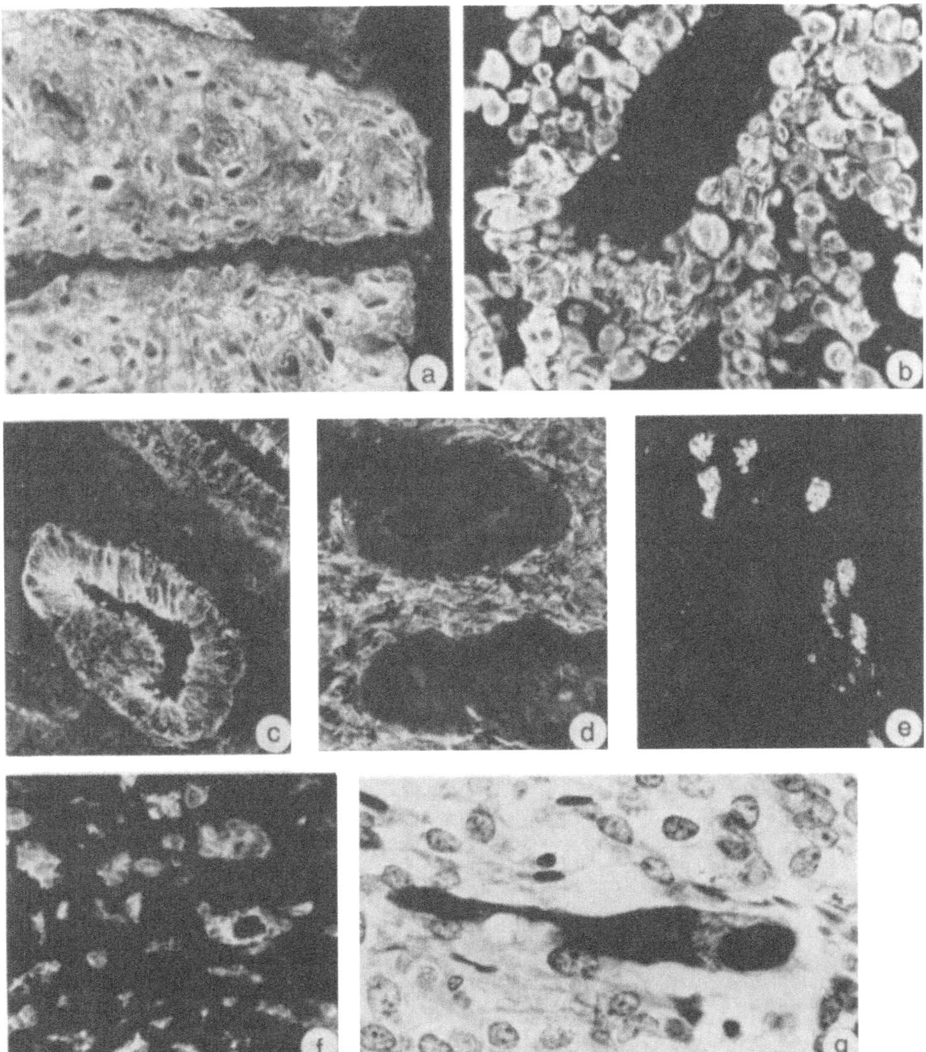

FIGURE 5. Application of intermediate filament antisera to human neoplasms in the indirect immunofluorescence technique on frozen sections (a-f) and the immunoperoxidase method on a paraffin section (g). A rabbit antibody to human skin keratins can be shown to react strongly with squamous cell carcinomas (a), mesotheliomas (b), adenocarcinomas (c; adenocarcinoma of colon) and metastatic carcinomas such as a lymph node metastasis of a lobular breast carcinoma (f). Vimentin (d) and desmin (e) are normally only found in stromal components, as shown in the case of adenocarcinomas of the colon. (g) Desmin antibodies react only with myogenic components, as shown for a rhabdomyosarcoma component in a mixed mesodermal tumor of the ovary.

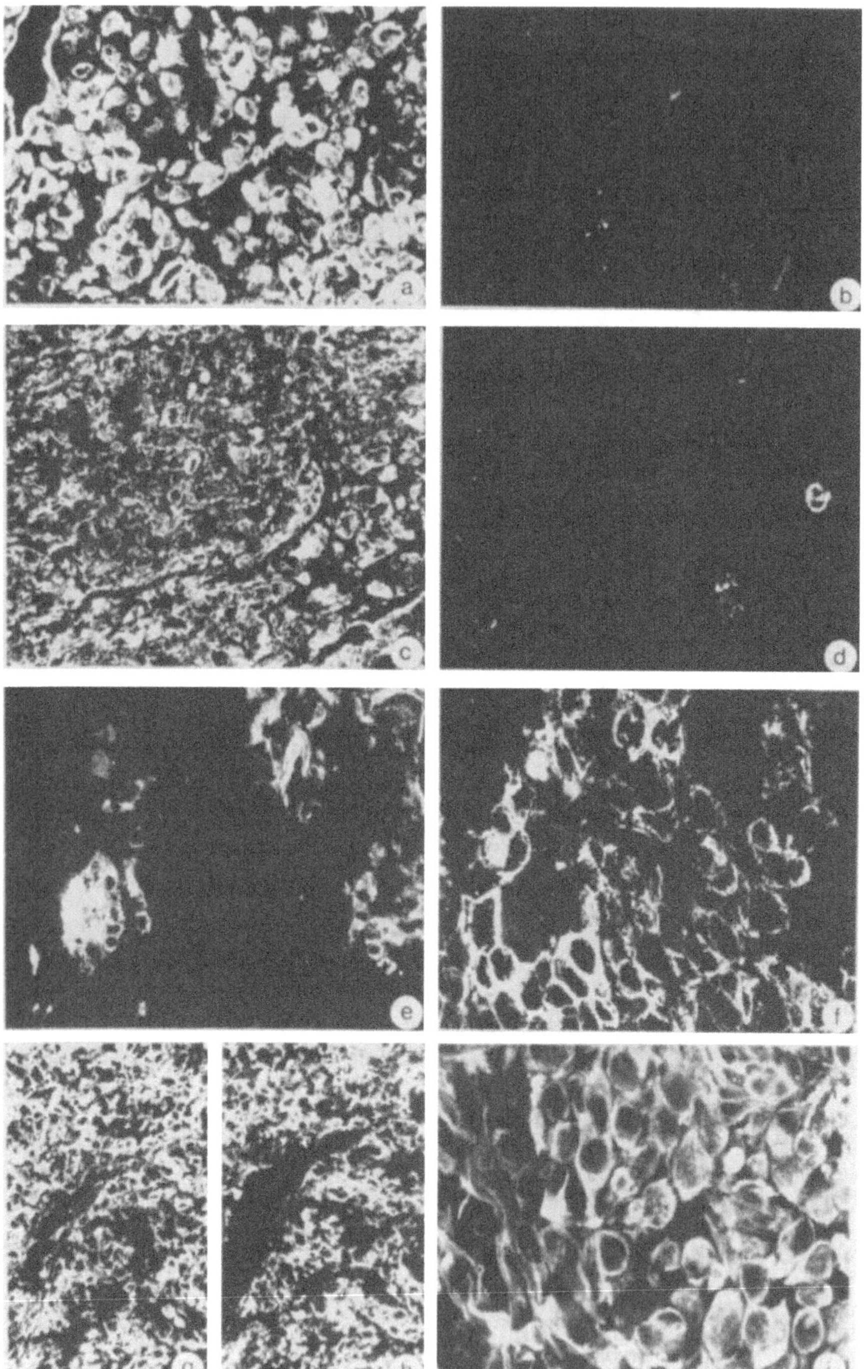

FIGURE 6.

TABLE 2. Problem cases in diagnostic histopathology where IFP antibodies may be helpfull.

Differential Diagnosis		Intermediate filament profile				
		CK	V	D	NF	GFAP
Metastatic/undiff. carcinoma	vs.	+	-	-	-	-
Lymphoma		-	+	-	-	-
Thymoma vs.		+	-	-	-	-
Lymphoma		-	+	-	-	-
Lymphepithelioma vs.		+	-	-	-	-
Lymphoma		-	+	-	-	-
Nephroblastoma	vs.	+	+	-	-	-
Lymphoma	vs.	-	+	-	-	-
Ewing's sarcoma	vs.	-	+	-	-	-
Embryonal rhabdomyosarcoma	vs.	-	+	+	-	-
Neuroblastoma		-	-	-	-/+	-
Spindle cell carcinoma	vs.	+	-	-	-	-
Spindle cell melanoma	vs.	-	+	-	-	-
Malignant fibrous histiocytoma	vs.	-	+	-	-	-
Leiomyosarcoma	vs.	-	+	+	-	-
Schwannoma	vs.	-	+	-	-	-
Spindle cell mesothelioma		+	+	-	-	-
Anaplastic seminoma vs.		-	+	-	-	-
Embryonal cell carcinoma		+	-	-	-	-
Glial tumors vs.		-	+	-	-	+
Meningioma		-	+	-	-	-
Meningial sarcoma		-	+	-	-	-
Chordoma vs.		+	-	-	-	-
Chondrosarcoma		-	+	-	-	-

FIGURE 6. Reaction pattern of vimentin antibodies (a,c,e,g,i) and cytokeratin antibodies (b,d,f,h) with frozen sections of lymphomas (a,b), seminomas (c,d), an embryonal cell carcinoma in the testis (e,f), a renal cell carcinoma (g,h) and a melanoma (i). Note reaction of lymphoma, seminoma, and melanoma with vimentin antibodies only (occasionally scattered cytokeratin-positive cells are observed in seminomas), positive reaction of the embryonal cell carcinoma for cytokeratin (f), and positive reaction of the stroma with vimentin antisera (e). Also note co-expression of cytokeratin (h) and vimentin (g) in the renal cell carcinoma.

desmin, while the mesothelioma co-expresses cytokeratins and vimentin and the leiomyosarcoma cells contain both desmin and vimentin.
From these latter two cases it may be obvious that in contrast to normal adult human tissues, certain neoplastic tissues may co-express different types of IFP. When tumor cells contain more than one IFP-type, in most cases vimentin is one of them. In the case of epithelial tumors vimentin IFP has, for example, been found next to cytokeratin IFP in pleomorphic adenomas of the parotid gland (28,29), in adenoid cystic carcinomas of the salivary gland and in the lung (see Chapter 10) , in mesotheliomas of the spindle cell type, in renal cell carcinomas (Grawitz tumor) (30) and nephroblastomas (Wilm's tumor) (31), and in thyroid tumors (32) and endometrial carcinomas.
Co-expression of vimentin and desmin is observed in most if not all rhabdomyosarcomas (23) and in leiomyosarcomas. We have observed that astrocytomas contain both GFAP and vimentin (unpublished observations). Co-expression of cytokeratins and neurofilament proteins has also been observed. This is the case in some neuroendocrine tumors, such as Merkel cell tumors (27) and some lung carcinoids (see Chapter 10) and pancreatic islet tumors (33). The fact that some tumor types co-express different types of IFP can be of help in the diagnosis of such tumors.

4. CYTOKERATIN DISTRIBUTION IN EPITHELIAL TISSUES

Antisera to cytokeratins are commonly produced against keratin proteins derived from human stratum corneum (4), but they have also been directed against hepatocyte cytokeratins or urinary bladder cytokeratins. These conventional rabbit antisera generally show a rather broad cross-reactivity and stain several types of epithelial tissues, although some antibodies raised in rabbits against isolated cytokeratin polypeptides show some specificity in their reaction (34). These reaction patterns are based on the fact that cytokeratins are a family of IFP. In contrast to other types of intermediate filaments, cytokeratin filaments are characterized by a remarkable biochemical diversity, represented in human epithelial tissues by at least 19 different cytokeratin polypeptides ranging in molecular weight between 40 and 68kDa (35). Moll et al (36) have published the catalog of human cytokeratins and designated them 1 to 19, cytokeratin 1 being the polypeptide with the highest molecular weight and highest isoelectric pH and cytokeratin 19 being the polypeptide with the lowest molecular weight and low isoelectric pH. These polypeptides are not expressed randomly throughout epithelia but occur in cell-type specific combinations (35,36). Also the diverse types of carcinomas differ in their cytokeratin polypeptide content. The polypeptide patterns of epithelial tumors are either identical with the cytokeratin pattern present in the cell of origin or at least closely related to it (see for

example 36,37). The cytokeratin polypeptide patterns (as obtained by two-dimensional gel electrophoresis) can be used for the identification or at least a subclassification of epithelial tissues and carcinomas (37-40).
Several monoclonal antibodies to different cytokeratins have been prepared and different reactivities of such antibodies with different subtypes of epithelial tissues and epithelial tumors have been noted (see for example Figures 7 and 8).

On the basis of their immunocytochemical reaction patterns with tissue frozen sections, the following types of monoclonal anti-cytokeratin antibodies can be distinguished, i.e.:

a) broadly cross-reacting antibodies, such as KG 8.13 (41), PKK1 (42), RCK 102 (43), CAM 5.2 (44),and AE1 (4), which stain virtually all types of epithelial tissues. These antibodies (see for example figure 8) have a reactivity pattern similar to that of many of the polyclonal cytokeratin antisera and cross-react with several cytokeratin polypeptides when tested in immunoblotting.
b) monoclonal antibodies which recognize several cytokeratin polypeptides in immunoblotting assays, but which react with certain subfamilies of epithelia (for review see 4).
c) Monoclonal cytokeratin antibodies, which cross-react with only one of the 19 cytokeratin polypeptides and which show a more tissue specific staining pattern. Sofar, chain-specific monoclonal antibodies have been described or prepared for cytokeratin 3, 4, 7, 8, 10, 13, 18 and 19 (43, 45-50). Some of these antibodies have been used in tumor characterization and it has been shown that they can be used to subdivide groups of carcinomas.

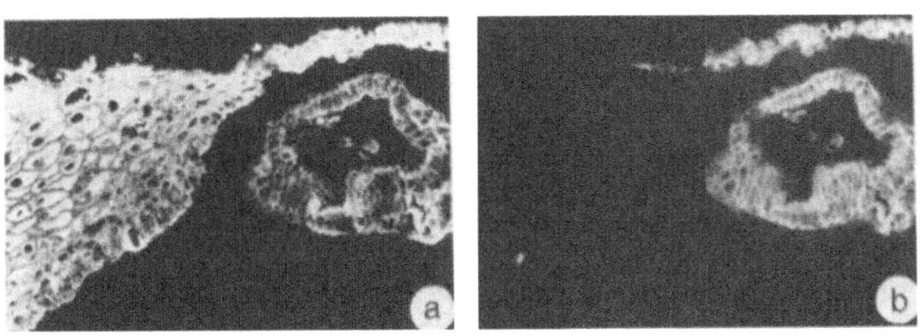

FIGURE 7. Monoclonal antibodies specific for certain individual cytokeratin proteins can distinguish between different types of epithelial tissues.
Double-label immunofluorescence micrographs of cervical epithelium (a,b; frozen sections) showing reactivity with a rabbit antiserum to skin keratins in both endocervical columnar- and ectocervical stratified epithelium (a), but a specific reaction of a monoclonal antibody to cytokeratin 18 (RGE 53) only with the endocervical columnar epithelium (b).

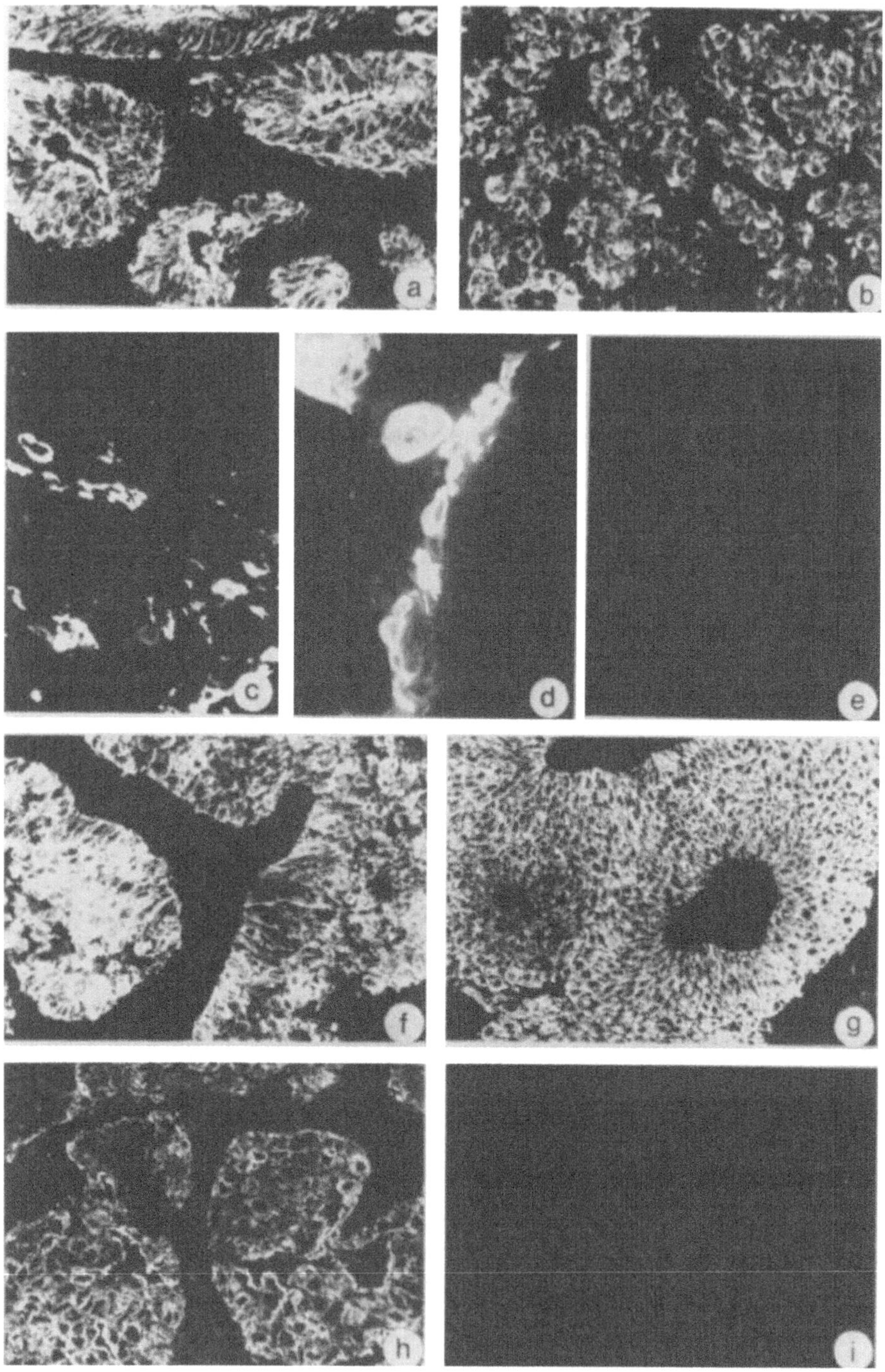

FIGURE 8.

Especially in cases of anaplastic carcinoma metastases these chain-specific antibodies can be of great help for tumor diagnosis. For example, monoclonal antibodies to cytokeratin 18 (45-48) can distinguish adenocarcinomas from squamous cell carcinomas (Figure 8). An antibody to cytokeratin 7 can distinguish adenocarcinomas of the gastrointestinal tract (most of which are negative with this antibody) from certain tumors of the urogenital- (Figure 8) and respiratory tract and breast tumors. The antibodies to cytokeratins 4 and 13 should in principle be able to recognize the tumors derived from non-keratinizing stratified epithelia and to distinguish them from tumors of bladder, lung, breast, and all adenocarcinomas and mesothelial cells. Not only can these antibodies refine carcinoma typing in frozen sections of surgically obtained material, they can also be applied succesfully to cytopathological preparations of fine needle aspiration biopsies obtained from palpable lymph nodes (51) (see below). Chain-specific cytokeratin antibodies have also been shown to be able to detect minor subpopulations of cells present in complex epithelial tissues or in heterogeneous carcinomas (see for example 49,52). Antibodies to cytokeratin 10 and 18 can detect different cell populations in for example squamous cell carcinomas of the lung (see Chapter 10) or in human- and rat transitional cell carcinomas. Thus, in the future, the use of an appropriate collection of monoclonal cytokeratin antibodies will not only allow tumors of epithelial origin to be distinguished from tumors of non-epithelial origin, but, in addition, will allow a further subdivision of carcinomas in relation to their histologic origin. Furthermore, such antibodies will be useful probes for the identification of subpopulations of tumor cells in heterogeneous neoplasms and for histogenetic studies.

FIGURE 8.
Application of monoclonal cytokeratin antibodies in the immunohistochemical recognition of certain subtypes of neoplastic epithelial differentiation (frozen sections; indirect immunofluorescence).
a,b) Prostate adenocarcinoma reactive with antibody RCK 102 (a), that cross-reacts with most epithelia, and antibody RGE 53 (b), specifically directed against cytokeratin 18 and reactive with adenocarcinomas but, in general, not with squamous cell carcinomas as shown in (e)
c,d) Reactivity pattern of the antibody to cytokeratin 10 (RKSE 60; see reference 5) with cornified cells in a transitional cell carcinoma (c), and in squamous metaplasia of the cervix (d).
f,g) Transitional cell carcinoma of the urinary bladder positive with antibody RCK 102 (f) and with monoclonal antibody RCK 105 (g), which specifically reacts with cytokeratin 7.
h,i) An adenomatous component within such a transitional cell carcinoma negative for cytokeratin 7 (i; RCK 105), but positive for cytokeratin 18 as detected by monoclonal antibody RCK 106 (h).

5. APPLICATION OF IFP ANTISERA IN CYTOLOGIC PREPARATIONS

It may be obvious from the foregoing that IFP antibodies may also have important applications in cytopathology. In this area of tumor diagnosis the pathologist is often confronted with severe problems concerning cell recognition and characterization since the tumor cell preparations are mostly devoid of any morphologic information from which the histogenesis of the aspirated tumor can be deduced.
Therefore, especially in this area of pathology tissue specific probes are needed. IFP antibodies have only incidentally been applied to cytologic tumor material (51,53-55).It is our experience that especially in cases of fine needle aspiration biopsies from palpable lymph nodes which are suspected for the presence of a tumor metastasis, application of cytokeratin antibodies may be of special importance and seems most promising. Chapter 15 will include data on the application of IFP antisera in cytologic specimens.

6. PITFALLS IN THE APPLICATION OF IFP ANTIBODIES FOR CELL AND TISSUE RECOGNITION

It is a well-known fact that formalin fixation of tissues and subsequent paraffin embedding may drastically decrease the immunocytochemical detectability of IFP, especially the cytokeratins, vimentin and desmin.
In general this means that these IFP can be detected only when present in relatively high concentrations or after proteolytic predigestion of paraffin sections. For example, we have noted that several leiomyosarcomas which are positive with desmin antibodies when tested in frozen sections, do not show this reaction anymore when fixed in formalin and embedded in paraffin. For this reason Altmannsberger et al. (56) have suggested to use ethanol fixed, paraffin embedded tissue blocks for the immunohistochemical detection of IFP. False negative results may, however, not only be obtained as a result of fixation but also because of a limited reaction spectrum of certain IFP-antibodies. This may be especially true for cytokeratin antisera. For example, antisera to human skin keratins often do not -or only weakly- react with certain types of adenocarcinomas (57,58). Therefore it is recommended to use methanol fixed frozen sections whenever possible and to elaborately test antisera for cross-reactivity with several different types of tissues. Furthermore, the use of a panel of IFP sera (for example cytokeratin- and vimentin antibodies) helps to avoid false negative results.

The use of monoclonal IFP antibodies may present special problems. First, as for the polyclonal antisera, only a part of the monoclonal IFP antibodies described sofar seems to react in routine formalin-fixed paraffin sections. Second, selective masking or unmasking of a certain epitope at certain stages of the cell cycle (59) or during differentiation or

neoplastic progression (60) should be ruled out when working with monoclonal antibodies. And finally, epitopes recognized by monoclonal antibodies may be sensitive not only to formalin fixation, but also to acetone, methanol or ethanol fixation.
However, when used with care and evaluated critically, immunohistochemical detection of IFP provides a powerful tool for the pathologist and cell biologist in the characterization of benign or malignant cells or tissues.

7. APPLICATION OF CYTOKERATIN ANTIBODIES IN THE FLOW CYTOMETRIC ANALYSIS OF HUMAN CARCINOMAS

To those investigators and clinicians dealing with DNA flow cytometric analysis of patient tumors it may be a daily experience that such analyses of carcinomas are in many instances disturbed or made impossible by the presence of stromal and inflammatory cells in the tumor cell suspensions. The variability of these admixtures makes it often difficult to determine the proliferative capacity or even to estimate the ploidy of a certain tumor. These parameters have, however, been shown to be of prognostic significance for several types of tumors.
In order to exclude the non-epithelial cell types from such analyses we have developed a two-parameter method using cytokeratin antibodies (61). For this purpose single cell suspensions from fresh tissues are fixed in 70% ethanol and stained with FITC for cytokeratin content using specific antibodies in the indirect immunofluorescence technique. Thereafter DNA is labeled with propidium iodide. Theoretically we can thus in a two-parameter analysis separate epithelial (cytokeratin positive) cells from non-epithelial (cytokeratin negative) cells (see figure 9).

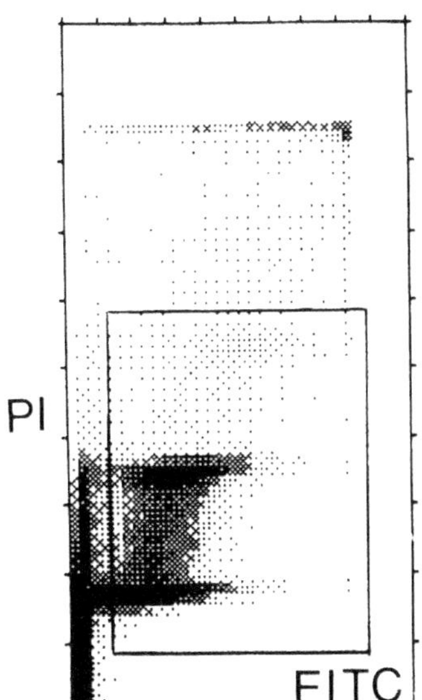

FIGURE 9. Two-parameter flow cytometric separation of epithelial tumor cells (present within the window) and stromal and inflammatory cells after labeling of the carcinoma cells with the monoclonal antibody RCK 102 and an FITC-conjugated second antibody. DNA was stained quantitatively with propidium iodide (PI).

Gating of the cytokeratin-positive cells then allows the estimation of ploidy and proliferative fraction of the epithelial tumor cells separately from stromal and inflammatory cells (62). This is especially helpful in those cases where only a low percentage of the cells present in a cell suspension consists of tumor cells. Furthermore, in cases of hypo- or hyperdiploid tumors this method can give a more precise estimation of the degree of aneuploidy.

8. CONCLUSION

From the foregoing it may be obvious that antibodies to IFP can discriminate between epithelial, mesenchymal, muscle, glial, and neural tissues and between the tumors derived from these different cell types. To obtain interpretable results, however, they should be applied with appropriate immunohistochemical techniques to optimally fixed tissue sections or cytologic preparations. In combination with other tissue-specific markers IFP antibodies can then serve as valuable tools in surgical pathology (63,64). Furthermore, monoclonal antibodies specific for individual cytokeratin polypeptides allow a further subdivision of epithelial tissues and carcinomas. Such antibodies are also useful in the detection of tumor cell heterogeneity. Next to their applicability in histopathology and cytopathology such IFP antibodies prove to be of great help in flow cytometry, where they allow a better analysis of tumor cell ploidy and proliferative capacity of a certain cancer.

ACKNOWLEDGEMENTS
The authors thank the following persons for their contributions in the work described in this chapter or in the preparation of the manuscript : Jose Aldeweireldt, Hans Beck, Jos Broers, Wout Feitz, Urbain van Haelst, Chester Herman, Arie Kant, Mirjam Klein Rot, Tineke Oostendorp, Peter Oud, Jo Puts, and Yvonne Stammes.
The work was supported in part by the Netherlands Cancer Foundation.

REFERENCES

1. Wang E, Fischman D, Liem RKH, Sun T-T (Eds) (1985) Intermediate filaments. Ann N Y Acad Sci, Volume 455.
2. Osborn M, Weber K (1983) Tumor diagnosis by intermediate filament typing: a novel tool for surgical pathology. Lab Invest 48, 372-394.
3. Miettinen M, Lehto V-P, Virtanen I (1984) Antibodies to intermediate filament proteins in the diagnosis and classification of human tumors. Ultrastructural Pathol. 7, 83-107.
4. Cooper D, Schermer A, Sun T-T (1985) Classification of human epithelia and their neoplasms using monoclonal antibodies to keratins: Strategies, applications and limitations. Lab Invest 52, 243-256.
5. Ramaekers FCS, Puts JJG, Moesker O, Kant A, Huysmans A, Haag D, Jap PHK, Herman CJ, Vooijs GP (1983) Antibodies to intermediate filament proteins in the immunohistochemical identification of human tumours: an overview. Histochem J 15, 691-713.
6. Franke WW, Grund C, Schmid E (1979) Intermediate-sized filaments in Sertoli cells are of the vimentin type. Eur J Cell Biol 19, 269-275.
7. Ramaekers F, Osborn M, Schmid E, Weber K, Bloemendal H, Franke WW (1980) Identification of the cytoskeletal proteins in lens-forming cells. A special epithelioid cell type. Exp Cell Res 127, 309-327.
8. LaRocca PJ, Rheinwald JG (1984) Coexpression of simple epithelial keratins and vimentin by human mesothelium and mesothelioma in vivo and in culture. Cancer Res 44, 2991-2999.
9. Czernobilsky B, Moll R, Levy R, Franke WW (1985) Co-expression of cytokeratin and vimentin filaments in mesothelial, granulosa and rete ovarii cells of the human ovary. Eur J Cell Biol 37, 175-190.
10. Sharp GA, Shaw G, Weber K (1982) Immunoelectron-microscopical localization of the three neurofilament triplet proteins along neurofilaments of cultured dorsal root ganglion cells. Exp Cell Res 137, 403-413.
11. Schmid E, Osborn M, Rungger-Brändle E, Gabbiani G, Weber K, Franke WW (1982) Distribution of vimentin and desmin filaments in smooth muscle tissues of mammalian and avian aorta. Exp Cell Res 137, 329-340.
12. Holtzer H, Bennett GS, Tapscott SJ, Croop JM, Toyama Y (1981) Intermediate-sized filaments: Changes in synthesis and distribution in cells of the myogenic and neurogenic lineages. Cold Spring Harbor Symp Quant Biol 46, 317-329.
13. Bignami A, Raju T, Dahl D (1982) Localization of vimentin, the non-specific intermediate filament protein, in embryonal glia and in early differentiating neurons. In vivo and in vitro immunofluorescence study of the rat embryo with vimentin and neurofilament antisera. Dev Biol 91, 286-295.
14. Holthöfer H, Miettinen A, Lehto V-P, Lethonen E, Virtanen

I (1984) Expression of vimentin and cytokeratin types of intermediate filament proteins in developing and adult human kidneys. Lab Invest 50, 552-559.
15. Franke WW, Schmid E, Winter S, Osborn M, Weber K (1979) Wide spread occurence of intermediate-sized filaments of the vimentin-type in cultured cells from diverse vertebrates. Exp Cell Res 123, 25-46.
16. Said JW, Nash G, Banks-Schlegel S, Sassoon AF, Shintaku IP (1984) Localized fibrous mesothelioma: An immunohistochemical and electronmicroscopic study. Hum Pathol 15, 440-443.
17. Ramaekers FCS, Vroom TM, Moesker O, Kant A, Scholte G, Vooijs GP (1985) The use of antibodies of intermediate filament proteins in the differential diagnosis of lymphoma versus metastatic carcinoma. Histochem J 17, 57-70.
18. Miettinen M, Lehto V-P, Badley RA, Virtanen I (1982) Expression of intermediate filaments in soft tissue sarcomas. Int J Cancer 30, 541-546.
19. Ramaekers FCS, Puts JJG, Moesker O, Kant A, Vooijs GP, Jap PHK (1983) Intermediate filaments in malignant melanomas. Identification and use as a marker in surgical pathology. J Clin Invest 71, 635-643.
20. Ramaekers F, Feitz W, Moesker O, Schaart G, Herman C, Debruyne F, Vooijs P (1985) Antibodies to cytokeratin and vimentin in testis tumour diagnosis. Virchows Arch (Pathol Anat) 408, 127-142.
21. Denk H, Krepler R, Artlieb U, Gabbiani G, Rungger-Brändle E, Leoncini P, Franke WW (1983) Proteins of intermediate filaments. An immunohistochemical and biochemical approach to the classification of soft tissue tumors. Am J Pathol 110, 193-208.
22. Altmannsberger M, Osborn M, Treuner J, Hölscher A, Weber K, Schauer A (1982) Diagnosis of human childhood rhabdomyosarcoma by antibodies to desmin, the structural protein of muscle specific intermediate filaments. Virchows Arch (Cell Pathol) 39, 203-215.
23. Molenaar WM, Oosterhuis JW, Oosterhuis AM, Ramaekers FCS (1985) Mesenchymal and muscle-specific intermediate filaments (vimentin and desmin) in relation to differentiation in childhood rhabdomyosarcomas. Human Pathol 16, 838-843.
24. Lehto V-P, Virtanen I, Miettinen M, Dahl D, Kahri A (1984) Neurofilaments in adrenal and extra-adrenal pheochromocytoma. Demonstration using immunofluorescence microscopy. Arch Pathol Lab Med 107, 492-494.
25. Lehto V-P, Miettinen M, Virtanen I (1985) A dual expression of cytokeratin and neurofilaments in bronchial carcinoid cells. Int J Cancer 35, 421-425.
26. Lehto V-P, Stenman S, Miettinen M, Dahl D, Virtanen I (1983) Expression of a neural type of intermediate filament as a distinguishing feature between oat cell carcinoma and other lung cancers. Am J Pathol 110, 113-118.
27. Gould VE, Moll R, Moll I, Lee I, Franke WW (1985)

Neuroendocrine (Merkel) cells of the skin: hyperplasias, dysplasias, and neoplasias. Lab Invest 52, 334-353.
28. Caselitz J, Osborn M, Seifert G, Weber K (1981) Intermediate-sized filament proteins (prekeratin, vimentin, desmin) in the normal parotid gland and parotid gland tumours. Virchows Arch (Pathol Anat) 393, 273-286.
29. Krepler R, Denk H, Artlieb U, Moll R (1982) Immunocytochemistry of intermediate filament proteins present in pleomorphic adenomas of the human parotid gland: characterization of different cell types in the same tumor. Differentiation 21, 191-199.
30. Herman CJ, Moesker O, Kant A, Huysmans A, Vooijs GP, Ramaekers FCS (1983) Is renal cell (Grawitz) tumor a carcinosarcoma? Evidence from analysis of intermediate filament types. Virchows Arch (Cell Pathol) 44, 73-83.
31. Altmannsberger M, Osborn M, Schäfer H, Schauer A, Weber K (1984) Distinction of nephroblastomas from other childhood tumors using antibodies to intermediate filaments. Virchows Arch (Cell Pathol) 45, 113-124.
32. Miettinen M, Franssila K, Lehto V-P, Paasivuo R, Virtanen I (1984) Expression of intermediate filament proteins in thyroid gland tumors. Lab Invest 50, 262-270.
33. Miettinen M, Lehto V-P, Dahl D, Virtanen I (1985) Varying expression of cytokeratin and neurofilaments in gastrointestinal neuroendocrine tumors. Lab Invest 52, 429-436.
34. Krepler R, Denk H, Wierich E, Schmid E, Franke WW (1981) Keratin-like proteins in normal and neoplastic cells of human and rat mammary gland as revealed by immunofluorescence microscopy. Differentiation 20, 242-252.
35. Quinlan RA, Schiller DL, Hatzfeld M, Achtstaetter T, Moll R, Jorcano JL, Magin TM, Franke WW (1985) Patterns of expression and organization of cytokeratin intermediate filaments. Ann N Y Acad Sci 455, 282-306.
36. Moll R, Franke WW, Schiller DL, Geiger B, Krepler R (1982) The catalog of human cytokeratins: patterns of expression in normal epithelia, tumors and cultured cells. Cell 31, 11-24.
37. Moll R, Levy R, Czernobilsky B, Hohlweg-Majert P, Dallenbach-Hellweg G, Franke WW (1983) Cytokeratins of normal epithelia and some neoplasms of the female genital tract. Lab Invest 49, 599-610.
38. Achtstaetter T, Moll R, Moore B, Franke WW (1985) Cytokeratin polypeptide pattern of different epithelia of the human male urogenital tract: Immunofluorescence and gel electrophoretic studies. J Histochem Cytochem 33, 415-426.
39. Moll R, Franke WW, Volc-Platzer B, Krepler R (1982) Different keratin polypeptides in epidermis and other epithelia of human skin: A specific cytokeratin of molecular weight 46000 in epithelia of the pilosebaceous tract and basal epitheliomas. J Cell Biol 95, 285-295.
40. Blobel G, Moll R, Franke WW, Vogt-Moykopf I (1984) Cytokeratins in normal lung and lung carcinomas. I:

Adenocarcinomas, squamous cell carcinomas and cultured cell lines. Virchows Arch (Cell Pathol) 45, 407-430.
41. Gigi O, Geiger B, Eshhar Z, Moll R, Schmid E, Winter S, Schiller DL, Franke WW (1982) Detection of cytokeratin determinant common to diverse epithelial cells by a broadly cross-reacting monoclonal antibody. EMBO J 1, 1429-1437.
42. Holthöfer H, Miettinen A, Paasivuo R, Lehto V-P, Linder E, Alfthan, O, Virtanen I (1983) Cellular origin and differentiation of renal carcinomas. A fluorescence microscopic study with kidney-specific antibodies, antiintermediate filament antibodies and lectins. Lab Invest 49, 317-326.
43. Broers JLV, Carney DN, Klein Rot M, Schaart G, Lane EB, Vooijs GP, Ramaekers FCS (1986) Intermediate filament proteins in classic- and variant-type small cell lung carcinoma cell lines. A biochemical and immunochemical analysis using a panel of monoclonal and polyclonal antibodies. J Cell Sci (in press).
44. Makin CA, Bobrow LG, Bodmer WF (1984) Monoclonal antibody to cytokeratin for use in routine histopathology. J Clin Pathol 37, 975-983.
45. Lane EB (1982) Monoclonal antibodies provide specific intramolecular markers for the study of epithelial tonofilament organization. J Cell Biol 92, 665-673.
46. Debus E, Weber K, Osborn M (1982) Monoclonal cytokeratin antibodies that distinguish simple from stratified squamous epithelia: characterization on human tissues. EMBO J 1, 1641-1647.
47. Ramaekers FCS, Huysmans A, Moesker O, Kant A, Jap P, Herman C, Vooijs P (1983) Monoclonal antibody to keratin filaments specific for glandular epithelia and their tumors: use in surgical pathology. Lab Invest 49, 353-361.
48. Debus E, Moll R, Franke WW, Weber K, Osborn M (1984) Immunohistochemical distinction of human carcinomas by cytokeratin typing with monoclonal antibodies. Am J Pathol 114, 121-130.
49. Muijen GNP van, Ruiter DJ, Franke WW, Achstaetter T, Haasnoot WHB, Ponec M, Warnaar SO (1986) Cell type heterogeneity of cytokeratin expression in complex epithelia and carcinomas as demonstrated by monoclonal antibodies specific for cytokeratins 4 and 13. Exp Cell Res 162, 97-113.
50. Tölle H-G, Weber K, Osborn M (1985) Micro-injection of monoclonal antibodies specific for one intermediate filament protein in cells containing multiple keratins allow insight into the composition of particular 10 nm filaments. Eur J Cell Biol 38, 234-244.
51. Ramaekers F, Haag D, Jap P, Vooijs GP (1984) Immunochemical demonstration of keratin and vimentin in cytologic aspirates. Acta Cytol 28, 285-292.
52. Ramaekers FCS, Moesker O, Huysmans A, Schaart G, Westerhof G, Wagenaar SjSc, Herman CJ, Vooijs GP (1985) Intermediate filament proteins in the study of tumor heterogeneity: an

in-depth study of tumors of the urinary and respiratory tract. Annals N Y Acad Sci 455, 614-634.
53. Kahn HJ, Hanna W, Yeger H, Baumal R (1982) Immunohistochemical localization of prekeratin filaments in benign and malignant cells in effusions. Am J Pathol 109, 206-214.
54. Droese M, Altmannsberger M, Kehl A, Lankisch PG, Weiss R, Weber K, Osborn M (1984) Ultrasound-guided percutaneous fine needle aspiration biopsy of abdominal and retroperitoneal masses. Accuracy of cytology in the diagnosis of malignancy, cytologic tumor typing and use of antibodies to intermediate filaments in selected cases. Acta Cytol 28, 368-384.
55. Ramaekers FCS, Haag D, Kant A, Moesker O, Jap PHK, Vooijs GP (1983) Coexpression of keratin and vimentin-type intermediate filaments in human metastatic carcinoma cells. Proc Natl Acad Sci USA 80, 2618-2622.
56. Altmannsberger M, Osborn M, Schauer A, Weber K (1981) Antibodies to different intermediate filament proteins. Cell type-specific markers on paraffin-embedded human tissues. Lab Invest 45, 427-434.
57. Schlegel R, Banks-Schlegel S, McLeod JA, Pinkus GS (1980) Immunoperoxidase localization of keratin in human neoplasms. Am J Pathol 101, 41-50.
58. Ramaekers F, Puts J, Moesker O, Kant A, Jap P, Vooijs P (1983) Demonstration of keratins in human adenocarcinomas. Am J Pathol 111, 213-223.
59. Franke WW, Schmid E, Wellsteed J, Grund C, Gigi O, Geiger B (1983) Change of cytokeratin filament organization during the cell cycle: Selective masking of an immunologic determinant in interphase PtK2 cells. J Cell Biol
97, 1255-1260.
60. Ramaekers F, Huysmans A, Moesker O, Schaart G, Herman C, Vooijs GP (1985) Cytokeratin expression during neoplastic progression of human transitional cell carcinomas as detected by a monoclonal and a polyclonal antibody. Lab Invest 52, 31-38.
61. Ramaekers FCS, Beck H, Vooijs GP, Herman CJ (1984) Flow cytometric analysis of mixed cell populations using intermediate filament antibodies. Exp Cell Res 153, 249-253.
62. Feitz WFJ, Beck HLM, Smeets AWGB, Debruyne FMJ, Vooijs GP, Herman CJ, Ramaekers FCS (1985) Tissue specific markers in flow cytometry of urological cancers: cytokeratins in bladder carcinoma. Int J Cancer 36, 349-356.
63. Battifora H (1985) Monoclonal antibodies in the histologic diagnosis of cancer. Laboratory Management 23 (vol. 5), 38-53).
64. Roholl PJM, de Jong ASM, Ramaekers FCS (1985) Application of markers in the diagnosis of soft tissue tumours. Histopathology 9, 1019-1035.

Immunological marker analysis of cells in the various hematopoietic differentiation stages and their malignant counterparts

J.J.M. van Dongen, H.J. Adriaansen and H. Hooijkaas

1. INTRODUCTION

The characterization of cells in the various hematopoietic differentiation stages can be performed morphologically. Additional characterization is obtained by immunological marker analysis (1-4). The expression of a particular set of immunological markers designates a cell to a particular differentiation stage. The various markers are detectable by means of antibodies or by rosette techniques (5-7).

Leukemias and non-Hodgkin lymphomas (NHL) can be regarded as malignant counterparts of cells in the various hematopoietic differentiation stages (8-10). Hematopoietic differentiation schemes as presented in Figure 1, are based upon knowledge concerning normal hematopoiesis as well as leukemias and NHL (1-4,8,9). Such differentiation schemes are hypothetic and cannot be complete. In addition, it should be realized that differentiation is a gradual procession of events and that differentiation stages are not as finite as suggested in the figure. However, such differentiation schemes provide an indication as to where the various leukemias and NHL can be located according to their maturation arrest (Fig. 2). It is noteworthy that a maturation arrest is not always restricted to one differentiation stage, but that several differentiation stages can occur within one malignancy.

It will be discussed which cells express the various immunological markers, how the expression of these markers can be detected and how immunological markers can be used for the characterization of normal hematopoietic cells as well as leukemic and NHL cells.

2. HEMATOPOIETIC DIFFERENTIATION STAGES AND IMMUNOLOGICAL MARKERS

Hematopoietic differentiation can be divided into a lymphoid and a myeloid lineage. The lymphoid differentiation consists of the B cell and T cell lineages. The B cell differentiation occurs partly in the bone marrow (BM) and partly in the lym-

Abbreviations: AET, 2-amino-ethylisothiouronium bromide; AIDS, acquired immunodeficiency syndrome; ALL, acute lymphoblastic leukemia; AML, acute myeloid leukemia; AP, alkaline phosphatase; ATG, anti-thymocyte globulin; BAL, bronchoalveolar lavage; BC, blast crisis; BM, bone marrow; BSA, bovine serum albumin; CALLA, common ALL antigen; CD, cluster of differentiation; cIg, cytoplasmic immunoglobulin; CLL, chronic lymphocytic leukemia; CML, chronic myeloid leukemia; CSF, cerebrospinal fluid; E, E rosette; FAB, French American British; FCS, fetal calf serum; FITC, fluorescein isothiocyanate; McAb, monoclonal antibody/antibodies; MNC, mononuclear cells; MRBC, mouse red blood cells; NHL, non-Hodgkin lymphomas; PB, peripheral blood; PBS, phosphate buffered saline; PE, phycoerythrin; PLL, prolymphocytic leukemia; PO, peroxidase; RT, room temperature; SmIg, surface membrane immunoglobulin; SRBC, sheep red blood cells; TdT, terminal deoxynucleotidyl transferase; TcR, T cell receptor; TRITC, tetramethylrhodamine isothiocyanate.

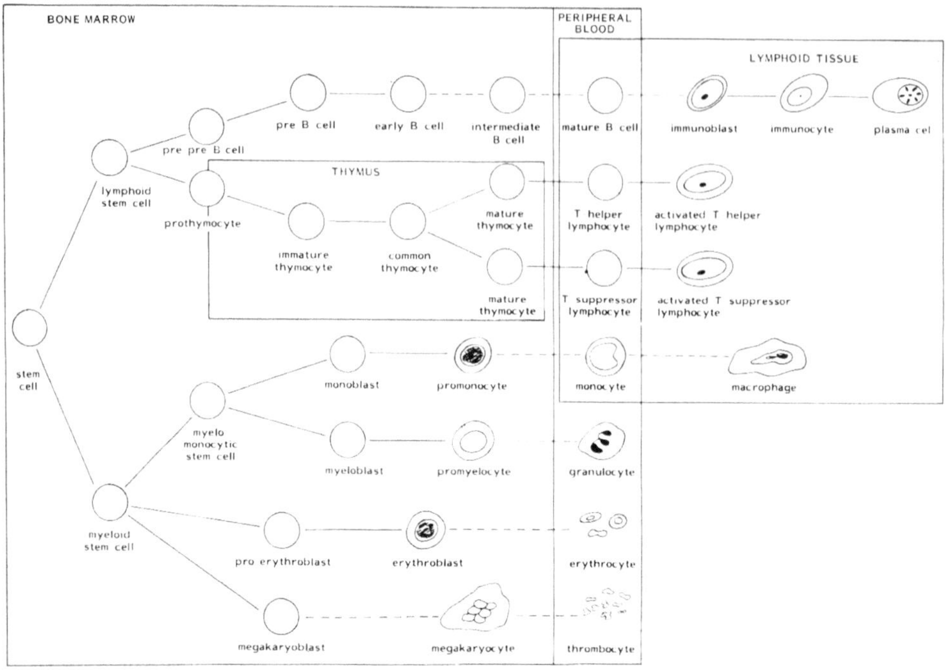

Figure 1. Hypothetical scheme of hematopoiesis. The different compartments, where cells in the various differentiation stages are located, are indicated.

phoid tissues, finally resulting in antibody secreting plasma cells. The major part of the T cell differentiation probably occurs in the thymus, finally resulting in the mature T helper lymphocytes and T suppressor lymphocytes, which are present in the peripheral blood (PB) and lymphoid tissues. The myeloid differentiation, consisting of the monocytic, granulocytic, erythroid, and thrombocytic lineages mainly takes place in the BM (Fig. 1).

Most hematopoietic differentiation stages can be characterized by the use of immunological markers (5-7). Although immunological markers represent differentiation antigens, they usually are not specific for one differentiation stage, but are expressed in several stages. However, a certain combination of markers can be specific for a particular differentiation stage. The expression of the various immunological markers per differentiation stage is summarized in the Figures 3 and 4. As is illustrated by these figures, at present, markers for the lymphoid differentiation lineage are more discriminating and more numerous than those for the myeloid lineage. Therefore, in particular, cells in the various lymphoid differentiation stages and their malignant counterparts can be characterized precisely. Detailed information about the markers presented in the Figures 3 and 4 is summarized in Table 1. In this table the markers are divided into groups according to their specificity: lymphoid markers (B cell markers and T cell markers), myeloid markers (myelomonocytic markers, erythroid markers and thrombocytic markers) and markers which are expressed by cells of several differentiation lineages.

2.1 Lymphoid markers

The enzyme terminal deoxynucleotidyl transferase (TdT) is present in the nucleus of immature lymphoid cells, but is absent in more mature differentiation stages (1,11,12). Early in B cell differentiation, in the pre-B cell stage, weak expression of cytoplasmic μ immunoglobulin heavy chains (weak cμ) takes place (13-16), while more mature B cells express both immunoglobulin heavy and light chains on their cell surface membrane (SmIg) (17,18). Finally, the plasma cell strongly expresses cytoplasmic immunoglobulin heavy and light chains (cIg) (19). Additional characterization of the various B cell differentiation stages can be performed by the use of other B cell markers such as the pan B cell marker B4 (20), the common acute lymphoblastic leukemia antigen (CALLA) (1,21-24) and the B cell markers BA-2, B1, B2, Y29/55 and FMC7 (23-32). The plasma cell is negative for these B cell markers, but expresses the PCA-1 antigen (Fig. 3) (33).

During T cell differentiation, several T cell markers appear on the cell surface membrane, resulting in the expression of many T cell antigens by functional T lymphocytes (2,3,34,35). The putative prothymocyte only expresses the Tp41 and T11 antigen (36-42). The T11 antigen represents the sheep red blood cell (SRBC) receptor (40,41,43). During further differentiation also the T1 antigen and finally the T4, T8, and also T3 antigens appear on the cell surface membrane (34,35,44-49). The T6 antigen or so-called 'common thymocyte antigen' is only temporarily expressed in the thymus (Fig. 3) (34,35,50). It is noteworthy that the mature T cell antigen T3 is closely associated with the T cell receptor (TcR) (51-54), which represents an antigen-specific receptor, comparable to SmIg, the antigen-specific receptor of the B cell (55-57). Within the protein complex formed by TcR and T3 (TcR-T3 complex), the T3 antigen probably plays an important role in the anchorage of TcR as well as in the transduction of signals from TcR to intracellular components (53,58).

2.2 Myeloid markers

Analogous to lymphoid markers, during myeloid differentiation also more or less characteristic markers appear on the cell surface membrane, while other markers disappear.

Almost all myelo-monocytic cells (immature and mature) are positive for My7 and My9 (59-62). In addition, monocytic cells express My4 and the more mature monocytes and macrophages may also express the markers Leu-M3 and Mo2/FMC17 (Fig. 4) (59-67).

The myeloid-granulocytic cells are positive for VIM-D5 and more mature granulocytic cells also express Leu-M4 (Fig. 4) (68,69).

Glycoforin A (GpA) and glycoprotein IIa and IIIa (GPIIa and GPIIIa) can be used as markers for the erythroid and thrombocytic differentiation lineages, respectively (Fig. 4) (70-74).

2.3 Markers which are not (or partly) restricted to one differentiation lineage

Several markers are not restricted to one differentiation lineage, but are expressed by cells of several differentiation lineages. The HLA-DR antigen is expressed by cells in immature hematopoietic differentiation stages, but also by B cells, monocytic cells and activated T lymphocytes (Fig. 3 and 4) (75-77). The transferrin receptor, the so-called T9 antigen, is expressed by almost all proliferating and activated cells (78-80).

Some markers, which initially seemed to be restricted to one differentiation line-

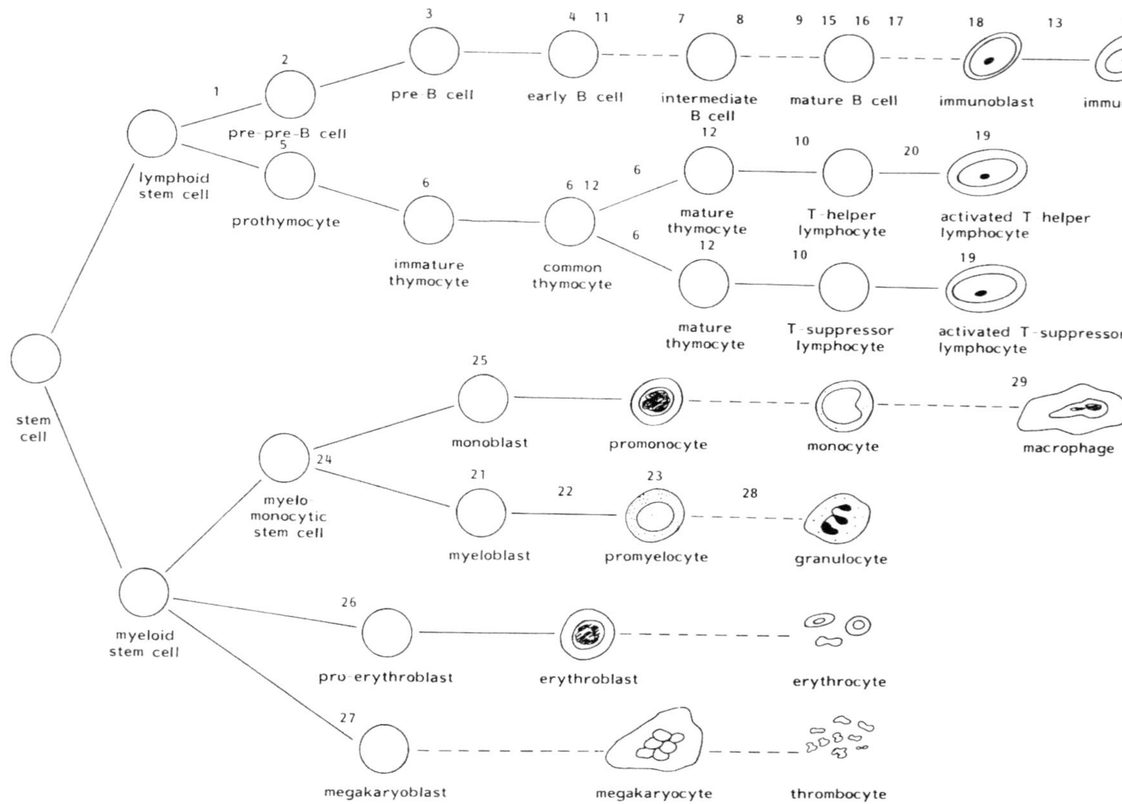

Figure 2. Hypothetical scheme of hematopoiesis. The numbers indicate as to where the various leukemias and NHL can be located according to their maturation arrest (c.f. section 5). 1: null ALL; 2: common ALL; 3: pre-B-ALL; 4: B-ALL; 5: prothymocytic ALL; 6: T-ALL; 7: B-CLL; 8: B-PLL; 9: hairy cell leukemia; 10: T-CLL; 11: B cell lymphoblastic lymphoma (e.g. Burkitt's lymphoma); 12: T cell lymphoblastic lymphoma (e.g. convoluted T cell lymphoma); 13: immunocytoma (e.g. M. Waldenström); 14: plasmacytoma (M. Kahler); 15: centroblastic lymphoma; 16: centroblastic - centrocytic lymphoma; 17: centrocytic lymphoma; 18: B cell immunoblastic lymphoma; 19: T cell immunoblastic lymphoma; 20: Sézary syndrome; 21: AML, M1 (myeloblastic leukemia without maturation); 22: AML, M2 (myeloblastic leukemia with maturation); 23: AML, M3 (hypergranular promyelocytic leukemia); 24: AML, M4 (myelomonocytic leukemia; AMML); 25: AML, M5 (monocytic leukemia; AMol); 26: AML, M6 (erythroleukemia); 27: megakaryoblastic leukemia; 28: CML; 29: true histiocytic lymphoma. The nomenclature of the NHL, indicated by numbers 11 to 19, is derived from the Kiel classification of NHL (111). The numbers 21 to 26 represent the various AML types according to the FAB classification (108).

age, later appeared to be expressed by certain cells of other lineages. This was especially the case for several T cell markers. The T6 antigen is not only expressed by thymocytes, but also by Langerhans cells in the skin (81). The T1 antigen appears to be expressed by a subpopulation of B cells (82-84) while very immature myeloid cells may express the Tp41 antigen (37). Some B cell markers are also not totally differentiation lineage restricted. For example, CALLA is also expressed by many cortical thymocytes and by granulocytes (85,86). Furthermore, the PCA-1 antigen is not only present on plasma cells, but is also weakly expressed by granulocytes and monocytes (33). Several of these 'aberrant' expressions are presented in Figures 3 and 4.

2.4 Additional markers

In order to prevent Figures 3 and 4 becoming too complex, five additional markers are not presented in these figures, but are described in Table 1, namely BA-1, Leu-14, the mouse red blood cell (MRBC) receptor, the C3bi receptor, and Monocyte-2.

The BA-1 antigen is expressed by most B cells from pre-pre-B cell to immunocyte (23,24,87), while more mature myeloid cells also express this antigen (87). Leu-14 is a B cell antigen, which is expressed by subpopulations of B cells. The MRBC receptor is expressed by a subpopulation of B cells, most probably the same B cell subpopulation, which also expresses the T1 antigen (83,88). The antibodies Mo1 and OKM1 recognize the C3bi receptor, which is expressed by all more mature myelo-monocytic cells and sometimes by B or T cells (60,62,64,65,89-91). Monocyte-2 is an antibody, which recognizes a monocytic antigen, expressed by a subpopulation of monocytes and macrophages (64,92).

Of course there exist more markers than are presented in Figures 3 and 4 and in Table 1. However, according to our experience the described panel of markers is generally very informative for immunological characterization of hematopoietic cells.

2.5 International nomenclature and classification of immunological markers

In order to classify the large number of immunological markers, an international nomenclature has been developed analogous to nomenclatures such as those for classifying HLA antigens and blood group antigens (6,7). The various immunological markers are classified in clusters of differentiation (CD). CD codes already exist for most B cell markers and T cell markers, but they are still lacking for the majority of the other immunological markers (6,7). The established CD codes are mentioned in Table 1.

3. DETECTION OF IMMUNOLOGICAL MARKERS OF CELLS IN SUSPENSION AND CELLS IN TISSUE SECTIONS

In recent years monoclonal antibodies (McAb) have increasingly been used for the detection of immunological markers in addition to conventional antisera (5-7). In order to visualize the reactivity of the antibodies, fluorochromes or enzymes are generally used as labels (93,94). Sometimes rosette techniques using erythrocytes are applied, e.g. for the detection of the T cell specific SRBC receptor (E rosette) (43) and the MRBC receptor (M rosette), which is expressed by a subpopulation of B cells (83,88). The staining techniques mentioned can be used for the detection of immunological markers on hematopoietic cells in suspension (Fig. 5-12) as well as on cells in tissue sections.

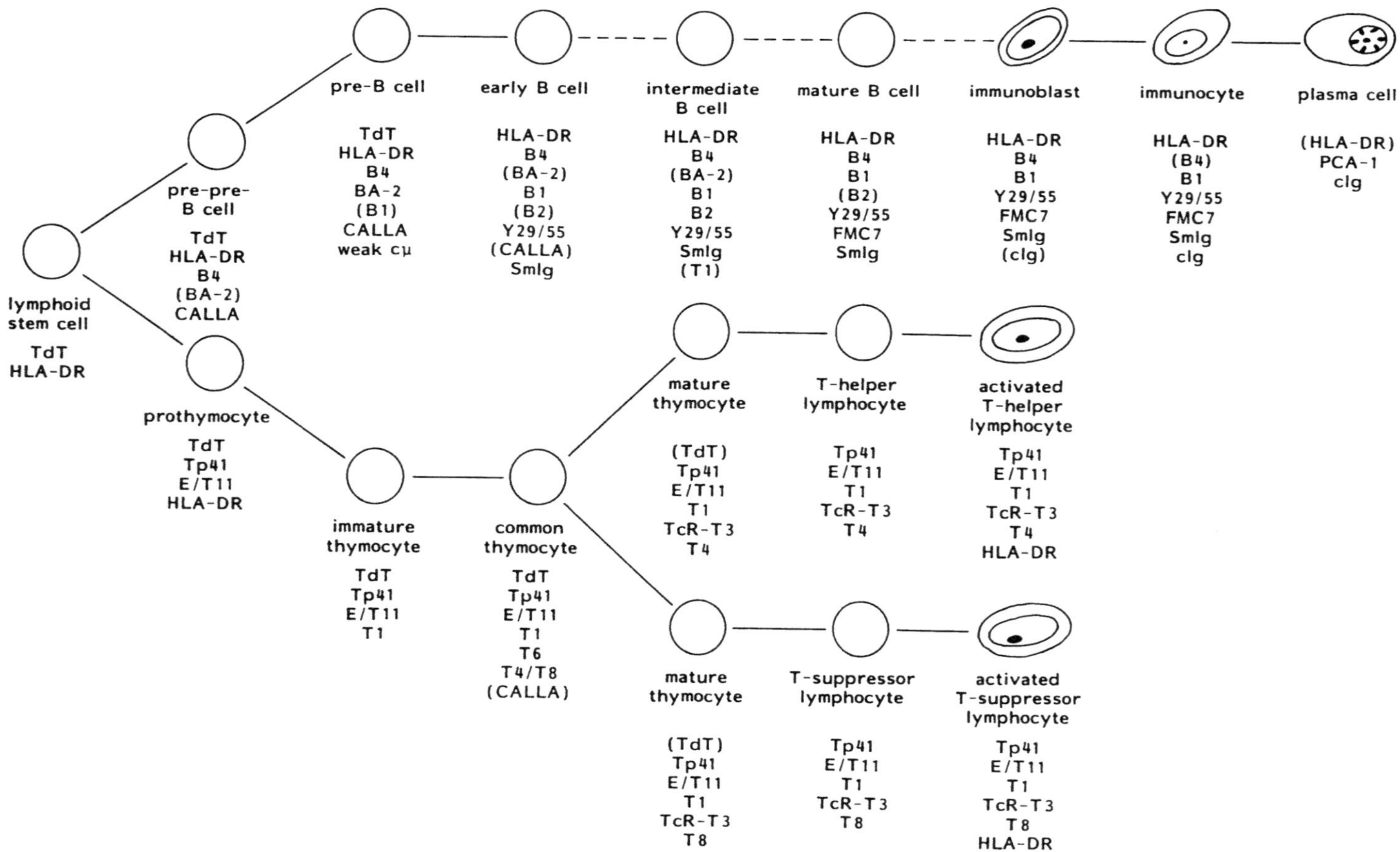

Figure 3. Hypothetical scheme of lymphoid differentiation. The expression of the various immunological markers by cells in the different stages of lymphoid differentiation are indicated. The markers in parentheses are not always expressed.

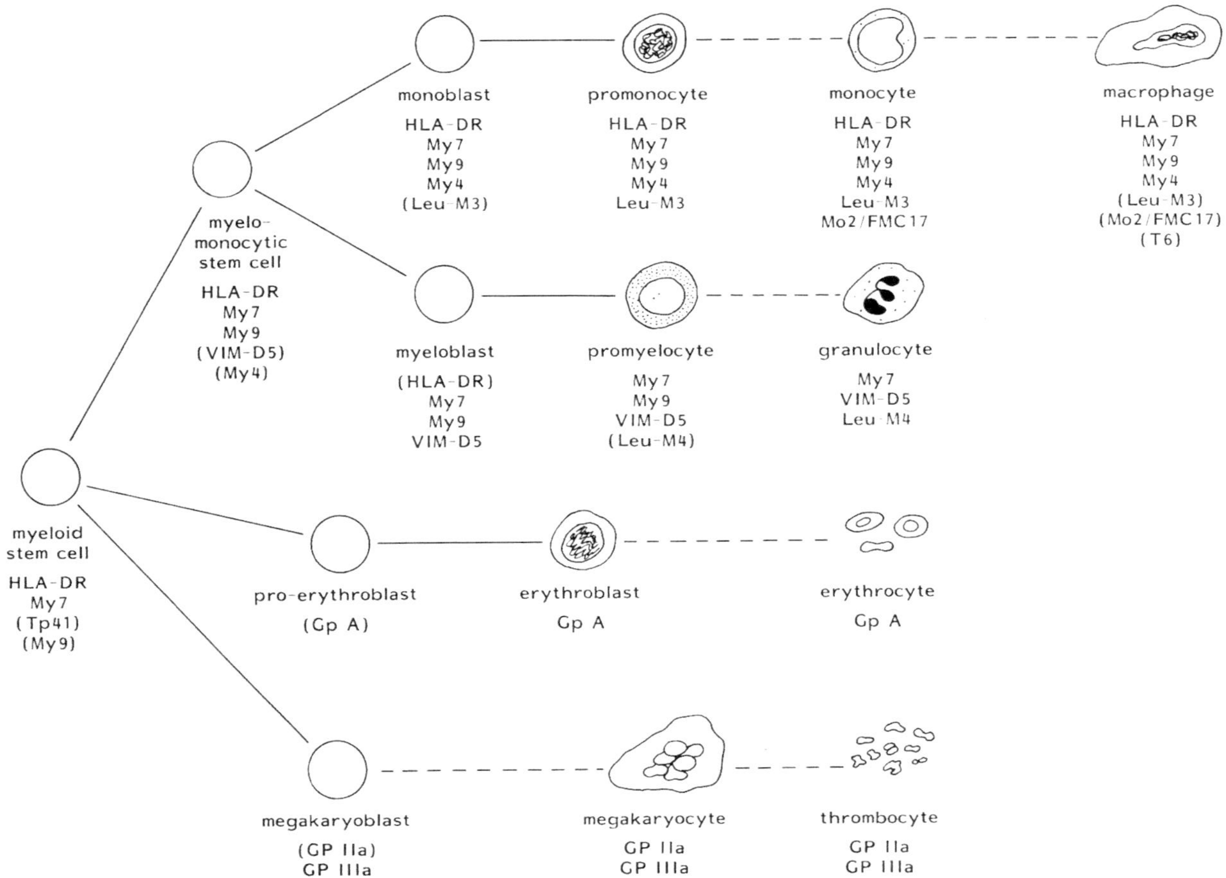

Figure 4. Hypothetical scheme of myeloid differentiation. The expression of the various immunological markers by cells in the different stages of myeloid differentiation are indicated. The markers in parentheses are not always expressed.

3.1 Immunological marker analysis of cells in suspension

Cells in suspension can be obtained from BM, PB, cerebrospinal fluid (CSF), bronchoalveolar lavage (BAL) fluid, pleural exudate, ascites, synovial fluid, etc. Generally, the granulocytes and erythrocytes are removed from the BM and PB samples by ficoll density centrifugation, which purification facilitates the analysis of the remaining mononuclear cells (MNC) (95).

For the detection of markers on the cell surface membrane the cells are incubated with the relevant antibodies in suspension, while for the detection of cytoplasmic or nuclear markers, cytocentrifuge preparations are made, which are subsequently incubated with the relevant antibodies. In our laboratory we mainly use direct and indirect fluorescence methods for the visualization of the reactivity of the antibodies (Fig. 5-7, 9-12). It is one of the advantages of a fluorochrome as label, that a double staining can be easily performed and evaluated (Fig. 5,7,9,10) (1,2,42). In general we use fluorescein isothiocyanate (FITC) and tetramethylrhodamine isothiocyanate (TRITC) as labels. TRITC can be replaced by phycoerythrin (PE) (96). Although PE has advantages for fluorescence activated cell sorting procedures, we prefer to use TRITC in fluorescence microscopy, because PE fades very quickly. If necessary, even a triple immunological staining can be performed using colloidal gold particles as the third label next to FITC and TRITC (Fig. 12) (93). Such double and triple immunological stainings allow the evaluation of two or three different markers at the single cell level. This is important for determining whether the markers are expressed by the same cell or by different cells (93,97). Detailed information concerning methods for immunological marker analysis of cells in suspension is described in section 4.

In our opinion it is necessary to use phase contrast facilities on a fluorescence microscope, since phase contrast morphology gives valuable information about the cells evaluated and allows the precise localization of the labels, which is important when intracellular antigens are stained, such as TdT (Fig. 5,9,12). In addition, this equipment allows optimal discrimination between labeled cells and contaminating autofluorescent particles.

3.2 Immunological marker analysis of cells in tissue sections

Cells in tissues such as obtained by biopsies from lymph nodes, tonsils, liver and spleen, can be characterized immunologically by the use of tissue sections. The tissue sections, usually frozen sections, are incubated with the relevant antibodies. The reactivity of the antibodies is visualized by the use of direct or indirect staining methods using an enzyme as label, such as peroxidase (PO) or alkaline phosphatase (AP) (9,98). Such enzymes transform a substrate into a colored precipitate. Double immunological stainings, using enzymes as labels (e.g. PO and AP) are possible if the detected antigens are expressed by different cells (94,97-99). Expression of two antigens by the same cell is difficult to prove by use of enzymes as labels (97), unless the antigens are expressed very strongly (100,101). Detailed information concerning methods for immunological marker analysis of cells in tissue sections are described in other chapters of this book.

The advantage of the use of tissue sections is that histological information can be combined with information about the expression of immunological markers (9). Nevertheless it may be necessary that a cell suspension is made from the tissue biopsy obtained for immunological marker analysis, especially if a part of the cell suspension is used for cytogenetic analysis.

Table 1. **Immunological markers, which can be used for the characterization of cells in the various hematopoietic differentiation stages and their malignant counterparts**

Antibody/technique	Cluster of differentiation[a]	Antigen recognized	Specificity	References
I LYMPHOID MARKERS				
anti-TdT[b,c]	–	terminal deoxy-nucleotidyl transferase	immature lymphoid cells (Fig. 3)	1, 11, 12
B CELL MARKERS				
B4[d] or Leu-12[c]	CD19	B cell antigen (p95)	all (precursor) B cells (Fig. 3)	20
VIL-A1[f] or J5[g] or BA-3[h]	CD10	common ALL antigen (CALLA) (gp100)	pre-pre-B cells, pre-B cells and a subpopulation of cortical thymocytes (Fig. 3); granulocytes	21-24, 85, 86
BA-1[h]	CD24	B cell antigen (p45,55,65)	most precursor B cells and all B cells; mature myeloid cells	23, 24, 87
BA-2[h]	CD9	B cell antigen (p24)	most precursor B cells and subpopulations of B cells (Fig. 3)	23-26
B1[d]	CD20	B cell antigen (p35)	all B cells (Fig. 3)	24, 27, 28
B2[d]	CD21	B cell antigen (p140)	subpopulations of B cells (Fig. 3)	24, 28, 29
Leu-14[c]	CD22	B cell antigen (p135)	subpopulations of B cells	
Y29/55[i]	–	B cell antigen	mature B cells (Fig. 3)	24, 30
FMC7[k]	–	B cell antigen	mature B cells (Fig. 3)	24, 31, 32
PCA-1[d]	–	plasma cell antigen	plasma cells (Fig. 3); granulocytes and monocytes	33
M rosette	–	mouse red blood cell (MRBC) receptor	small subpopulation of B cells ('resting B cells'); B-CLL cells	83, 88
SmIg[l,m] (κ,λ,μ,δ,γ,α,ε)	–	surface membrane immunoglobulin	SmIg positive B cells (Fig. 3); each B cell (clone) expresses only one Ig light chain isotype (κ or λ), but can express multiple Ig heavy chain isotypes	17, 18
cIg[l,m] (κ,λ,μ,δ,γ,α,ε)	–	cytoplasmic immunoglobulin	cIg positive cells (Fig. 3); each cIg positive B cell (clone) expresses only one Ig light chain isotype and one Ig heavy chain isotype	19
weak cμ (pre-B)[l,m]	–	weak expression of cytoplasmic μ heavy chain	pre-B-cells (Fig. 3); only μ heavy chain is weakly expressed in the cytoplasm (no light chain expression)	13-16
κ/λ ratio			the normal κ/λ ratio ranges from 0.7 to 5.5 (mean: 2)	17, 109, 110

Antibody/technique	Cluster of differentiation[a]	Antigen recognized	Specificity	References
T CELL MARKERS				
3A1[n] or WT1[o]	CD7	Tp41 antigen (p41)	all T cells (Fig. 3); 5% of AML (Fig. 4)	34-39
E (rosette)	–	sheep red blood cell (SRBC) receptor	all T cells (Fig. 3)	43
T11[d] or Leu-5[c] or OKT11[g]	CD2	T11 antigen; SRBC receptor (p50)	all T cells (Fig. 3)	34, 35, 40,41
T1[d] or Leu-1[c] or OKT1[g]	CD5	T1 antigen (p67)	thymocytes and mature T cells (Fig. 3); small subpopulation of B cells (Fig. 3); B-CLL	34, 35, 44, 45, 82, 84
T6[d] or Leu-6[c] or OKT6[g] or 66IIC7[p]	CD1	T6 antigen (common thymocyte antigen) (p45-12)	cortical thymocytes (Fig. 3); Langerhans cells in the skin (Fig. 4)	34, 35, 50, 81
T4[d] or Leu-3[c] or OKT4[g] or RIV6[o]	CD4	T4 antigen (p55)	T helper cells (Fig. 3)	34, 35, 46
T8[d] or Leu-2[c] or OKT8[g] or FK18[o] or SPV-T8[p]	CD8	T8 antigen (p32-33)	T suppressor cells (Fig. 3)	34, 35, 46, 47
T3[d] or Leu-4[c] or OKT3[g] or WT32[o] or SPV-T3b[p]	CD3	T3 antigen (p19-29)	mature T cells (Fig. 3)	34, 35, 48, 49, 52
WT31[q]	–	T cell receptor (TcR) (gp37-44)	mature T cells (Fig. 3)	52, 54
2 MYELOID MARKERS				
MYELOMONOCYTIC MARKERS				
My7[d]	CDw13	myelo-monocytic antigen (p160)	all myeloid and monocytic cells (Fig. 4)	59 - 61
My9[d]	–	myelo-monocytic antigen (p72)	almost all myeloid and monocytic cells, except granulocytes (Fig. 4)	62
Mo1[d] or OKM1[g]	CD11	C3bi receptor (p95-150)	myeloid and monocytic cells	60, 62, 64, 65, 89 - 91
VIM-D5[f] or B4.3[r]	CD15	myeloid antigen (p105-150)	immature and mature myeloid cells (Fig. 4)	68, 69
Leu-M4[c]	–	myeloid antigen	mature myeloid cells (Fig. 4)	
My4[d]	–	monocytic antigen (p55)	monocytic cells and macrophages (Fig. 4)	59 - 61
Leu-M3[c]	–	monocytic antigen	monocytic cells and macrophages (Fig. 4)	63, 64
Mo2[d] or FMC17[k]	CDw14	monocytic antigen	monocytes and macrophages (Fig. 4)	62, 65 - 67
Monocyte-2[b]	–	monocytic antigen (p75)	monocytes and macrophages	64, 92
ERYTHROID MARKERS				
VIE-G4[f]	–	glycophorin A (GpA) (gp41)	erythroid cells (Fig. 4)	70, 71

Antibody/technique	Cluster of differentiation[a]	Antigen recognized	Specificity	References
THROMBOCYTIC MARKERS				
C8.13[f]	-	glycoprotein IIa (GPIIa)	megakaryocytic cells and thrombocytes (Fig. 4)	72
C17.27[f]	-	glycoprotein IIIa (GPIIIa) (gp110)	megakaryocytic cells and thrombocytes (Fig. 4)	72 - 74
3. MARKERS WHICH ARE NOT RESTRICTED TO ONE DIFFERENTIATION LINEAGE				
anti-HLA-DR[c] or OKIa[g]	-	HLA-DR non-polymorphic antigen (p29-34)	hematopoietic precursor cells, B cells, activated T lymphocytes, monocytic cells and macrophages (Fig. 3 and 4)	75 - 77
T9[d] or OKT9[g] or 66IG10[p]	-	T9 antigen; transferrin receptor (p90)	proliferating cells; activated cells	78 - 80

a CD = cluster of differentiation, as proposed by the first and second International Workshops on Human Leukocyte Differentiation Antigens, (Paris, France, 1982; Boston, MA, 1984) (c.f. references 6 and 7)
b Bethesda Research Laboratories, Gaithersburg, MD
c Supertechs, Bethesda, MD
d Coulter Clone, Hialeah, FL
e Becton Dickinson, Sunnyvale, CA
f Dr. W. Knapp, Vienna, Austria
g Ortho Diagnostic Systems, Raritan, NJ
h Hybritech, San Diego, CA
i Dr. H.K. Forster, Hoffman-La Roche, Basel, Switzerland
k Sera-Lab, Crawley Down, England
l Kallestad Laboratories, Austin, TX
m DAKO, Kopenhagen, Danmark
n American Type Culture Collection, Rockville, MD
o National Institute of Public Health and Environmental Hygiene, Bilthoven, The Netherlands
p Monosan/Sanbio, Nistelrode, The Netherlands
q Dr. W. Tax, St. Radboud Hospital, University of Nijmegen, The Netherlands
r Central Laboratory of the Blood Transfusion Service, Amsterdam, The Netherlands

4. METHODS FOR IMMUNOLOGICAL MARKER ANALYSIS OF CELLS IN SUSPENSION

4.1 Preparation of cell suspensions

MNC from BM and PB are isolated by ficoll density centrifugation (Ficoll Paque; density 1.077 g/cm^3; Pharmacia, Uppsala, Sweden) for 15 min at room temperature (RT) with a centrifugal force of 1000 g. All standard washings of cells in suspension derived from BM, PB, CSF, pleural exudate, ascites, etc., are performed with phosphate-buffered saline (PBS) (300 mosmol; pH 7.8), supplemented with 0.5% bovine serum albumin (BSA; Organon Teknika, Oss, The Netherlands) and 0.05% sodium azide. Washing centrifugations are performed for 5 min at 4°C with a force of 400 g. If the cells are incubated in suspension for the detection of surface membrane markers by use of antibodies, the cell concentration is adjusted to 10^7 cells per ml. Cytocentrifuge preparations are made using cell suspensions with a concentration of 0.5 to 2 x 10^6 cells per ml, depending on the size of the cells; in the case of a BM or PB cell sample a concentration of 2 x 10^6 cells per ml is generally used. If the cell suspension is used for rosette techniques, the cell concentration is also adjusted to 2 x 10^6 cells per ml.

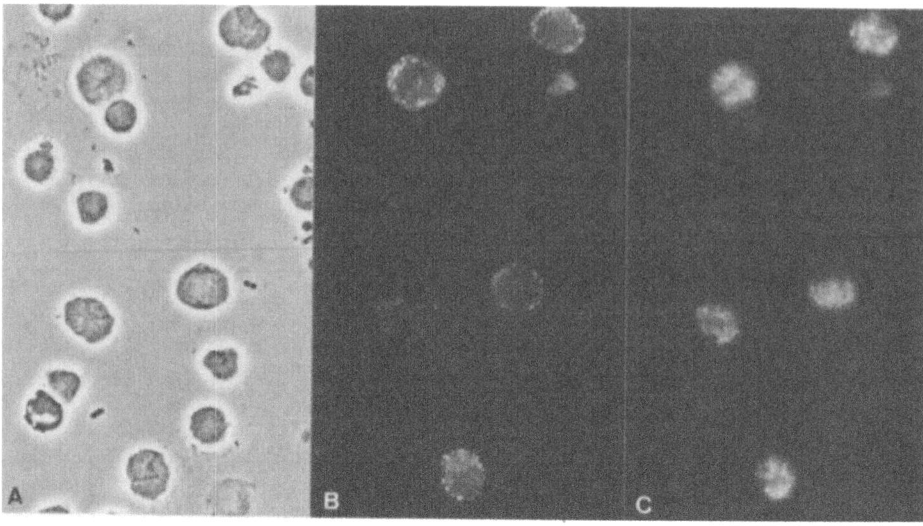

Figure 5. Double immunological staining for CALLA and TdT on MNC of PB from a patient in early relapse of an ALL.
A: phase contrast picture; B: CALLA positive cells (TRITC labeled); C: TdT positive cells (FITC labeled). All TdT positive cells in the PB sample appeared to express CALLA, indicating that it concerned a CALLA positive ALL.

4.2 General remarks concerning immunological stainings

Most immunological markers are detected by the use of antibodies. Commercially available McAb generally can be diluted 1:50 to 1:200, while commercially available conventional antisera can be diluted 1:20 to 1:80. However, each batch of antibodies has to be optimally titrated for the different applications. The labeled cells or cytocentrifuge preparations are mounted in glycerol/PBS (9:1), containing 1 mg *p*-phenylenediamine per ml (BDH Chemicals, Poole, UK) to prevent fading of fluorochromes (102). Coverslips are sealed with paraffin wax with ceresin (BDH Chemicals). Some immunological markers are detected by rosette techniques. Such rosette tests generally are evaluated by the use of a counting chamber.

We will describe several single, double and triple immunological staining methods as well as the microscopes, which we use for the evaluation of the immunological stainings.

4.3 Single immunological stainings

In single staining methods using antibodies, we generally use FITC as fluorochrome. Several single staining methods using antibodies or rosette techniques will be described.

4.3.1 *Detection of cell surface membrane markers by the use of antibodies*
In the case of a direct immunological staining (e.g. using FITC-conjugated anti-human-Ig antisera) 50 μl of the cell suspension (10^7 cells per ml) is incubated for 30 min at 4°C with 50 μl of the relevant, optimally titrated, FITC-conjugated antibody.

After this incubation the cells are washed twice. In the case of an indirect immunological staining (e.g. using mouse McAb), the cells undergo an additional incubation (30 min, 4°C) with the relevant FITC-conjugated second step antiserum (a FITC-conjugated goat anti-mouse-Ig antiserum, if mouse McAb are used). After the second incubation, the cells are washed twice and the cell pellet is mounted in glycerol.

4.3.2 *Detection of cIg*
Fifty μl of the cell suspension (2 x 10^6 cells per ml) is centrifuged on slides in a cytocentrifuge (Nordic, Tilburg, The Netherlands). The cytocentrifuge preparations are air-dried for at least 15 min and the location of the cells is marked by encircling with a glass pencil. The preparations are fixed in acid ethanol (ethanol with 5% acetic acid) for 15 min at −20°C. The preparations are then washed in PBS (pH 7.8) for 15 min, dried, and incubated with 15 μl of a FITC-conjugated anti-human-Ig heavy or light chain antiserum (Table 1) in a moist chamber (30 min, RT) (19). Subsequently the slides are washed again in PBS (15 min), mounted in glycerol, covered with a coverslip and sealed (Fig. 6,7,10).

4.3.3 *Detection of TdT*
Cytocentrifuge preparations are made, air-dried, fixed in methanol (30 min, 4°C) and washed in PBS. The preparations are incubated with 15 μl of optimally titrated rabbit anti-TdT antiserum (Table 1) in a moist chamber (30 min, RT) and washed in PBS. Subsequently, the preparations are incubated with 15 μl of a FITC-conjugated goat anti-rabbit-Ig antiserum and washed again (12,42). Afterwards the preparations are mounted in glycerol, covered with a coverslip and sealed (Fig. 5,9,12).

4.3.4 *E rosette test*
SRBC are washed five times with PBS; washing centrifugations are performed for 10 min at RT with a centrifugal force of 1500 g. Subsequently, the SRBC are incubated with 2-amino-ethylisothiouronium bromide (AET) (40 mg per ml; pH 9.0) for 15 min at 37°C. Afterwards these AET-treated SRBC are washed several times with PBS and finally are resuspended in PBS, supplemented with 10% fetal calf serum (FCS) (43).

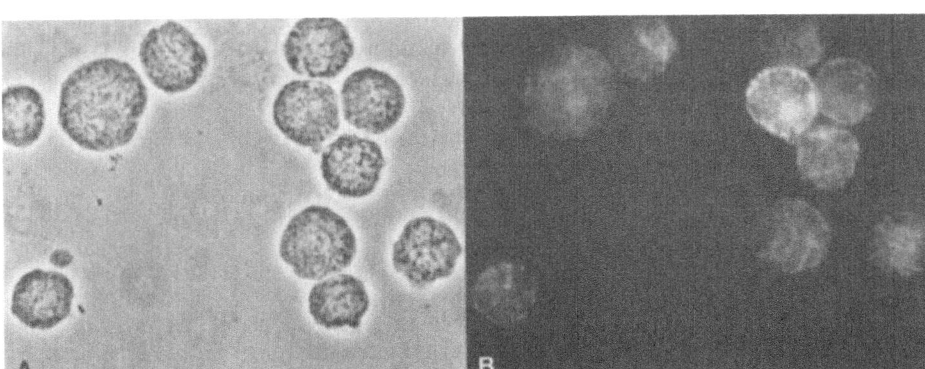

Figure 6. Immunological staining for cytoplasmic μ Ig heavy chain on MNC of BM from an ALL patient at diagnosis.
A: phase contrast picture; B: weak cμ positive cells (FITC labeled). Most MNC of BM appeared to be weakly positive for cμ, indicating that it concerned a pre-B-ALL.

One hundred μl of the cell suspension (2 x 10^6 cells per ml) is mixed with 100 μl AET-treated SRBC (2 x 10^8 SRBC per ml), and centrifuged for 5 min at 4°C with a centrifugal force of 300 g. The pellet is incubated for at least 15 min at 4°C. After this incubation the pellet is very carefully resuspended in the supernatant. Fifty μl of acridine orange (5 μg per ml) is added to stain the DNA of the nucleated cells. The cell suspension is carefully mounted into a counting chamber and evaluated by combining epi-illumination (using the FITC filter combination) with trans-illumination (c.f. section 4.6.1 and Fig. 8). A nucleated cell is regarded as positive, if three or more erythrocytes are attached to the cell (Fig. 8).

4.3.5 *M rosette test*
Fresh collected MRBC are washed five times with PBS. Fifty μl of the cell suspension (2 x 10^6 cells per ml), 50 μl of the MRBC suspension (1 x 10^8 MRBC per ml) and 100 μl FCS are mixed. This mixture is incubated for 15 min at 37°C and subsequently centrifuged for 5 min at 4°C with a centrifugal force of 300 g. The pellet is incubated at 4°C for 18 hours without being disturbed (83,88). After this incubation 100 μl of the supernatant is removed and the pellet is very carefully resuspended. Acridine orange is added to the cell suspension and the percentage M rosette forming cells is determined in a counting chamber (c.f. section 4.3.4).

4.4 Double immunological stainings

All of the various single immunological stainings, described in section 4.3, can be combined. When antibodies are used in double immunological stainings, we use FITC and TRITC as labels. In our laboratory the double stainings with antibodies are performed in four different ways:

- *Combination of two fluorochrome-conjugated antibodies*
  The advantage of fluorochrome-conjugated antibodies is that these antibodies can be mixed and that therefore only one incubation step is needed for the double staining. However, weakly expressed antigens might be insufficiently stained in a direct staining method, so that positivity is not always detectable.
- *Combination of a fluorochrome-conjugated mouse McAb and an unconjugated mouse McAb*
  In such combinations, the cell suspension is first incubated with the unconjugated McAb, followed by an incubation with a fluorochrome-conjugated anti-mouse-Ig antiserum. Subsequently, the cells are incubated with normal mouse serum to block free antigen binding sites of the anti-mouse-Ig antiserum (c.f. section 4.5). Finally, the fluorochrome-conjugated McAb is used.
- *Combination of two unconjugated mouse McAb with different isotypes*
  Indirect staining methods using McAb can be performed by selecting pairs of mouse McAb on the basis of their different isotypes (e.g. IgM and IgG or IgG1 and IgG2). This application is restricted by the availability of FITC- and TRITC-conjugated anti-mouse-Ig-(sub)class specific antisera.
- *Combination of antibodies from different species*
  Antibodies, raised in different species, can be combined very easily. E.g. a rabbit antiserum can be combined with a mouse McAb, using a FITC-conjugated goat anti-rabbit-Ig antiserum and a TRITC-conjugated goat anti-mouse-Ig antiserum, respectively (c.f section 4.4.3).

By the use of these four possibilities or their combinations, many different double immunofluorescence stainings can be performed. Additional possibilities for double immunological stainings can be obtained by using biotin-conjugated or arsanilic-

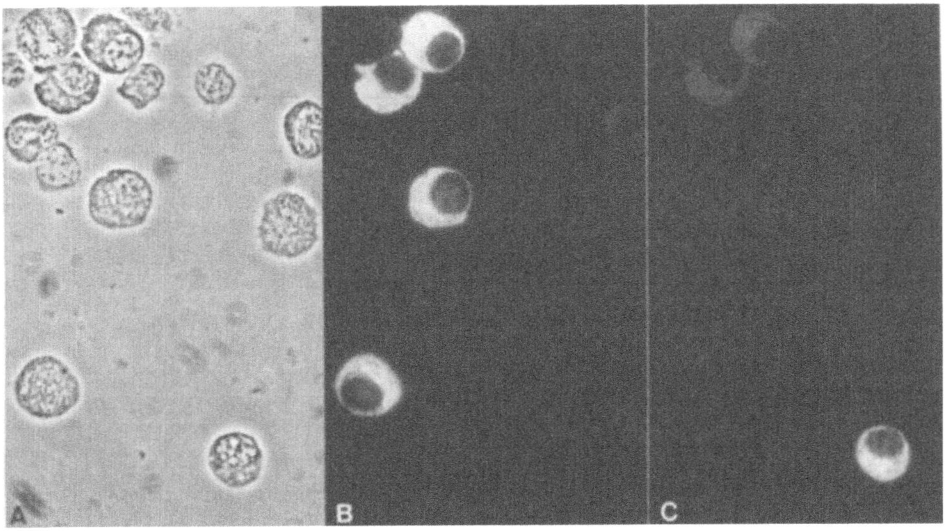

Figure 7. Double immunological staining for cκ and cλ on BM cells from a patient with a plasmacytoma.
A: phase contrast picture; B: cκ positive cells (TRITC labeled); C: cλ positive cell (FITC labeled). The majority of the cIg positive cells appeared to be positive for cκ; only a few cλ positive cells were detectable in the cytocentrifuge preparation. This indicates that the plasmacytoma cells were cκ positive.

acid-conjugated McAb; the reactivity of such McAb is visualized by the use of fluorochrome-conjugated avidin molecules or a fluorochrome-conjugated anti-arsanilic-acid antiserum, respectively (103,104). In the combined detection of a cell surface membrane antigen and a cytoplasmic antigen, we prefer to use FITC as label for the detection of the cytoplasmic antigen and TRITC as label for the detection of the cell surface membrane antigen. In our experience the use of TRITC for the labeling of cytoplasmic antigens generally results in a higher background staining as compared with FITC. In addition to double stainings with antibodies, an antibody staining can be combined with a rosette technique. Several double immunological stainings will be described.

4.4.1 *Double immunofluorescence staining for Smκ and Smλ*
The cell suspension is incubated with a mixture of a TRITC-conjugated anti-human-κ antiserum and a FITC-conjugated anti-human-λ antiserum (Table 1) (30 min at 4°C). After the incubation the cells are washed and a suspension preparation is made (c.f. section 4.3.1).

4.4.2 *Double immunofluorescence staining for cκ and cλ*
A cytocentrifuge preparation is made, fixed in acid ethanol and subsequently incubated with 15 μl of a mixture of a TRITC-conjugated anti-human-κ antiserum and a FITC-conjugated anti-human-λ antiserum (30 min, RT) (c.f. section 4.3.2) (Fig. 7).

4.4.3 *Double immunofluorescence staining for a cell surface membrane antigen and TdT*
Fifty μl of the cell suspension is incubated with the relevant antibody, which is directly or indirectly labeled with TRITC (c.f. section 4.3.1). After the incubation

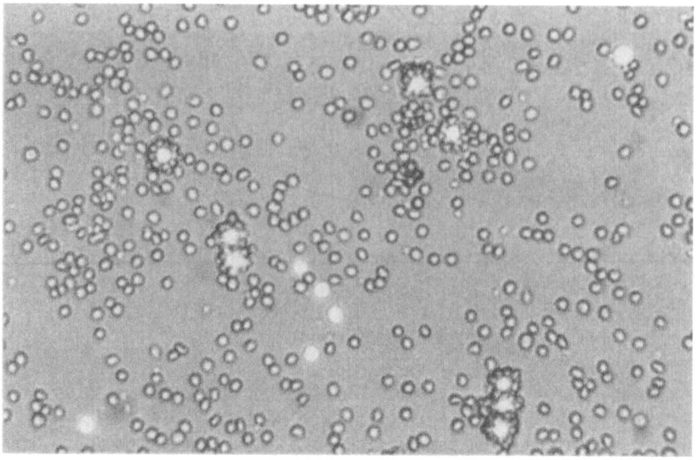

Figure 8. E rosette test on MNC of PB from a healthy adult.
The nucleated cells were stained with acridine orange and evaluated by combining epi-illumination (using a FITC filter combination) with trans-illumination (c.f. section 4.3.4). Eight cells in the presented field form rosettes, while six cells do not.

and washings, 200 µl of PBS/0.5% BSA is added to the cell pellet. Subsequently cytocentrifuge preparations are made (50 µl of the cell suspension per preparation), which are fixed in methanol (30 min, 4°C). The cytocentrifuge preparations are subjected to the indirect TdT staining with a rabbit anti-TdT antiserum and a FITC-conjugated goat anti-rabbit-Ig antiserum (c.f. section 4.3.3) (Fig. 5,9).

4.4.4 *Double immunofluorescence staining for a cell surface membrane antigen and cIg*
The cell suspension is incubated with the relevant antibody, which is directly or indirectly labeled with TRITC. Subsequently cytocentrifuge preparations are made (c.f. section 4.4.3). The cytocentrifuge preparations are fixed in acid ethanol (15 min, −20°C) and subjected to a direct cIg staining, using a FITC-conjugated anti-human-Ig antiserum (c.f. section 4.3.2) (Fig. 10).

4.4.5 *Double immunological staining for SmIg and the MRBC receptor*
Fifty µl of the cell suspension is incubated with a FITC-conjugated anti-human-Ig antiserum (c.f. section 4.3.1). After the incubation and washings, the cell suspension is subjected to the M rosette test (c.f. section 4.3.5). Subsequently the concentration of the cell suspension (MRBC plus nucleated cells) is adjusted to 2 x 10^6 cells per ml and cytocentrifuge preparations are made (50 µl of the cell suspension per preparation). The cytocentrifuge preparations are fixed in methanol (5 min, 4°C), mounted in glycerol, covered with a coverslip and sealed (Fig. 11).

4.5 Triple immunological staining

In the triple immunological staining we use colloidal gold particles of 30 nm as the third label next to FITC and TRITC (93). Colloidal gold can be visualized in the same epi-illumination system, which is used for the evaluation of fluorescence (c.f. section 4.6.2). Although colloidal gold particles of 30 nm can easily be used as label for the detection of cytoplasmic markers of cells in tissue sections (105), this is more difficult when cytocentrifuge preparations are used. Therefore we use the colloidal gold technique for staining cell surface membrane markers. One example of a triple immunological staining will be described.

Triple immunological staining for T3, HLA-DR and TdT
Fifty µl of the cell suspension is incubated with the anti-T3 antigen McAb Leu-4 (Table 1), washed and subsequently incubated with 50 µl of an undiluted goat anti-mouse-Ig antiserum, conjugated with colloidal gold particles of 30 nm (G30; Janssen Pharmaceutica, Beerse, Belgium). Afterwards the cells are incubated with normal mouse serum (diluted 1 in 100) to block free antigen binding sites of the goat anti-mouse-Ig antiserum. Subsequently the cells are incubated with a TRITC-conjugated anti-HLA-DR McAb (Becton Dickinson, Sunnyvale, CA). After the incubation and washings, 200 µl of PBS/0.5% BSA is added to the cell pellet. Finally, cytocentrifuge preparations are made, which are subjected to the indirect TdT staining using FITC as label (c.f. section 4.3.3) (Fig. 12).

4.6 Microscopes

4.6.1 Evaluation of single and double immunological stainings, using fluorochromes
For the evaluation of fluorescence (FITC, TRITC and acridine orange), we use Zeiss Standard 16 microscopes (Carl Zeiss, Oberkochen, FRG), equipped with a IV FL Fluoreszenz-Auflichtkondensor (epi-illumination condensor) and phase contrast facilities. The epi-illumination system contains two filter combinations: Zeiss filter combination 14 (BP 510-560; FT 580; LP 590) for the evaluation of TRITC labeling and Zeiss filter combination 19 (BP 485/20; FT 510; LP 515) combined with a KP 560 filter for the evaluation of FITC labeling and acridine orange staining. The

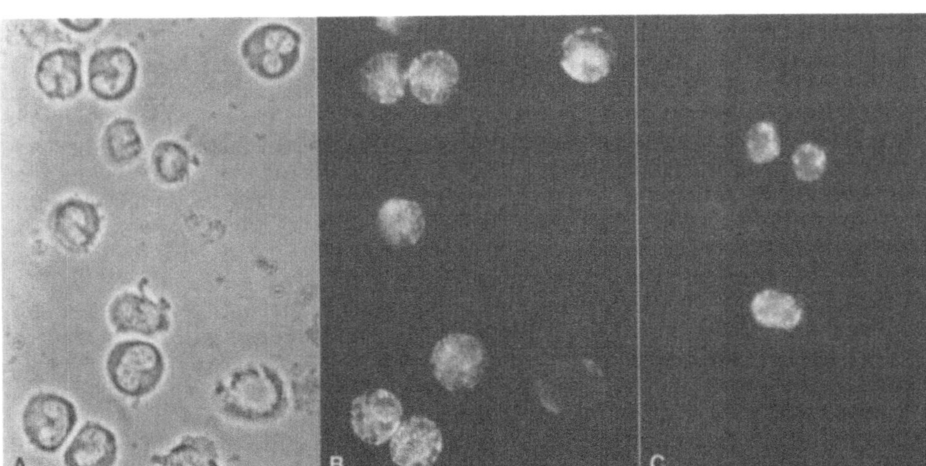

Figure 9. Double immunological staining for VIM-D5 and TdT on MNC of BM from a CML patient in early lymphoid BC.
A: phase contrast picture; B: VIM-D5 positive cells (TRITC labeled); C: TdT positive cells (FITC labeled). The three TdT positive cells do not express the myeloid marker VIM-D5.

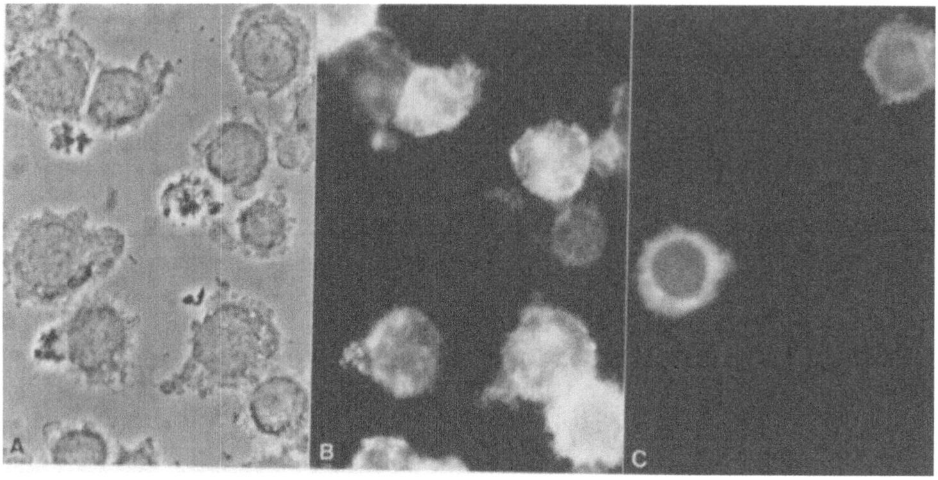

Figure 10. Double immunological staining for HLA-DR and cμ on cells of a Burkitt lymphoma derived cell line.
A: phase contrast picture; B: HLA-DR positive cells (TRITC labeled); C: cμ positive cells (FITC labeled). The HLA-DR positive cells did not express cμ.

microscopes are equipped with at least three Zeiss objectives: a neofluar 63/1.25 Oel Ph3 for evaluation of surface membrane staining, TdT staining, etc.; a plan-apochromat 40/1.0 Oel Ph3 for evaluation of strong expression of cIg and a neofluar 16/0.40 Ph2 for evaluation of the rosette tests. These objectives are used in combination with the Zeiss wide-field oculars Kpl-W10x/18.

4.6.2 *Evaluation of the triple immunological staining, using colloidal gold as the third label*

We use two different microscopes for the evaluation of colloidal gold in combination with FITC and TRITC: a Zeiss Universal II (Carl Zeiss, Oberkochen, FRG) and a Leitz Orthoplan (Ernst Leitz, Wetzlar, FRG). The Zeiss Universal II is equipped with a III RS Fluoreszenz-Auflichtkondensor, phase contrast facilities and the same filtercombinations, objectives and oculars as described for the Zeiss Standard 16 microscopes (c.f. section 4.6.1). The Leitz Orthoplan is equipped with a Ploemopak 2 epi-illumination system, phase contrast facilities and the following two filter combinations: Leitz filter combination I2 (BP 450-490; RKP 510; LP 515) for the evaluation of FITC and Leitz filter combination N2 (BP 530-560; RKP 580; LP 580) for the evaluation of TRITC. The most frequently used objective of the Leitz microscope is the PL APO 63/1.40 Oel PHACO 4 in combination with the wide-field oculars Periplan GW 10xM.

For the evaluation of colloidal gold, we use a polarization filter combination in both microscopes, consisting of a polarizer for the excitation light, a beamsplitter and an analyzer, which extinguishes the reflected light that has the same polarization as the excitation beam. The objectives which are used for evaluation of colloidal gold should not contain phase contrast rings. According to our experience the best objective is the Zeiss Antiflex-Neofluar 63/1.25 Oel, which contains a rotable quarter-wave plate (93).

5. IMMUNOLOGICAL PHENOTYPES OF LEUKEMIAS AND NHL

Immunological marker analysis can be applied not only to the characterization of normal hematopoietic cells, but also to the characterization of leukemias and NHL (Fig. 2).

The maturation-arrest of the acute leukemias is localized in the immature differentiation stages (e.g. acute lymphoblastic leukemias (ALL) and acute myeloid leukemias (AML)). Chronic leukemias are the malignant counterparts of cells in more mature differentiation stages (e.g. chronic lymphocytic leukemias (CLL) and chronic myeloid leukemias (CML)). Generally, NHL have a mature immunological phenotype.

Several differentiation stages may occur within one malignancy. This indicates that malignant cells are capable of further maturation and that their maturation-arrest is not restricted to a single differentiation stage. This especially occurs in AML and NHL.

5.1 Lymphoid malignancies

ALL can be divided into at least five different types according to their immunological phenotype: null ALL, common ALL, pre-B-ALL, B-ALL and T-ALL (1,2,8,106). These immunological phenotypes are summarized in Table 2. T-ALL can be subdivided into several immature and more mature subtypes, as is indicated in Figures 2 and 3 (2,8,34,42,107). The morphological 'French American British' (FAB) classification of ALL recognizes three ALL types: L1, L2 and L3 (108). This FAB classification does not correlate well with the immunological classification. L1 and L2 morphology can be found in most immunological ALL types; only L3 morphology seems to be restricted to the seldom occurring B-ALL.

Normally about 60% of the B cells expresses κ light chain, while about 30% expresses λ light chain; the normal κ/λ ratio varies from 0.7 to 5.5 (109). Since a B cell malignancy represents a clonal expansion of B cells, only one type Ig light chain (κ or λ) is expressed. Therefore, the κ/λ ratio is used for the detection of a B cell malignancy and may give an impression of the number of malignant cells

Table 2. **Immunological phenotypes of ALL**

	TdT	HLA-DR	B4	CALLA	weak cμ	SmIg	T cell marker
null ALL	+	+	(+)[a]	–	–	–	–
common ALL	+	+	+	+	–	–	–
pre-B-ALL	+	+	+	+	+	–	–
B-ALL	–	+	+	(+)[a]	–	+	–
T-ALL[b]	+	–[c]	–	–[d]	–	–	+

a Not always expressed
b Several subtypes of T-ALL can be recognized, based on their positivity for the various T cell markers
c The rare prothymocytic T-ALL is HLA-DR positive
d Some T-ALL express CALLA.

Table 3. **Immunological phenotypes of some B cell malignancies**

	HLA-DR	B1	SmIg	cIg	PCA-1	T1
B-CLL	+	+	±[a]	–	–	+
B-PLL	+	+	++[b]	–	–	–[c]
M. Waldenström	+	+	±[a]	+	–	–
M. Kahler	–	–	–	++[b]	+	–

a Weak expression
b Strong expression
c Some B-PLL express the T1 antigen

(17,109,110). Several B cell malignancies can be distinguished by the use of additional B cell markers. B cell CLL (B-CLL) can be discriminated from other B cell malignancies by their weak expression of SmIg and positivity for the T1 antigen (82,83). On the other hand, a B cell pro-lymphocytic leukemia (B-PLL) strongly expresses SmIg and is generally negative for the T1 antigen (8). The immunological phenotypes of several B cell malignancies are summarized in Table 3.

Immunological marker analysis of NHL does not result in a classification comparable to the detailed morphological classifications, such as the Kiel classification (111). However, immunological marker analysis is still valuable in the diagnosis of NHL. It is possible to determine whether a B cell or T cell malignancy is involved and to prove the clonality of the tumor by means of the κ/λ ratio in the case of a B cell malignancy (Fig. 7) (17,109,110). In addition, more and more immunological markers (especially B cell markers) are becoming available, which may result in a better immunological classification of NHL (c.f. other chapters of this book).

5.2 Myeloid malignancies

The myeloid markers at present available can be used for the classification of the myeloid malignancies, although they are not as discriminating as the lymphoid markers (Fig. 4).

The morphological FAB classification of AML and the immunological classification of AML are both based on differentiation characteristics (60,62,108). Although Figures 2 and 4 suggest that the FAB classification and immunological classification of AML are similar, this is only true in the case of more mature AML (i.e. acute monocytic leukemia and acute promyelocytic leukemia) (62). AML often appear to consist of several subpopulations, which hampers the immunological marker analysis of AML. Only double immunofluorescence stainings for the various myeloid markers allow the immunological marker analysis of the subpopulations. CML cells express granulocytic markers such as VIM-D5 (Fig. 4). When a CML transforms into a blastic crisis (BC), immunological marker analysis can reveal whether it concerns a myeloid or lymphoid BC (Fig. 9). The immunological phenotypes of a myeloid BC are comparable to those of the various AML, while the phenotype of a lymphoid BC is generally similar to the phenotype of a common ALL or pre-B-ALL (8,112).

The true histiocytic NHL is very rare. By using the various monocytic-macrophage markers (indicated in Figure 4 and Table 1) it is possible to characterize these NHL.

6. APPLICATION OF IMMUNOLOGICAL MARKER ANALYSIS

6.1 Immunological marker analysis of cells in normal hematopoietic differentiation stages

Immunological marker analysis can be used for the characterization of hematopoietic cell populations, such as in patients with primary immunodeficiencies (113). It can also provide information concerning diseases, where the balance between various (sub)populations is disturbed (114,115). In patients with the acquired immunodeficiency syndrome (AIDS) the T4/T8 ratio in PB becomes extremely low (116,117). In patients with active sarcoidosis the percentage T lymphocytes in BAL fluid is about 22% and sometimes up to 80% with high T4/T8 ratios, while in BAL fluid from normal controls, low percentages T lymphocytes are detected (118,119). The monitoring of percentages of T lymphocytes and T4/T8 ratios may be useful during follow-up of patients, that have undergone an organ transplantation (e.g. during anti-thymocyte globuline (ATG) treatment) (120,121) (Table 4).

In addition, immunological marker analysis is used to determine the nature of cells in culture, such as in lymphocyte proliferation tests.

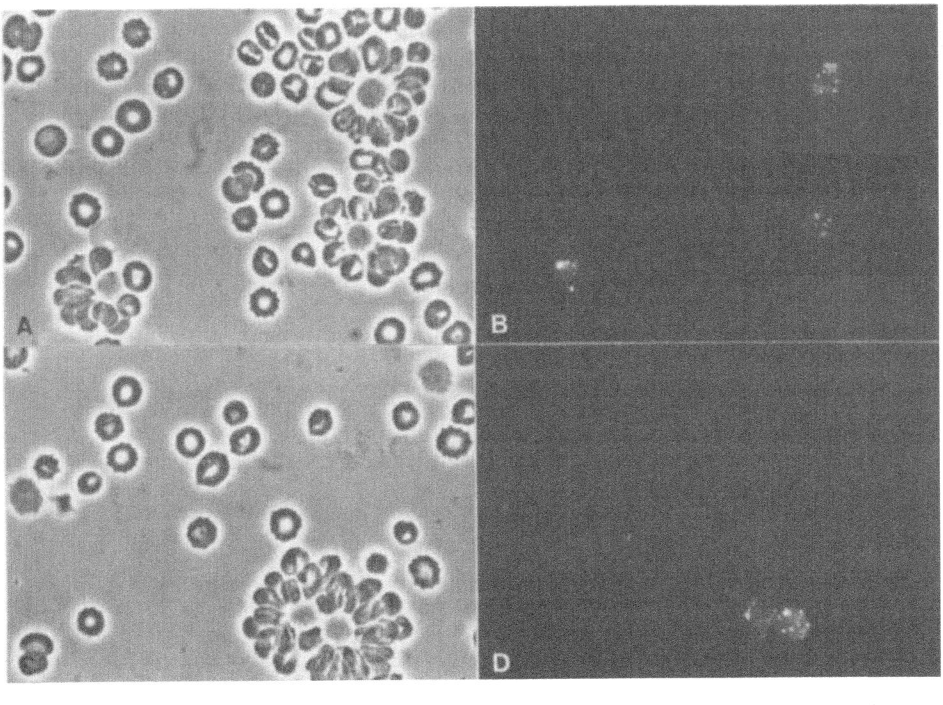

Figure 11. Double immunological staining for Smλ and M rosette on MNC of PB from a CLL patient.
A and C: phase contrast pictures; B and D: Smλ positive cells (FITC labeled). A and B represent the same field and C and D represent the same field. The M rosette forming cells also weakly expressed Smλ, while the Smλ negative cells did not form M rosettes.

6.2 Immunological marker analysis of leukemias and NHL

Immunological marker analysis of leukemias and NHL enables a reproducable classification of these malignancies. By means of clinical trials it may be possible to recognize immunological subtypes of leukemias and NHL, which differ in clinical behaviour and therapy sensitivity (122). Therefore it is necessary to characterize these malignancies according to clinical, morphological and immunological criteria, allowing adaptation of treatment protocols. Furthermore, immunological marker analysis is important for the detection of associations between immunological phenotypes and chromosome aberrations, to gain more insight in oncogenesis (123,124). In addition immunological marker analysis allows the detection of two malignancies in one patient (125) and the characterization of subpopulations within one malignancy (126) (Table 4).

During maintenance therapy and even after termination of therapy it remains uncertain whether malignant cells are still present. The application of immunological marker analysis can be used for the detection of low numbers of malignant cells, but is hampered by the presence of their normal counterparts (127). Therefore, cells positive for a certain marker or marker combination can only be regarded as malignant if these positive cells are present in higher frequencies than normal or if they are detected outside their normal homing areas. Since TdT positive cells are normally not detectable in CSF and since most ALL are positive for TdT, the TdT determination is valuable for the early detection of central nervous system leukemia in ALL patients (128). Another example of immunological detection of low numbers of malignant cells is the double immunofluorescence staining for a T cell marker and TdT on cell samples from patients suffering from a TdT positive T cell malignancy (129-131). This approach is based on the fact that $T1^+/TdT^+$, $T6^+/TdT^+$, and $T3^+/TdT^+$ cells normally occur in the thymus only (42,129-131). The application of these double stainings for analysis of BM and PB samples of T-ALL patients allows early detection of relapse (127,131).

Table 4. **Application of immunological marker analysis**

A. Immunological marker analysis of cells in normal hematopoietic differentiation stages is important for:

- determination of percentages of T lymphocytes and T4/T8 ratios in cell samples from patients with diseases such as sarcoidosis, AIDS, etc.
- analysis of cell populations in BM, PB and lymphoid tissues from patients with (primary) immunodeficiencies.
- analysis of cultured cells, e.g. in the case of lymphocyte proliferation tests.

B. Immunological marker analysis of leukemias and NHL is important for:

- classification of leukemias and NHL
- recognition of subtypes of leukemias and NHL, which differ in clinical behaviour and therapy resistance
- recognition of association between immunological phenotypes of leukemias and NHL and chromosomal aberrations
- detection of two malignancies in one patient
- characterization of subpopulations within one malignancy
- detection of low numbers of malignant cells.

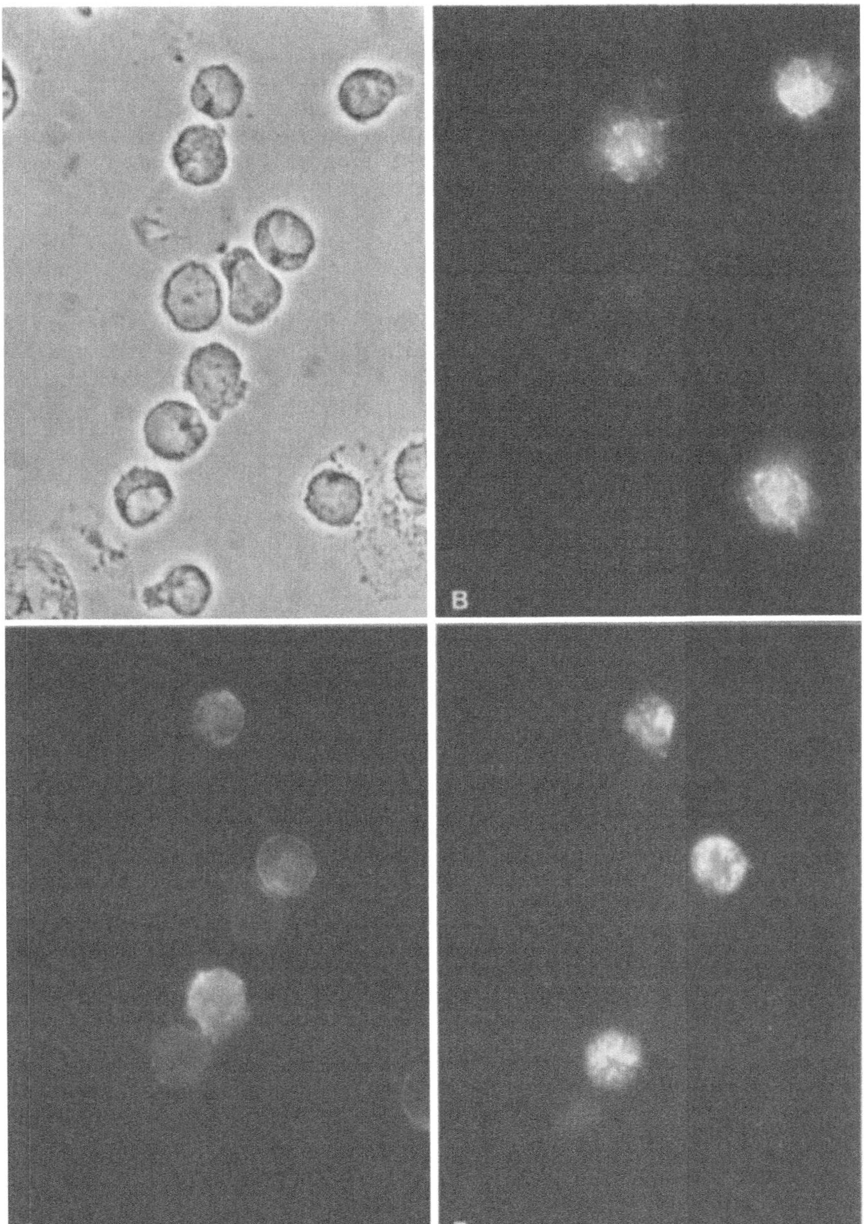

Figure 12. Triple immunological staining for T3, HLA-DR and TdT on MNC of BM from a child with ALL in complete remission under maintenance treatment.
A: phase contrast picture; B: T3 positive cells (colloidal gold labeled); C: HLA-DR positive cells (TRITC labeled); TdT positive cells (FITC labeled). The three TdT positive cells are also positive for HLA-DR, but negative for the T3 antigen. The former cells probably represent precursor B cells, while the T3 positive cells represent mature T lymphocytes.

7. CONCLUSION

Immunological marker analysis of normal hematopoietic cells and their malignant counterparts is an important tool for diagnostic use. It allows a precise analysis of leucocyte subpopulations in various diseases, such as immunodeficiencies. Moreover, it results in a reproducable classification of leukemias and NHL and allows the detection of low numbers of malignant cells. Finally, it may be used not only for diagnostic purposes, but also for clinical research.

ACKNOWLEDGMENTS

We gratefully acknowledge Prof. Dr. R. Benner for his continuous support, Mrs. A.P. Tio-Gillen and Dr. A.C. Knulst for critical reading of the manuscript, Mr. R. van den Beemd, Mrs. K. Benne, Mrs. W.M. Comans-Bitter, Mrs. E.G.M. Cristen, Mrs. A.A. van der Linde-Preesman, Mrs. A.F. Wieringa-Wolf, Mrs. A. Wijdenes-de Bresser and Mrs. I.L.M. Wolvers-Tettero for their technical assistance, Mr. C.J. van Dijk and Mr. T.M. van Os for their excellent photographic assistance and Mrs. J. de Goey-van Dooren for help in preparing the manuscript.
This work was supported by the Netherlands Cancer Foundation (Koningin Wilhelmina Fonds) and the Sophia Foundation for Medical Research (Sophia Children's Hospital, Rotterdam).

REFERENCES

1. Janossy, G., Bollum, F.J., Bradstock, K.F. and Ashley, J. (1980). Cellular phenotypes of normal and leukemic hemopoietic cells determined by analysis with selected antibody combinations. *Blood* **56**: 430-441.
2. Janossy, G., Tidman, N., Papageorgiou, E.S., Kung, P.C. and Goldstein, G. (1981). Distribution of T lymphocyte subsets in the human bone marrow and thymus: An analysis with monoclonal antibodies. *J. Immunol.* **126**: 1608-1613.
3. Tidman, N., Janossy, G., Bodger, M., Granger, S., Kung, P.C. and Goldstein, G. (1981). Delineation of human thymocyte differentiation pathways utilizing double-staining techniques with monoclonal antibodies. *Clin. exp. Immunol.* 45: 457-467.
4. Hokland, P., Ritz, J., Schlossman, S.F. and Nadler, L.M. (1985). Orderly expression of B cell antigens during the in vitro differentiation of nonmalignant human pre-B cells. *J. Immunol.* **135**: 1746-1751.
5. Knapp, W. (ed.) (1981). *Leukemia markers.* Academic Press, London.
6. Bernard, A., Boumsell, L., Dausset, J., Milstein, C. and Schlossman, S.F. (eds.) (1984). *Leucocyte typing. Human leucocyte differentiation antigens detected by monoclonal antibodies.* Springer-Verlag, Berlin.
7. Reinherz, E.L., Haynes, B.F., Nadler, L.M. and Bernstein, I.D. (eds.) (1986). *Leucocyte typing II.* Volume 1: Human T lymphocytes; Volume 2: Human B lymphocytes; Volume 3: Human myeloid and hematopoietic cells. Springer-Verlag, Berlin.
8. Foon, K.A., Schroff, R.W. and Gale, R.P. (1982). Surface markers on leukemia and lymphoma cells: Recent advances. *Blood* **60**: 1-19.
9. Van der Valk, P., Jansen, J., Daha, M.R. and Meijer, C.J.L.M. (1983). Characterization of B-cell non-Hodgkin's lymphomas. A study using a panel of monoclonal and heterologous antibodies. *Virchows Arch.* **401**: 289-305.
10. Chan, L.C., Pegram, S.M. and Greaves, M.F. (1985). Contribution of immunophenotype to the classification and differential diagnosis of acute leukaemia. *Lancet* i: 475-479.

11. Bollum, F.J. (1979). Terminal deoxynucleotidyl transferase as a hematopoietic cell marker. *Blood* **54**: 1203-1215.
12. Goldschneider, I., Gregoire, K.E., Barton, R.W. and Bollum, F.J. (1977). Demonstration of terminal deoxynucleotidyl transferase in thymocytes by immunofluorescence. *Proc. Natl. Acad. Sci. USA* **74**: 734-738.
13. Raff, M.C., Megson, M., Owen, J.J.T. and Cooper, M.D. (1976). Early production of intracellular IgM by B-lymphocyte precursors in mouse. *Nature* **259**: 224-226.
14. Burrows, P., LeJeune, M. and Kearney, J.F. (1979). Evidence that murine pre-B cells synthesise μ heavy chains but no light chains. *Nature* **280**: 838-840.
15. Vogler, L.B., Crist, W.M., Bockman, D.E., Pearl, E.R., Lawton, A.R. and Cooper, M.D. (1978). Pre-B-cell leukemia: A new phenotype of childhood lymphoblastic leukemia. *New Engl. J. Med.* **298**: 872-878.
16. Vogler, L.B., Crist, W.M., Sarrif, A.M., Pullen, D.J., Bartolucci, A.A., Falletta, J.M., Dowell, B., Humphrey, G.B., Blackstock, R., Van Eys, J., Metzgar, R.S. and Cooper, M.D. (1981). An analysis of clinical and laboratory features of acute lymphocytic leukemias with emphasis on 35 children with pre-B leukemia. *Blood* **58**: 135-140.
17. Teodorescu, M. and Mayer, E.P. (1978). Surface immunoglobulin in immunoproliferative diseases. *Ann. Clin. Lab. Sci.* **8**: 353-365.
18. Vessière-Louveaux, F.M.Y.R., Hijmans, W. and Schuit, H.R.E. (1981). Multiple heavy chain isotypes on the membrane of the small B lymphocytes in human blood. *Clin. exp. Immunol.* **43**: 149-156.
19. Hijmans, W., Schuit, H.R.E. and Klein, F. (1969). An immunofluorescence procedure for the detection of intracellular immunoglobulins. *Clin. exp. Immunol.* **4**: 457-472.
20. Nadler, L.M., Anderson, K.C., Marti, G., Bates, M., Park, E., Daley, J.F. and Schlossman, S.F. (1983). B4, a human B lymphocyte-associated antigen expressed on normal, mitogen-activated, and malignant B lymphocytes. *J. Immunol.* **131**: 244-250.
21. Ritz, J., Pesando, J.M., Notis-McConarty, J., Lazarus, H. and Schlossman, S.F. (1980). A monoclonal antibody to human acute lymphoblastic leukaemia antigen. *Nature* **283**: 583-585.
22. Knapp, W., Majdic, O., Bettelheim, P. and Liszka, K. (1982). VIL-A1, a monoclonal antibody reactive with common acute lymphatic leukemia cells. *Leuk. Res.* **6**: 137-147.
23. LeBien, T., Kersey, J., Nakazawa, S., Minato, K. and Minowada, J. (1982). Analysis of human leukemia/lymphoma cell lines with monoclonal antibodies BA-1, BA-2 and BA-3. *Leuk. Res.* **6**: 299-305.
24. McKenzie, I.F.C. and Zola, H. (1983). Monoclonal antibodies to B cells. *Immunol. Today* **4**: 10-15.
25. Kersey, J.H., LeBien, T.W., Abramson, C.S., Newman, R., Sutherland, R. and Greaves, M. (1981). p24: A human leukemia-associated and lymphohemopoietic progenitor cell surface structure identified with monoclonal antibody. *J. Exp. Med.* **153**: 726-731.
26. Ash, R.C., Jansen, J., Kersey, J.H., LeBien, T.W. and Zanjani, E.D. (1982). Normal human pluripotential and committed hematopoietic progenitors do not express the p24 antigen detected by monoclonal antibody BA-2: Implications for immunotherapy of lymphocytic leukemia. *Blood* **60**: 1310-1316.
27. Stashenko, P., Nadler, L.M., Hardy, R. and Schlossman, S.F. (1980). Characterization of a human B lymphocyte-specific antigen. *J. Immunol.* **125**: 1678-1685.
28. Stashenko, P., Nadler, L.M., Hardy, R. and Schlossman, S.F. (1981). Expression of cell surface markers after human B lymphocyte activation. *Proc. Natl. Acad. Sci. USA* **78**: 3848-3852.
29. Nadler, L.M., Stashenko, P., Hardy, R., Van Agthoven, A., Terhorst, C. and Schlossman, S.F. (1981). Characterization of a human B cell-specific antigen (B2) distinct from B1. *J. Immunol.* **126**: 1941-1947.
30. Forster, H.K., Gudat, F.G., Girard, M.F., Albrecht, R., Schmidt, J., Ludwig, C. and Obrecht, J.P. (1982). Monoclonal antibody against a membrane antigen characterizing leukemic human B-lymphocytes. *Cancer Res.* **42**: 1927-1934.
31. Brooks, D.A., Beckman, I.G.R., Bradley, J., McNamara, P.J., Thomas, M.E. and Zola, H. (1981). Human lymphocyte markers defined by antibodies derived from somatic cell hybrids. IV. A monoclonal antibody reacting specifically with a subpopulation of human B lymphocytes. *J. Immunol.* **126**: 1373-1377.
32. Catovsky, D., Cherchi, M., Brooks, D., Bradley, J. and Zola, H. (1981). Heterogeneity of B-cell leukemias demonstrated by the monoclonal antibody FMC7. *Blood* **58**: 406-408.
33. Anderson, K.C., Park, E.K., Bates, M.P., Leonard, R.C.F., Hardy, R., Schlossman, S.F. and Nadler, L.M. (1983). Antigens on human plasma cells identified by monoclonal antibodies. *J. Immunol.* **130**: 1132-1138.

34. Janossy, G. and Prentice, H.G. (1982). T cell subpopulations, monoclonal antibodies and their therapeutic applications. *Clin. Haematol.* **11**: 631-660.
35. Hansen, J.A., Martin, P.J., Beatty, P.G., Clark, E.A. and Ledbetter, J.A. (1984). Human T lymphocyte cell surface molecules defined by the workshop monoclonal antibodies ('T cell protocol'). In *'Leucocyte typing'*, A. Bernard, L. Boumsell, J. Dausset, C. Milstein, and S.F. Schlossman (eds.). Springer-Verlag, Berlin. p. 195-212.
36. Haynes, B.F., Mann, D.L., Hemler, M.E., Schroer, J.A., Shelhamer, J.H., Eisenbarth, G.S., Strominger, J.L., Thomas, C.A., Mostowski, H.S. and Fauci, A.S. (1980). Characterization of a monoclonal antibody that defines an immunoregulatory T cell subset for immunoglobulin synthesis in humans. *Proc. Natl. Acad. Sci. USA* **77**: 2914-2918.
37. Vodinelich, L., Tax, W., Bai, Y., Pegram, S., Capel, P. and Greaves, M.F. (1983). A monoclonal antibody (WT1) for detecting leukemias of T-cell precursors (T-ALL). *Blood* **62**: 1108-1113.
38. Tax, W.J.M., Tidman, N., Janossy, G., Trejdosiewicz, L., Willems, R., Leeuwenberg, J., De Witte, T.J.M., Capel, P.J.A. and Koene, R.A.P. (1984). Monoclonal antibody (WT1) directed against a T cell surface glycoprotein: Characteristics and immunosuppressive activity. *Clin. exp. Immunol.* **55**: 427-436.
39. Sutherland, D.R., Rudd, C.E. and Greaves, M.F. (1984). Isolation and characterization of a human T lymphocyte-associated glycoprotein (gp40). *J. Immunol.* **133**: 327-333.
40. Howard, F.D., Ledbetter, J.A., Wong, J., Bieber, C.P., Stinson, E.B. and Herzenberg, L.A. (1981). A human T lymphocyte differentiation marker defined by monoclonal antibodies that block E-rosette formation. *J. Immunol.* **126**: 2117-2122.
41. Verbi, W., Greaves, M.F., Schneider, C., Koubek, K., Janossy, G., Stein, H., Kung, P. and Goldstein, G. (1982). Monoclonal antibodies OKT11 and OKT11A have pan-T reactivity and block sheep erythrocyte 'receptors'. *Eur. J. Immunol.* **12**: 81-86.
42. Van Dongen, J.J.M., Hooijkaas, H., Comans-Bitter, M., Hählen, K., De Klein, A., Van Zanen, G.E., Van 't Veer, M.B., Abels, J. and Benner, R. (1985). Human bone marrow cells positive for terminal deoxynucleotidyl transferase (TdT), HLA-DR, and a T cell marker may represent prothymocytes. *J. Immunol.* **135**: 3144-3150.
43. Moore, A.L. and Zusman, J. (1978). Conditions enhancing the percentage and size of E rosettes formed by T lymphocytes. *J. Immunol. Methods* **23**: 275-284.
44. Engleman, E.G., Warnke, R., Fox, R.I., Dilley, J., Benike, C.J. and Levy, R. (1981). Studies of a human T lymphocyte antigen recognized by a monoclonal antibody. *Proc. Natl. Acad. Sci. USA* **78**: 1791-1795.
45. Martin, P.J., Hansen, J.A., Siadak, A.W. and Nowinski, R.C. (1981). Monoclonal antibodies recognizing normal human T lymphocytes and malignant human B lymphocytes: A comparative study. *J. Immunol.* **127**: 1920-1923.
46. Engleman, E.G., Benike, C.J., Glickman, E. and Evans, R.L. (1981). Antibodies to membrane structures that distinguish suppressor/cytotoxic and helper T lymphocyte subpopulations block the mixed leukocyte reaction in man. *J. Exp. Med.* **153**: 193-198.
47. Ledbetter, J.A., Evans, R.L., Lipinski, M., Cunningham-Rundles, C., Good, R.A. and Herzenberg, L.A. (1981). Evolutionary conservation of surface molecules that distinguish T lymphocyte helper/inducer and cytotoxic/suppressor subpopulations in mouse and man. *J. Exp. Med.* **153**: 310-323.
48. Borst, J., Prendiville, M.A. and Terhorst, C. (1982). Complexity of the human T lymphocyte-specific cell surface antigen T3. *J. Immunol.* **128**: 1560-1565.
49. Tax, W.J.M., Willems, H.W., Reekers, P.P.M., Capel, P.J.A. and Koene, R.A.P. (1983). Polymorphism in mitogenic effect of IgGl monoclonal antibodies against T3 antigen on human T cells. *Nature* **304**: 445-447.
50. Lerch, P.G., Van de Rijn, M., Schrier, P. and Terhorst, C. (1983). Biochemical comparison of the T6 antigen and HLA-A,B antigens. *Hum. Immunol.* **6**: 13-30.
51. Meuer, S.C., Fitzgerald, K.A., Hussey, R.E., Hodgdon, J.C., Schlossman, S.F. and Reinherz, E.L. (1983). Clonotypic structures involved in antigen-specific human T cell function. *J. Exp. Med.* **157**: 705-719.
52. Borst, J., Coligan, J.E., Oettgen, H., Pessano, S., Malin, R. and Terhorst, C. (1984). The δ- and ε-chains of the human T3/T-cell receptor complex are distinct polypeptides. *Nature* **312**: 455-458.
53. Owen, M.J. (1984). T-cell receptor companions. *Nature* **312**: 406.
54. Spits, H., Borst, J., Tax, W., Capel, P.J.A., Terhorst, C. and De Vries, J.E. (1985). Characteristics of a monoclonal antibody (WT-31) that recognizes a common epitope on the human T cell receptor for antigen. *J. Immunol.* **135**: 1922-1928.
55. Hood, L., Kronenberg, M. and Hunkapiller, T. (1985). T cell antigen receptors and the immunoglobulin supergene family. *Cell* **40**: 225-229.

56. Acuto, O. and Reinherz, E.L. (1985). The human T-cell receptor: Structure and function. *New Engl. J. Med.* **312**: 1100-1111.
57. Marrack, P. and Kappler, J. (1986). The T cell and its receptor. *Sci. Am.* **254(2)**: 36-45.
58. Weiss, A., Imboden, J., Shoback, D. and Stobo, J. (1984). Role of T3 surface molecules in human T-cell activation: T3-dependent activation results in an increase in cytoplasmic free calcium. *Proc. Natl. Acad. Sci. USA* **81**: 4169-4173.
59. Griffin, J.D., Ritz, J., Nadler, L.M. and Schlossman, S.F. (1981). Expression of myeloid differentiation antigens on normal and malignant myeloid cells. *J. Clin. Invest.* **68**: 932-941.
60. Griffin, J.D., Mayer, R.J., Weinstein, H.J., Rosenthal, D.S., Coral, F.S., Beveridge, R.P. and Schlossman, S.F. (1983). Surface marker analysis of acute myeloblastic leukemia: Identification of differentiation-associated phenotypes. *Blood* **62**: 557-563.
61. Griffin, J.D., Larcom, P. and Schlossman, S.F. (1983). Use of surface markers to identify a subset of acute myelomonocytic leukemia cells with progenitor cell properties. *Blood* **62**: 1300-1303.
62. Sabbath, K.D., Ball, E.D., Larcom, P., Davis, R.B. and Griffin, J.D. (1985). Heterogeneity of clonogenic cells in acute myeloblastic leukemia. *J. Clin. Invest.* **75**: 746-753.
63. Dimitriu-Bona, A., Burmester, G.R., Waters, S.J. and Winchester, R.J. (1983). Human mononuclear phagocyte differentiation antigens. I. Patterns of antigenic expression on the surface of human monocytes and macrophages defined by monoclonal antibodies. *J. Immunol.* **130**: 145-152.
64. Hance, A.J., Douches, S., Winchester, R.J., Ferrans, V.J. and Crystal, R.G. (1985). Characterization of mononuclear phagocyte subpopulations in the human lung by using monoclonal antibo-
dies: Changes in alveolar macrophage phenotype associated with pulmonary sarcoidosis. *J. Immunol.* **134**: 284-292.
65. Todd III, R.F., Nadler, L.M. and Schlossman, S.F. (1981). Antigens on human monocytes identified by monoclonal antibodies. *J. Immunol.* **126**: 1435-1442.
66. Brooks, D.A., Zola, H., McNamara, P.J., Bradley, J., Bradstock, K.F., Hancock, W.W. and Atkins, R.C. (1983). Membrane antigens of human cells of the monocyte/macrophage lineage studied with monoclonal antibodies. *Pathol.* **15**: 45-52.
67. Hancock, W.W., Zola, H. and Atkins, R.C. (1983). Antigenic heterogeneity of human mononuclear phagocytes: Immunohistologic analysis using monoclonal antibodies. *Blood* **62**: 1271-1279.
68. Majdic, O., Liszka, K., Lutz, D. and Knapp, W. (1981). Myeloid differentiation antigen defined by a monoclonal antibody. *Blood* **58**: 1127-1133.
69. Geurts van Kessel, A.H.M., Tetteroo, P.A.T., Von dem Borne, A.E.G. Kr., Hagemeijer, A. and Bootsma, D. (1983). Expression of human myeloid-associated surface antigens in human-mouse myeloid cell hybrids. *Proc. Natl. Acad. Sci. USA* **80**: 3748-3752.
70. Andersson, L.C., Gahmberg, C.G., Teerenhovi, L. and Vuopio, P. (1979). Glycophorin A as a cell surface marker of early erythroid differentiation in acute leukemia. *Int. J. Cancer* **23**: 717-720.
71. Liszka, K., Majdic, O., Bettelheim, P. and Knapp, W. (1983). Glycophorin A expression in malignant hematopoiesis. *Am. J. Hematol.* **15**: 219-226.
72. Knapp, W., Majdic, O., Bettelheim, P., Liszka, K. and Stockinger, H. (1984). Antigenic heterogeneity in acute leukemia. *Contr. Oncol.* **19**: 75-87.
73. Rabellino, E.M., Levene, R.B., Leung, L.L.K. and Nachman, R.L. (1981). Human megakaryocytes. II. Expression of platelet proteins in early marrow megakaryocytes. *J. Exp. Med.* **154**: 88-100.
74. Tetteroo, P.A.T., Lansdorp, P.M., Leeksma, O.C. and Von dem Borne, A.E.G.Kr. (1983). Monoclonal antibodies against human platelet glycoprotein IIIa. *Brit. J. Haematol.* **55**: 509-522.
75. Reinherz, E.L., Kung, P.C., Pesando, J.M., Ritz, J., Goldstein, G. and Schlossman, S.F. (1979). Ia determinants on human T-cell subsets defined by monoclonal antibody. Activation stimuli required for expression. *J. Exp. Med.* **150**: 1472-1482.
76. Lampson, L.A. and Levy, R. (1980). Two populations of Ia-like molecules on a human B cell line. *J. Immunol.* **125**: 293-299.
77. Falkenburg, J.H.F., Jansen, J., Van der Vaart-Duinkerken, N., Veenhof, W.F.J., Blotkamp, J., Goselink, H.M., Parlevliet, J. and Van Rood, J.J. (1984). Polymorphic and monomorphic HLA-DR determinants on human hematopoietic progenitor cells. *Blood* **63**: 1125-1132.
78. Hercend, T., Ritz, J., Schlossman, S.F. and Reinherz, E.L. (1981). Comparative expression of T9, T10, and Ia antigens on activated human T cell subsets. *Hum. Immunol.* **3**: 247-259.

79. Sutherland, R., Delia, D., Schneider, C., Newman, R., Kemshead, J. and Greaves, M. (1981). Ubiquitous cell-surface glycoprotein on tumor cells is proliferation-associated receptor for transferrin. *Proc. Natl. Acad. Sci. USA* **78**: 4515-4519.
80. Van de Rijn, M., Geurts van Kessel, A.H.M., Kroezen, V., Van Agthoven, A.J., Verstijnen, K., Terhorst, C. and Hilgers, J. (1983). Localization of a gene controlling the expression of the human transferrin receptor to the region q12→qter of chromosome 3. *Cytogenet. Cell Genet.* **36**: 525-531.
81. Fithian, E., Kung, P., Goldstein, G., Rubenfeld, M., Fenoglio, C. and Edelson, R. (1981). Reactivity of Langerhans cells with hybridoma antibody. *Proc. Natl. Acad. Sci. USA* **78**: 2541-2544.
82. Royston, I., Majda, J.A., Baird, S.M., Meserve, B.L. and Griffiths, J.C. (1980). Human T cell antigens defined by monoclonal antibodies: The 65,000-dalton antigen of T cells (T65) is also found on chronic lymphocytic leukemia cells bearing surface immunoglobulin. *J. Immunol.* **125**: 725-731.
83. Caligaris-Cappio, F., Gobbi, M., Bofill, M. and Janossy, G. (1982). Infrequent normal B lymphocytes express features of B-chronic lymphocytic leukemia. *J. Exp. Med.* **155**: 623-628.
84. Burns, B.F., Warnke, R.A., Doggett, R.S. and Rouse, R.V. (1983). Expression of a T-cell antigen (Leu-1) by B-cell lymphomas. *Am. J. Pathol.* **113**: 165-171.
85. Neudorf, S.M.L., LeBien, T.W. and Kersey, J.H. (1984). Characterization of thymocytes expressing the common acute lymphoblastic leukemia antigen. *Leuk. Res.* **8**: 173-179.
86. Braun, M.P., Martin, P.J., Ledbetter, J.A. and Hansen, J.A. (1983). Granulocytes and cultured human fibroblasts express common acute lymphoblastic leukemia-associated antigens. *Blood* **61**: 718-725.
87. Abramson, C.S., Kersey, J.H. and LeBien, T.W. (1981). A monoclonal antibody (BA-1) reactive with cells of human B lymphocyte lineage. *J. Immunol.* **126**: 83-88.
88. McGraw, D.J., Kurec, A.S. and Davey, F.R. (1981). Mouse erythrocyte formation. A marker for resting B lymphocytes. *Am. J. Clin. Pathol.* **77**: 177-183.
89. Sanchez-Madrid, F., Nagy, J.A., Robbins, E., Simon, P. and Springer, T.A. (1983). A human leukocyte differentiation antigen family with distinct α-subunits and a common β-subunit: The lymphocyte function-associated antigen (LFA-1), the C3bi complement receptor (OKM1/Mac-1), and the p150,95 molecule. *J. Exp. Med.* **158**: 1785-1803.
90. Arnaout, M.A., Tod III, R.F., Dana, N., Melamed, J., Schlossman, S.F. and Colten, H.R. (1983). Inhibition of phagocytosis of complement C3- or immunoglobulin G-coated particles and of C3bi binding by monoclonal antibodies to a monocyte-granulocyte membrane glycoprotein (Mol). *J. Clin. Invest.* **72**: 171-179.
91. Wright, S.D., Rao, P.E., Van Voorhis, W.C., Craigmyle, L.S., Iida, K., Talle, M.A., Westberg, E.F., Goldstein, G. and Silverstein, S.C. (1983). Identification of the C3bi receptor of human monocytes and macrophages by using monoclonal antibodies. *Proc. Natl. Acad. Sci. USA* **80**: 5699-5703.
92. Ugolini, V., Nunez, G., Smith, R.G., Stastny, P. and Capra, J.D. (1980). Initial characterization of monoclonal antibodies against human monocytes. *Proc. Natl. Acad. Sci. USA* **77**: 6764-6768.
93. Van Dongen, J.J.M., Hooijkaas, H., Comans-Bitter, W.M., Benne, K., Van Os, T.M. and De Josselin de Jong, J. (1985). Triple immunological staining with colloidal gold, fluorescein and rhodamine as labels. *J. Immunol. Methods* **80**: 1-6.
94. Moir, D.J., Ghosh, A.K., Abdulaziz, Z., Knight, P.M. and Mason, D.Y. (1983). Immunoenzymatic staining of haematological samples with monoclonal antibodies. *Brit. J. Haematol.* **55**: 395-410.
95. Böyum, A. (1968). Isolation of mononuclear cells and granulocytes from human blood. Isolation of mononuclear cells by one centrifugation, and of granylocytes by combining centrifugation and sedimentation at 1 g. *Scand. J. Clin. Lab. Invest.* **21**: 77-89.
96. Oi, V.T., Glazer, A.N. and Stryer, L. (1982). Fluorescent phycobiliprotein conjugates for analyses of cells and molecules. *J. Cell Biol.* **93**: 981-986.
97. Janossy, G. and Campana, D. (1985). Immunofluorescence studies in leukaemia diagnosis. In: *Methods in haematology: Monoclonal antibodies.* P. Beverley (ed.). Churchill Livingstone, Edinburgh. p.97-131.
98. Mason, D.Y., Stein, H., Naiem, M. and Abdulaziz, Z. (1981). Immunohistological analysis of human lymphoid tissue by double immunoenzymatic labelling. *J. Cancer Res. Clin. Oncol.* **101**: 13-22.
99. Feller, A.C. and Parwaresch, M.R. (1983). Simultaneous enzyme-immunocytochemical detection of antigens in monocellular specimens with monoclonal antibodies. *J. Immunol. Methods* **63**: 273-279.

100. Van Rooijen, N. and Kors, N. (1985). Double immunocytochemical staining in the study of antibody-producing cells in vivo. Combined detection of antigen specificity (anti-TNP) and (sub)class of intracellular antibodies. *J. Histochem. Cytochem.* **33**: 175-178.
101. Van Rooijen, N., Kors, N., Claassen, E. and Boorsma, D.M. (1985). Binding of different antigen-enzyme and antibody-enzyme conjugates by intracellular antibodies in cytoplasm and Golgi complex of plasma cells. A double immunocytochemical study. *Histochem.* **83**: 61-63.
102. Johnson, G.D. and De C. Nogueira Araujo, G.M. (1981). A simple method of reducing the fading of immunofluorescence during microscopy. *J. Immunol. Methods* **43**: 349-350.
103. Guesdon, J.L., Ternynck, T. and Avrameas, S. (1979). The use of avidin-biotin interaction in immunoenzymatic techniques. *J. Histochem. Cytochem.* **27**: 1131-1139.
104. Simmonds, R.G., Smith, W. and Marsden, H. (1982). 3-Phenylazo-4-hydroxyphenylisothiocyanates: Reagents for efficient haptenation of immunoglobulin and other carrier molecules. *J. Immunol. Methods* **54**: 23-30.
105. De Mey, J. (1983). Colloidal gold probes in immunocytochemistry. In: *Immunocytochemistry: Practical applications in pathology and biology.* J.M. Polak and S. Van Noorden (eds.). Wright PSG, Bristol. p. 82-112.
106. Van der Reijden, H.J., Van Wering, E.R., Van de Rijn, J.M., Melief, C.J.M., Van 't Veer, M.B., Behrendt, H. and Von dem Borne, A.E.G.Kr. (1983). Immunological typing of acute lymphoblastic leukaemia. *Scand. J. Haematol.* **30**: 356-366.
107. Greaves, M.F., Rao, J., Hariri, G., Verbi, W., Catovsky, D., Kung, P. and Goldstein, G. (1981). Phenotypic heterogeneity and cellular origins of T cell malignancies. *Leuk. Res.* **5**: 281-299.
108. Bennett, J.M., Catovsky, D., Daniel, M.T., Flandrin, G., Galton, D.A.G., Gralnick, H.R. and Sultan, C. (1976). Proposals for the classification of the acute leukaemias. *Brit. J. Haematol.* **33**: 451-458.
109. Samoszuk, M.K., Krailo, M., Han Yan, Q., Lukes, R.J. and Parker, J.W. (1985). Limitations of numerical ratios for defining monoclonality of immunoglobulin light chains in B-cell lymphomas. *Diagnostic Immunol.* **3**: 133-138.
110. Smith, B.R., Weinberg, D.S., Robert, N.J., Towle, M., Luther, E., Pinkus, G.S. and Ault, K.A. (1984). Circulating monoclonal B lymphocytes in non-Hodgkin's lymphoma. *New Engl. J. Med.* **311**: 1476-1481.
111. Lennert, K. (ed.) (1978). *Malignant lymphomas other than Hodgkin's disease.* Springer-Verlag, Berlin.
112. Canellos, G.P. and Griffin, J.D. (1985). Chronic granulocytic leukemia: The heterogeneity of stem cell differentiation within a single disease entity. *Semin. Oncol.* **12**: 281-289.
113. Haynes, B.F., Warren, R.W., Buckley, R.H., McClure, J.E., Goldstein, A.L., Henderson, F.W., Hensley, L.L. and Eisenbarth, G.S. (1983). Demonstration of abnormalities in expression of thymic epithelial surface antigens in severe cellular immunodeficiency diseases. *J. Immunol.* **130**: 1182-1188.
114. Bach, M.A. and Bach, J.F. (1981). The use of monoclonal anti-T cell antibodies to study T cell imbalances in human diseases. *Clin. exp. Immunol.* **45**: 449-456.
115. Goodwin, J.S. (1981). OKT3, OKT4, and all that. *J.A.M.A.* **246**: 947-948.
116. Gottlieb, M.S., Schroff, R., Schanker, H.M., Weisman, J.D., Thim Fan, P., Wolf, R.A. and Saxon, A. (1981). Pneumocystis carinii pneumonia and mucosal candidiasis in previously healthy homosexual men. *New Engl. J. Med.* **305**: 1425-1431.
117. Gottlieb, M.S., Groopman, J.E., Weinstein, W.M., Fahey, J.L. and Detels, R. (1983). The acquired immunodeficiency syndrome. *Ann. Int. Med.* **99**: 208-220.
118. Crystal, R.G., Roberts, W.C., Hunninghake, G.W., Gadek, J.E., Fulmer, J.D. and Line, B.R. (1981). Pulmonary sarcoidosis: A disease characterized and perpetuated by activated lung T-lymphocytes. *Ann. Int. Med.* **94**: 73-94.
119. Crystal, R.G., Bitterman, P.B., Rennard, S.I., Hance, A.J. and Keogh, B.A. (1984). Interstitial lung diseases of unknown cause. Disorders characterized by chronic inflammation of the lower respiratory tract. *New Engl. J. Med.* **310**: 235-244.
120. Cosimi, A.B., Colvin, R.B., Burton, R.C., Rubin, R.H., Goldstein, G., Kung, P.C., Hansen, W.P., Delmonico, F.L. and Russell, P.S. (1981). Use of monoclonal antibodies to T-cell subsets for immunologic monitoring and treatment in recipients of renal allografts. *New Engl. J. Med.* **305**: 308-314.
121. Shen, S.Y., Weir, M.R., Kosenko, A., Revie, D.R., Ordonez, J.V., Dagher, F.J., Chretien, P. and Sadler, J.H. (1985). Reevaluation of T cell subset monitoring in cyclosporine-treated renal allograft recipients. *Transpl.* **40**: 620-623.

122. Greaves, M.F., Janossy, G., Peto, J. and Kay, H. (1981). Immunologically defined subclasses of acute lymphoblastic leukaemia in children: Their relationship to presentation features and prognosis. *Brit. J. Haematol.* **48**: 179-197.
123. Chaganti, R.S.K. (1983). Significance of chromosome change to hematopoietic neoplasms. *Blood* **62**: 515-524.
124. Williams, D.L., Look, A.T., Melvin, S.L., Roberson, P.K., Dahl, G., Flake, T. and Stass, S. (1984). New chromosomal translocations correlate with specific immunophenotypes of childhood acute lymphoblastic leukemia. *Cell* **36**: 101-109.
125. Van Dongen, J.J.M., Hooijkaas, H., Michiels, J.J., Grosveld, G., De Klein, A., Van der Kwast, Th.H., Prins, M.E.F., Abels, J. and Hagemeijer, A. (1984). Richter's syndrome with different immunoglobulin light chains and different heavy chain gene rearrangements. *Blood* **64**: 571-575.
126. Van Dongen, J.J.M., Hooijkaas, H., Hagemeijer, A., Hählen, K., Van Zanen, G.E. and Lansdorp, P.M. (1984). Characterization and monitoring of the malignant cells in the blastic and chronic phase of chronic myeloid leukemia. In: *Protides of the biological fluids.* Vol 31. H. Peeters (ed.). Pergamon Press, Oxford. p. 711-714.
127. Van Dongen, J.J.M., Hooijkaas, H., Adriaansen, H.J., Hählen, K. and Van Zanen, G.E. (1986). Detection of minimal residual acute lymphoblastic leukemia by immunological marker analysis: Possibilities and limitations. In: *Minimal residual disease in acute leukemia 1986.* A. Hagenbeek and B. Löwenberg (eds.). Martinus Nijhoff Publishers, Boston. p. 113-133.
128. Hooijkaas, H., Van Dongen, J.J.M., Hählen, K. and Van Zanen, G.E. (1984). Immunological characterisation of cells in cerebrospinal fluid from patients with lymphoid malignancies. *Lancet* i: 518-519.
129. Bradstock, K.F., Janossy, G., Hoffbrand, A.V., Ganeshaguru, K., Llewellin, P., Prentice, H.G. and Bollum, F.J. (1981). Immunofluorescent and biochemical studies of terminal deoxynucleotidyl transferase in treated acute leukaemia. *Brit. J. Haematol.* **47**: 121-131.
130. Bradstock, K.F., Janossy, G., Tidman, N., Papageorgiou, E.S., Prentice, H.G., Willoughby, M. and Hoffbrand, A.V. (1981). Immunological monitoring of residual disease in treated thymic acute lymphoblastic leukaemia. *Leuk. Res.* **5**: 301-309.
131. Van Dongen, J.J.M., Hooijkaas, H., Hählen, K., Benne, K., Bitter, W.M., Van der Linde-Preesman, A.A., Tettero, I.L.M., Van de Rijn, M., Hilgers, J., Van Zanen, G.E. and Hagemeijer, A. (1984). Detection of minimal residual disease in TdT positive T cell malignancies by double immunofluorescence staining. In: *Minimal residual disease in acute leukemia.* B. Löwenberg and A. Hagenbeek (eds.). Martinus Nijhoff Publishers, Boston. p. 67-81.

7. MONOCLONAL ANTIBODIES IN LYMPHOMA DIAGNOSIS AND CLASSIFICATION

S. POPPEMA, H. HOLLEMA

1. INTRODUCTION

The availability of monoclonal antibodies reactive with antigens present on leukocytes and leukocyte subpopulations has enabled a more reliable diagnosis and a more precise subclassification of malignant lymphomas. The wide application of monoclonal antibodies on frozen tissue sections makes one almost forget that the first monoclonal anti T cell reagents were described in 1979 (1), and the first applications of such antibodies on human lymph nodes by immunoperoxidase techniques were in 1981 (2). Since 1973 there had been a significant progress in the histological classification of malignant lymphomas, that was partly based on careful cytological comparisons between the cells of malignant lymphomas and of normal lymphoid tissues, an partly on the results of immunological marker studies, derived from basic immunology (3, 4). Among these first immunological studies were the demonstration of complement receptors by rosetting techniques on frozen tissue sections of follicular lymphomas in 1974 (5) and the demonstration of cytoplasmic immunoglobulin by immunoperoxidase staining of paraffin tissue sections in 1974 (6). In subsequent years both techniques appeared to have drawbacks, such as the inability to distinguish between complement receptors on the dendritic reticulum cells and those on the lymphoid cells, and the finding that cytoplasmic immunoglobulin, e.g. in Reed-Sternberg cells, may be the result of non specific uptake or diffusion of immunoglobulin into cells (7). A further improvement was the introduction of aceton fixation of frozen tissue sections, which permitted the demonstration of membrane immunoglobulins and T cell antigens, employing rabbit antisera and a three step immunoperoxidase technique (18). This technique could then easily be adapted to a four step immunoperoxidase technique for the demonstration of T cell antigens with monoclonal mouse hybridoma derived antibodies on aceton fixed frozen tissue sections (2).

All subsequent techniques and improvements are based on the use of aceton fixed frozen tissue sections. The most simple technique is a two step immunoperoxidase technique employing mouse monoclonal antibodies and peroxidase conjugated rabbit anti

D.J. Ruiter et al. (eds), Application of Monoclonal Antibodies in Tumor Pathology
© 1987, Martinus Nijhoff Publishers, Dordrecht, The Netherlands, ISBN 0-89838-853-8

mouse immunoglobulin antibodies. Other popular techniques employ biotin-avidin reagents (9) and alkaline phosphatase conjugates or complexes (10). The findings described and illustrated in this chapter were obtained with the two step immunoperoxidase method on frozen tissue sections. This method has now been used in our department of pathology for 5 years and has proven to be reliable and diagnostically significant. In this chapter we will review the litterature on the immunophenotyping of lymphomas and summarize our findings with a series of anti B cell reagents on frozen tissue sections of 124 non Hodgkin lymphomas of B cell origin.

A more recent development is the preparation of monoclonal antileukocyte antibodies reactive with antigens resistent to routine fixation and paraffin embedment procedures. Such reagents are of great value since the use of frozen tissue sections has some disadvantages. Firstly, in cases where a lymphoma is not suspected at the moment of surgery, tissue will usually be fixed in formalin. Secondly, immunohistology on formalin fixed paraffin embedded sections will enable a better cytomorphological analysis of positive or negative staining cell populations than in aceton fixed frozen tissue sections. So far, a limited number of such reagents is available. These reagents do allow the distinction between non Hodgkin lymphomas and tumors of non lymphoid origin and in addition they distinguish between lymphomas of B cell and T cell origin.

In our opinion, paraffin tissue reactive monoclonal antibodies will find a broad application in routine immunohistological diagnosis of malignant lymphomas.

In this chapter we will demonstrate the feasibility of lymphoma diagnosis and subclassification employing these new reagents.

2. DISTINCTION OF MALIGNANT LYMPHOMAS FROM OTHER NEOPLASMS, AND IMMUNOPHENOTYPING OF LYMPHOMAS BY THE USE OF PARAFFIN REACTIVE ANTIBODIES

Usually, malignant lymphomas can be distinguished from other neoplasms on morphological criteria. However, some poorly differentiated carcinomas may show a morphology which can not be distinguished from large cell lymphomas with certainty. The development of monoclonal reagents that can distinguish between leukocytes and epithelial cells has provided the tools to solve these difficult cases. In many cases the diagnosis can even be double checked since one reagent should be positive and the other negative. The basis of this method is the use of antibodies against leukocyte commonantigens in combination with antibodies reactive with cytoskeletal proteins.

TABLE I. Monoclonal reagents in the differential diagnosis of large cell undifferentiated tumors (simplified scheme, see chapters 5 and 17)

	Lymphoma	Carcinoma	Sarcoma
leukocyte common antigens	+	-	-
vimentin	+	-	+
cytokeratin	-	+	-

Over the past few years different groups have described monoclonal anti leukocyte common antigen reagents which will be reactive on routine paraffin sections. These antibodies recognize a group of antigens with molecular weights near 200.000 Dalton (T 200 antigens). We have also produced reagents,not only reactive with lymphocytes,but with all haematopoietic cells.Mixtures of two of these antibodies were found to be useful for the differentiation of haematopoietic neoplasms from non lymphoid tumors (11). More recently,Epstein et al.(12) and our group (13) produced monoclonal reagents reactive with lymphocyte subsets on paraffin embedded tissue sections. In addition,monoclonal antibodies Leu M1 and Tü9 were found to be reactive with myeloid cells and Sternberg-Reed cells in paraffin tissue sections (14,15). The paraffin reactive antibodies are summarized in table II.

Monoclonal antibody MB1 is reactive with all B cells and with about 50% of small,mature,unactivated T cells.Immature T cells are not reactive.MB2 is reactive with all B cells and not with T cells (fig. 1A). The antigen appears to be cytoplasmic.MB3 is reactive with a cytoplasmic antigen in all HLA-Dr positive cells and therefore is present in all B cells,but also in interdigitating cells in lymph nodes and in reticulo-epithelial cells of the thymus.

TABLE II. Paraffin tissue reactive antileukocyte antibodies

			T cells		B cells	
Ig	subclass	M.W.	immature	mature	mantle zone	germ. center
MAL	IgG1	200,110,100	+	+	+	+
MB1	IgG1	200,110,100	-	50%	+	+
MB2	IgG1	28	-	-	+	+
MB3	IgG2b	31	-	-	+	+
MT1	IgG1	190,110,100	+	+	-	-
MT2	IgG1	200,190	-	+	+	-
LN1	IgM	45-85	-	-	-	+
LN2	IgG1	31	-	-	+	+
LN3	IgG2a	28,32	-	-	+	+

It is similar to LN2 and both antibodies recognize an antigen with molecular weight of 31 KD. Its relation to HLA-Dr is unknown at present. Antibody MT1 is reactive with a membrane antigen on all T lymphocytes,myeloid cells,monocytes,macrophages and erythroid precursors, but not with B lymphocytes (fig. 1B). However, B lymphoblastic lymphomas, some B lymphocytic lymphomas, and centrocytic lymphomas also show a weak reactivity with MT1. Centroblastic-centrocytic lymphomas, centroblastic lymphomas and B-immunoblastic lymphomas are MT1 negative. MT2 is reactive with mature T cells, but not with activated T cells and immature T cells.

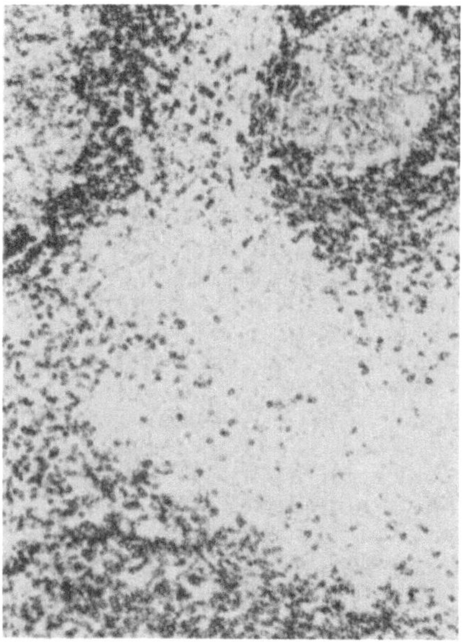

FIG. 1A. Reactive lymph node stained with MB2. Strong staining of small mantle zone B cells, weaker staining of germinal center cells and negative T cell areas. (paraffin section, B5 fixation).

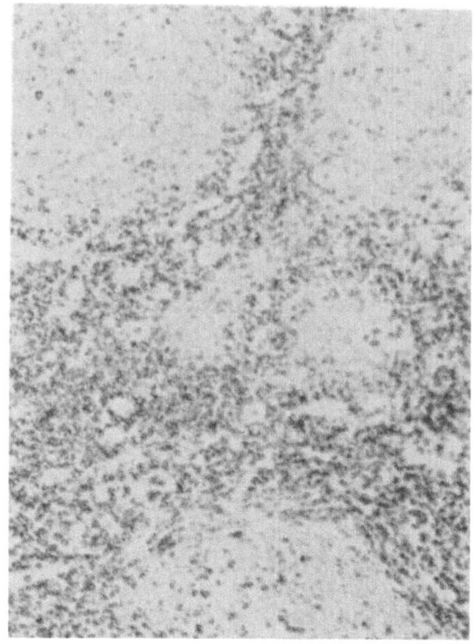

FIG. 1B. Same lymph node as in fig. 1A stained with MT1. Strong staining of small interfollicular T cells. No staining of B cells. (paraffin section, B5 fixation).

In addition, it is reactive with small mantle zone B cells, but not with germinal center cells. So far, only a limited number of lymphomas have been studied, but it appears that centroblastic-centrocytic lymphomas, unexpectedly, are MT2 positive. The LN1 antibody is strongly reactive with germinal center B cells, but not with mantle zone B cells and T cells. It is also reactive with most B cell lymphomas. Antibody LN3 is reactive with HLA-Dr membrane antigens on B cells, interdigitating cells and reticulo-epithelial cells of the thymus. These antibodies promise to be of great value in the diagnosis of reactive and neoplastic disorders of the lymphoid system. A possible flow sheet for the differentiation of B and T cell lymphomas with these antibodies is illustrated in fig. 2.

3. IMMUNOPHENOTYPING OF MALIGNANT LYMPHOMAS EMPLOYING MONOCLONAL ANTIBODIES REACTIVE WITH B CELLS ON FROZEN TISSUE SECTIONS

In addition to antibodies reactive with immunoglobulin heavy chains ($\gamma, \alpha, \mu, \delta, \varepsilon$) and light chains ($\kappa$, λ)a series of monoclonal antibodies reactive with antigens either on all B cells or on B cell subsets has been described. These reagents

FIGURE 2. Lymphoma analysis with paraffin tissue reactive antibodies.

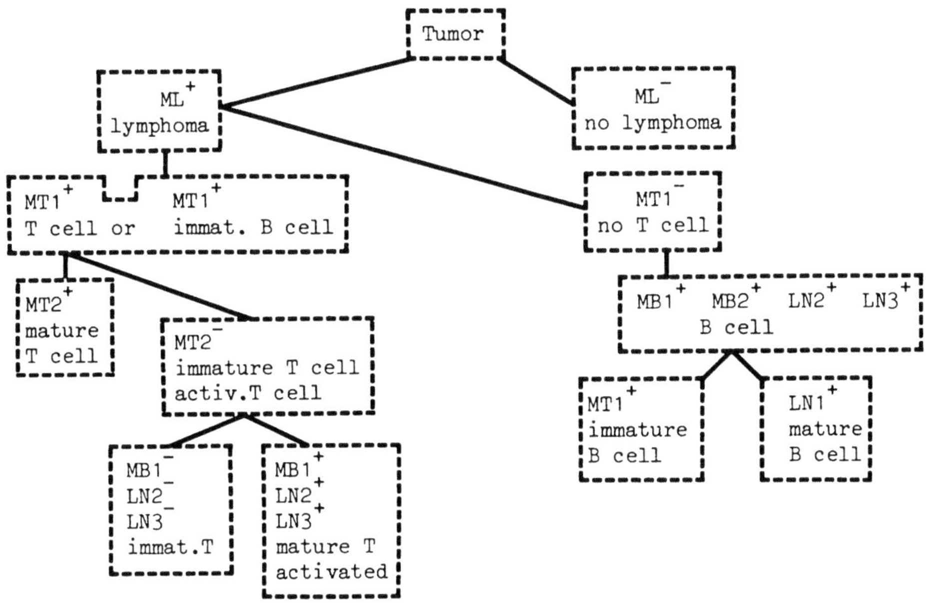

are summarized in table III. The results with these reagents on a series of 124 non Hodgkin lymphomas of B cell origin are shown in table IV. As a practical approach to lymphoma diagnosis we employ a panel with antibody 64-1B9 (CD20), 32-4A2 (CD21), T1 (CD5), CALLA (CD10), 89-1B11 (antiLFA3) and monoclonal anti IgG antibodies (κ, λ, G, A, M, D). The diagnostic implications of staining with these reagents are indicated in figure 3. When employing this panel, T-cell lymphomas can be recognized by absence of staining, except with T1(CD5) and histiocytic tumors can be identified by 89-1B11 staining only. In such cases, appropriate panels of anti T cell or anti monocyte reagents can be applied. Hairy cell leukemia can be recognized by a combined reactivity with CD20 and 1B11.

3.1. C.L.L. and immunocytoma (C.L.L. and I.C.)

Malignant lymphoma, small lymphocytic of the Working Formulation includes chronic lymphocytic leukemia of B cell origin and lymphocytic lymphoma with plasmacytoid differentiation (immunocytoma) in the Kiel Classification.
In both types of lymphoma a diffuse infiltration of atypical lymphocytes with more or less pronounced so called pseudofollicles or proliferation centers can be seen. These pseudofollicles contain prolymphocytes and lymphoblasts. The main difference between B-CLL and immunocytoma is the presence of lymphocytes with plasmacytoid differentiation and/or of plasma-

FIGURE 3. Diagnostic implications of marker analysis on frozen tissue sections of B cell lymphomas.

CD10	M.L. pre pre B
CD20; CD10 cytopl. μ	M.L. pre B
CD20; CD10 membr.M + D, M	M.L. B lymphoblastic
CD20; $CD21^{m}$; CD5 membr.M + D, M	M.L. lymphocytic (immunocytoma, C.L.L.)
CD20; $CD21^{m + DRC}$; CD5 membr. M + D, M	M.L. centrocytic
CD20; $CD21^{DRC}$; CD10 membr. M + D, M, G, A, O	M.L. centroblastic-centrocytic
CD20; $CD21^{m+/-}$; $CD10^{+/-}$ membr. M + D, M, G, A, O	M.L. centroblastic
CD20 membr. M, G, A, O and cytopl.	M.L. immunoblastic
CD20 cytopl. G, A	M.L. plasmacytic

$CD21^{m}$ = membrane staining of lymphoma cells
$CD21^{DRC}$ = staining of dendritic reticulumcell network.

cells in immunocytoma (fig. 4). Both types of lymphoma are usually IgM^{+}, or IgD^{+} and IgM^{+}. They are reactive with pan B cell reagents, most cases have C3d receptors and less than half of the cases have C3b receptors. There is a striking, relatively weak reactivity with Leu1/T1 antibodies, suggesting that these lymphomas are related to or derived from a small subpopulation of B cells present in the mantle zones of reactive follicles.

A small minority of immunocytomas is not reactive with pan B cell reagents.

TABLE III

	B-cell reagents	M.W.	
CD19	B4[C]	p 95	pan B
CD20	B1[C], 64-1B9[*]	p 30	pan B
CD22	Leu 14[B&D], 89-1G8[*]	p 135	pan B
CD21	B2[C], 32-4A2[*]	p 140	C3d receptor
-	C3b rec[D]	p 205	C3b receptor
CD24	BA1[H]	p 45,55,65	B subpopulation
CD5	Leu 1[B&D], OKTI[O.D.],T1[*]	p 67	T plus B subpopulation
CD10	CALLA[B&D], J5[C]	p 100	B subpopulation
	Leu M5[B&D], 89-1B11[*]	p 150,90	macrophages, B and T subpopulation
-	89-2A9[**]	-	B subpopulation (hairy cell leuk.)
-	1H3[**]	-(cytopl.)	B subpopulation (mantle zone)

H = Hybritech
D = Dakopatts
C = Coulter
B&D = Becton & Dickinson
O.D.= Ortho Diagnostics
* = equivalent antibodies produced in our laboratory
** = new reagents produced in our laboratory

TABLE IV. Immunophenotype of B cell lymphomas

	κ/λ	M+D	M	G	A	O	B1	Leu 14	C3d	C3b	89-1B11	Leu 1	CALLA	89-2Ag	Leu M1	K1-1
8 CLL	4:4	2	6	0	0	0	8	6	7	3	0	8	0	0	0	0
10 IC	7:3	7	1	1	0	1	10	10	9	5	3	10	0	0	0	0
4 HCL	2:2	1	1	2	0	0	4	4	0	0	4	0	0	4	0	0
21 CB/CC	10:11	4	5	8	2	2	21	17	3	4	0	0	16	0	1	1
10 CC	4:6	8	1	0	0	1	10	10	9	9	0	10	0	0	0	0
8 CC large	4:4	5	3	0	0	0	8	8	0	0	0	4	0	0	0	0
26 CB	14:8	4	10	5	4	3	26	19	10	5	0	3	9	0	1	3
17 IB	9:8	0	9	2	3	3	17	17	1	1	0	0	4	0	2	2
10 LB	1:7	6	2+1	0	0	1	10	8	0	0	0	0	8	0	0	?
6 PL	2:4	0	0	2	1	3	(2*)	0	0	0	0	0	0	0	0	0
4 Multilob.	1:1	0	0	0	0	0	4	3	0	0	0	1	0	0	0	0

*minority of cells

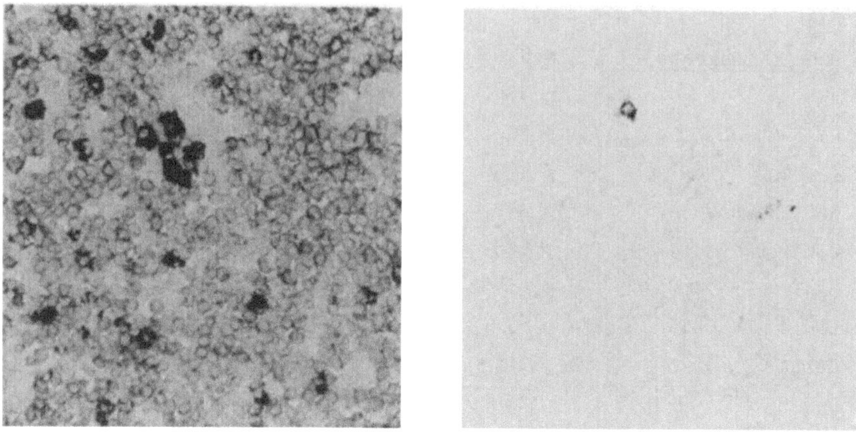

FIG. 4. Immunocytoma; clear membrane staining of majority of lymphocytes and several cells with intense cytoplasmic positivity for kappa light chains on the left and only one positive small lymphocyte stained for lambda light chains on the right. (frozen sections, aceton fixation).

3.2. Hairy cell leukemia (H.C.L.)

Hairy cell leukemia (HCL) is a type of B cell leukemia with characteristic clinical and morphological features. The bone marrow and spleen are heavily infiltrated by lymphoid cells with long, hairy, surface extensions, which can usually be identified in phase contrast microscopy. Morphologically, hairy cell leukemia differs from other types of B cell lymphoma since it infiltrates the red pulp of the spleen instead of the white pulp. Enzymecytochemical staining for tartrate-resistant acid phosphatase is a useful diagnostic adjunct, though it is not entirely specific for hairy cell leukemia.

The long standing dispute on the origin of hairy cells, i.e. B cell or monocyte, has been solved by the demonstration that hairy cells show Ig gene rearrangement (16).

In addition, hairy cells were shown to be reactive with anti B cell monoclonal antibodies. A number of groups has produced monoclonal antibodies with a restricted specificity for hairy cells. Antibodies S-HCL3 (17), and 89- 1B11 (18) are reactive with hairy cells and with macrophages. Therefore, reactivity with pan B cell reagents and Leu M5 (or 89- 1B11) is highly suggestive for HCL (fig. 5 A,B). However, we have found a few cases of immunocytoma with a similar marker pattern. Recently we produced another monoclonal antibody, 89- 2A9 (18), which is reactive with hairy cell leukemia and a smal normal lymphocyte population in the interfollicular area in normal lymph nodes (fig. 5 C). In normal peripheral blood less than 1% of positive cells is present. Other lymphomas, including the Leu M5 positive immunocytomas, were found to be not reactive with 89- 2A9. Other findings distinguishing HCL from other lymphocytic lymphomas are the absence of C3b and C3d receptors and the absence of Leu1 reactivity.

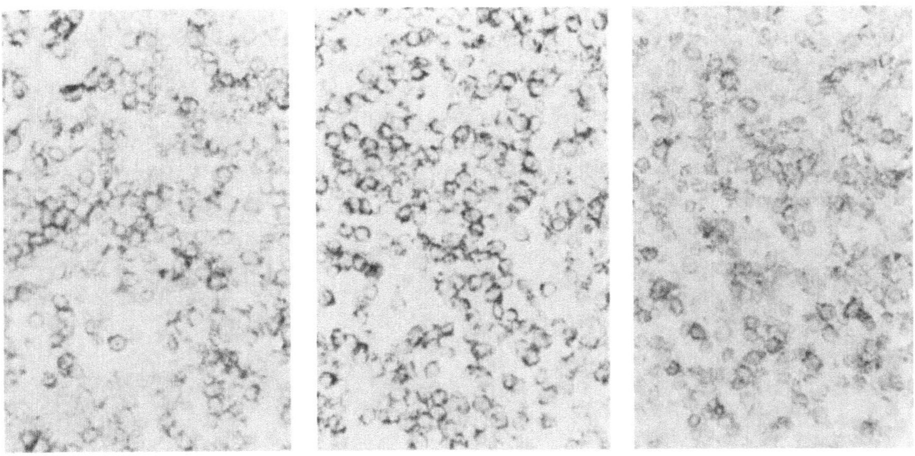

FIG. 5. Hairy cell leukemia; clear staining of the majority of cells in spleen involved by hairy cell leukemia with 1G8 (left), 1B11 (middle), and 2A9 (right) (frozen sections, aceton fixation, see table III for origin of antibodies).

3.3. Centroblastic-centrocytic lymphomas (C.B.-C.C.)

The Working Formulation distinguishes four different types of follicular and/or diffuse follicular center cell lymphomas with cleaved cells (centrocytes) and non cleaved cells (centroblasts) (19). Similar proposals for a subdivision of centroblastic-centrocytic lymphomas were made by our group (20). It should be stressed that these subtypes are not different entities, but rather represent different forms or even stages of the same disease. Morphological studies by Lennert demonstrated the presence of centroblasts and centrocytes in normal germinal centers as well as in the nodules of follicular lymphomas. In addition, dendritic reticulum cells were shown to be present in the reactive as well as in the neoplastic nodules by electron microscopy. By immunohistological studies the most striking feature is the nodularity, even in cases which show only faintly distinguishable nodules in conventional light microscopy. This can be noted particularly after staining with anti complement receptor antibodies (B2, aC3br 32- 4A2). The neoplastic cell population is monoclonal or in very unusual cases biclonal. The cells express IgG in about 50% of the cases and IgA in about 5% of our cases (fig. 6 A, B). The other cases express IgM or IgM and IgD. In several cases the same monoclonal immunoglobulin can be demonstrated on small centrocytes localized in the interfollicular areas where no dendritic cells are found. The neoplastic cells are always reactive with pan B cell reagents, but show variable and frequently weak reactivity with the anti C3d and anti C3b receptor reagents. Leu1 is not reactive with CB/CC lymphomas. However, CALLA is clearly reactive with the large majority of cases of follicular lymphoma, whereas this antibody has also reactivity in normal germinal centers (fig. 6 C). In addition, sometimes CALLA reactivity can be found also in the small interfollicular centrocytes. Another similarity between reactive and neoplastic germinal centers is the presence of an intrafollicular population of $Leu3^+$, $Leu7^+$ T cells, not found in other types of lymphomas.

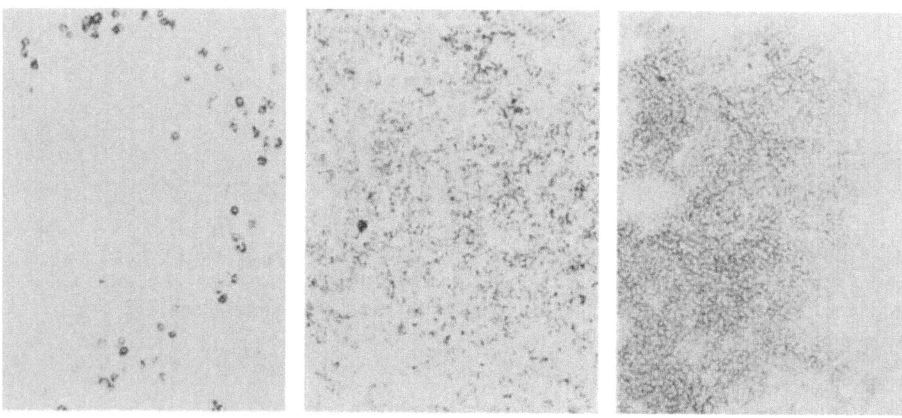

FIG. 6. Centroblastic-centrocytic lymphoma; nodule stained for IgM, showing small reactive mantle zone B cells (left), for IgG, showing relatively weak membrane staining of the lymphoma cells (middle), and for CALLA, showing clear staining of all lymphoma cells (right). (frozen sections, aceton fixation).

3.4. Centrocytic lymphomas (C.C.)

Centrocytic lymphomas exclusively contain centrocytes (cleaved cells) and no centroblasts (non cleaved cells). Different sizes of the centrocytes have lead to a subtyping of small centrocytic versus large (anaplastic) centrocytic lymphomas. Another category of lymphomas, the so called intermediate lymphocytic lymphomas, including so called mantle zone lymphomas are strikingly similar to the small centrocytic lymphomas. Small centrocytic lymphomas typically are IgM^+, IgD^+, are reactive with pan B cell reagents, are clearly reactive with anti C3d receptor and anti C3b receptor reagents

and also with Leu1/T1. In addition, centrocytic lymphomas usually have networks, frequently nodular, of dendritic reticulum cells, that are staining with anti C3d or C3b receptor antibodies and anti DRC antibodies.
Large centrocytic lymphomas in this series were not reactive with anti C3d and anti C3b receptor antibodies and had Leu1 reactivity in 50% of the cases. None of the cases of centrocytic lymphoma was reactive with anti CALLA antibody. The findings indicate that the centrocytes of CB/CC lymphomas and of CC lymphomas have clearly different immunophenotypes, despite their morphological resemblance, see table V.
This strongly supports the existence of centrocytic lymphomas as an entity as has been done in the Kiel classification. However, we also conclude that centrocytic lymphoma is derived from transformed small lymphocytes early in germinal center reaction and not from the centrocytes as found in the light zones of late germinal center reaction, that give rise to centroblastic-centrocytic lymphomas. Therefore we propose a B cell differentiation scheme with two types of centrocytes, one early in germinal center reaction, as proposed by Lukes (3), and one late in germinal center reaction as proposed by Lennert (4). The differences in malignancy grade between CB-CC and CC lymphomas, being of low and intermediate grade, respectively, certainly justifies a strict separation as can be achieved with immunohistology. The differences in biological behaviour are explained by the origin from transformed,proliferating cells of CC lymphoma, and the origin from cells differentiating towards memory B cells of CB-CC lymphoma. The malignancy grade of CB-CC lymphoma is dependent on the percentage of centroblasts, being the predominantly proliferating cells in this type of lymphoma.

TABLE V. Different types of centrocytes.

	in CB-CC	in CC
IgM/IgD	±	+
IgG/IgA	+	-
Leu1	-	+
CALLA	+	-

3.5. Centroblastic and B-immunoblastic lymphomas (C.B. and B-I.B.)

Centroblastic lymphomas contain a majority of centroblasts. Only few cases are pure centroblastic lymphomas. Most cases also contain centrocytes, immunoblasts and plasmablasts and are termed polymorphic centroblastic lymphomas. The transition between centroblastic and immunoblastic lymphomas is a gradual one, since immunoblastic lymphomas can be defined as containing a majority of immunoblasts. Many cases of immunoblastic lymphoma have plasmablastic differentiation. In our series more

than 50% of the cases had IgM or IgM and IgD, about 30% had IgG or IgA and 15% had no detectable surface or cytoplasmic immunoglobulins. However, all cases were reactive with pan B cell reagents, although about 25% of the centroblastic cases was not reactive with Leu14. About 40% of the centroblastic lymphomas showed reactivity with anti C3d receptor reagents, whereas only 6% of the immunoblastic lymphomas stained with anti C3d receptor antibodies.
A recently recognized type of large cell germinal center cell lymphoma is the so called multilobated lymphoma of B cell origin. In our series 4 cases were found, that had absence of heavy chain staining in common. All 4 cases were reactive with pan B cell reagents and none had complement receptors. One case was reactive with Leu1.

3.6. B-lymphoblastic lymphomas (B-L.B.)

Lymphoblastic lymphomas contain medium sized blast cells, with a small rim of basophilic cytoplasm. The B-lymphoblastic lymphomas can be subdivided in Burkitt (type), non Burkitt type, and unclassified cases. In our series most cases are Burkitt type lymphomas. Six cases had membrane IgM and IgD and two cases had membrane IgM. Two cases had a pre B cell phenotype, having cytoplasmic   chains only, and two cases had pre-pre B phenotype, having no detectable Ig. CALLA reactivity was found in all Burkitt typecases, and in the pre B cell and pre-pre B cell cases. Surprisingly, antibody B2, reactive with C3d receptor antigen, gave a characteristic cytoplasmic dot like staining in all Burkitt type B-lymphoblastic lymphomas.

4. CONCLUSIONS

During the past five years significant progress has been made in the immunophenotyping of non Hodgkin lymphomas. The application of monoclonal antibodies on frozen tissue sections allows for a precise determination of the stage of differentiation of B-cells, and consequently, to a reliable immunohistological diagnosis. This also facilitates the detection of dissemination, residual disease and relapse of these lymphomas. In the past two years new reagents have been developed that allow for the identification of lymphocyte subsets in paraffin tissue sections. In the years to come, we should try to produce additional paraffin tissue reactive reagents, reagents discriminating between large cell lymphomas with relatively favourable and unfavourable prognosis and reagents and methods useful for in vivo imaging and immunotherapy of B cell lymphomas.

REFERENCES

1. Reinherz EL, Kung PC, Goldstein G, Schlossman SF: Separation of functional subsets of human T cells by a monoclonal antibody. Proc. Natl. Acad. Sci. USA 76:4061, 1979.
2. Poppema S, Bhan AK, Reinherz EL, McCluskey RT, Schlossman SF: Distribution of T cell subsets in human lymph nodes. J. Exp. Med. 153:3041, 1981.
3. Lukes RJ, Collins RD: Immunologic characterization of human malignant lymphomas. Cancer 34:1488-1503, 1974.
4. Gérard-Marchant R, Hamlin I, Lennert K, Rilke F, Stansfeld AG, van Unnik JAM: Classification of non-Hodgkin's lymphomas. Lancet 1974; ii, 406.
5. Jaffe ES, Shevach EM, Frank MM: Nodular lymphoma, evidence of origin from follicular B lymphocytes. New Engl. J. Med. 290:813-819, 1974.
6. Taylor CR: The nature of Reed-Sternberg cells and other malignant "reticulum" cells. Lancet ii:802-807, 1974.
7. Poppema S, Elema JD, Halie MR: The significance of intra-cytoplasmic proteins in Reed-Sternberg cells. Cancer 42: 1793-1803, 1978.
8. Poppema S, Elema JD, Halie MR: The localization of Hodgkin's disease in lymph nodes. A study with immunohistological, enzyme histochemical and rosetting techniques on frozen sections. Int. J. Cancer 24:532-540, 1979.
9. Hsu SM, Raine L, Fanger H: Use of avidin-biotin-peroxidase complex (ABC) in immunoperoxidase procedures. J.Histochem. Cytochem. 29:577-580, 1981.
10. Cordell JL, Falini B, Erber WN, Ghosh AK, Abdulaziz Z, Macdonald S, Pulford KAF, Stein H, Mason DY: Immunoenzymatic labeling of monoclonal antibodies using immune complexes of alkaline phosphatase and monoclonal anti alkaline phosphatase. J. Histochem. Cytochem. 32:219-229, 1984.
11. Warnke RA, Gatter KC, Phil D, Falini B, Hildreth P, Woolston RE, Pulford K, Cordell JL, Cohen B, De Wolf-Peeters C, Mason DY: Diagnosis of human lymphoma with monoclonal antileukocyte antibodies. N. Engl. J. Med. 309:1275, 1983.
12. Epstein AL, Marder RJ, Winter JN, Fox RI: Two new monoclonal antibodies (LN-1, LN-2) reactive in B5 formalin-fixed paraffin embedded tissues with follicular center and mantle zone human B lymphocytes and derived tumors. J. Immunol. 133:1028-1036, 1984.
13. Poppema S, Hollema H, Visser L, Vos H: Monoclonal antibodies reactive with lymphocyte subsets in paraffin embedded tissue sections. 1986, Submitted.
14. Hsu SM, Jaffe ES: Leu M1 and peanut agglutinin stain the neoplastic cells of Hodgkin's disease. Am. J. Clin. Pathol. 82:29-32, 1984.
15. Stein H, Uchanska-Ziegler B, Gerdes J, Ziegler A, Wernet P: Hodgkin- and Sternberg-Reed cells contain antigens specific

to late cells of granulopoiesis. Int. J. Cancer 29: 283-290, 1982.
16. Korsmeyer SJ, Greene WC, Cossman J, Hsu SM, Jensen JP, Neckers LM, Marshall SL, Bakshi A, Depper JM, Leonard WJ, Jaffe ES, Waldmann TA: Rearrangement and expression of immunoglobulin genes and expression of Tac antigen in hairy cell leukemia. Proc. Natl. Acad. USA 80:4522-4530, 1983.
17. Schwarting R, Stein H, Wang CY: Monoclonal antibodies S-HCL1 and S-HCL3 allow the diagnosis of hairy cell leukemia. Blood 65:974-983, 1985.
18. Poppema S, Visser L: Monoclonal antibody reactive with hairy cell leukemia and a minor normal lymphocyte sub-population. Lab. Invest. 54:50A, 1986.
19. The non-Hodgkin's lymphoma pathologic classification project. National Cancer Institute sponsored study of classifications of non-Hodgkin's lymphomas. Cancer 49: 2112-2135, 1982.
20. Molenaar WM, van den Berg HM, Halie MR, Poppema S: The heterogeneity of follicular center cell lymphomas. I Cytohistologic, immunlogic, and enzymehistochemical aspects. Cancer 52:2269-2276, 1983.

8. MONOCLONAL ANTIBODIES RECOGNIZING MELANOMA-ASSOCIATED ANTIGENS

D.J. RUITER, E-B. BROECKER, C. VENNEGOOR AND S. FERRONE.

1. INTRODUCTION

Cutaneous melanoma accounts for roughly 1% of cancers in the United States (1). It has been reported repeatedly that its incidence in western countries is rising rapidly (1). Accordingly, its mortality is rising, but less rapidly than its incidence because an increasing proportion of cases is diagnosed in an early phase of tumor growth. The most common types of cutaneous melanoma are superficial spreading melanoma (SSM), nodular melanoma (NM) and lentigo malignant melanoma (LMM). In SSM and LMM early melanomas show a horizontal (radial) growth pattern (1). More advanced tumors show superimposed a vertical growth pattern as a result of further neoplastic progression (1).

In addition to the large congenital nevocellular nevus in the last decade another precursor lesion for cutaneous melanoma has been described that was labeled dysplastic nevus (2). Dysplastic nevi occur either as familial or sporadic types. The life-time risk for cutaneous melanoma may approach 100% for individuals with the familial dysplastic nevus syndrome (1).Therefore, cutaneous human melanoma and precursor lesions are particularly suited for studies on neoplastic progression.

The prognosis of cases with cutaneous melanoma correlates inversely to the microscopically assessed tumor thickness (1). Locoregional metastases most often are localized in lymph nodes and skin;distant metastases in skin, lung, liver, central nervous system or gastro-intestinal tract. Although most primary cutaneous melanomas produce melanin, metastatic melanomas often are oligo- or amelanotic, which may give rise to diagnostic problems.

Monoclonal antibodies (MoAbs) have been developed against differentiation antigens on human melanoma cells, and against determinants on human melanoma cells that may be a marker for neoplastic progression (3). Analysis with MoAbs that recognize HLA antigens has revealed expression of HLA class II antigens on certain melanoma cells and absence of HLA class I antigens on others (4,5). In this chapter a review will be given on melanoma-associated antigens as well as the application of MoAbs in the phenotyping of melanocytic lesions in diagnostic histopathology and tumor biology. Furthermore, the use of MoAbs for the quantitative detection of melanoma-associated antigens in serum, the localization of melanomas in vivo, approaches to therapy of melanoma patients, and the possible mechanism of therapy with MoAbs as examined in experimental tumor models are surveyed. In addition some future developments in the field will be discussed.

2. MELANOMA-ASSOCIATED ANTIGENS.

Melanoma-associated antigens recognized by MoAbs can be divided into three groups: 1) differentiation markers, 2) markers associated with certain stages of neoplastic progression, and 3) markers associated with cell function (6). This classification is somewhat artificial, and overlap between categories of markers is therefore unavoidable. These markers will be reviewed in the following paragraphs.

2.1 Differentiation markers.

To the best of our knowledge no differentiation marker absolutely specific for melanocytic lesions has been described. The differentiation markers described have a broad distribution in melanocytic lesions, but may also be present in a variable number of other normal cells and other tumors. A list of representative markers and the corresponding antibodies is given in Table 1.

TABLE 1. Melanoma-associated antigens: differentiation markers.

			Distribution*		
Antigen	Monoclonal antibody	Tissue preparation	Melanoma	Other malignant tumors	Reference
gp90-34	NKI/C3	p	132/140	43/297	Vennegoor et al. (7)
					Van Duinen et al. (8)
S-100	anti-S-100+	p, f	44/47	31/145	Nakijima et al. (9)
p60-30 p92, p200	ME series	p	1/7-5/8	NT	Atkinson et al. (10)
gp280 500	653.40S	f	41/41	6/111	Natali et al. (11)
gp280 440 (proteo-glycan)	225.28S	f	59/59	5/10	Wilson et al. (12)
p97	96.5	f	14/17	0/5	Garrigues et al. (13)
GD3	R-24	f	58/58	2/38	Dippold et al. (14)
		f	58/61	18/81	Real et al. (15)
mw?	M-2-2-4	f	64/70	2/15	Suter et al. (16)

* number of lesions positive/number of lesions examined

NT = not tested

p = paraffin sections

f = frozen sections

\+ = polyvalent antiserum

mw? = molecular weight not known

2.1.1 Antigens detectable in paraffin sections.
Antigens detectable in formalin fixed paraffin sections are gp 90-34 recognized by NKI/C3 (7), S-100 protein (9) and a variety of proteins with a molecular weight ranging from 30 to 200 kD, recognized by MoAbs of the ME-series (10). Because the reported number of melanoma lesions tested with MoAbs of the ME-series is limited they will not be discussed further. Both gp 90-34 and S-100 protein can be demonstrated in a high proportion of melanocytic lesions. The immunohistochemical staining results are illustrated in Figs. 1 and 2, respectively.

In addition to melanoma gp 90-34 is often found in other neuroendocrine tumors especially carcinoid tumors (Tables 2A and 2B).

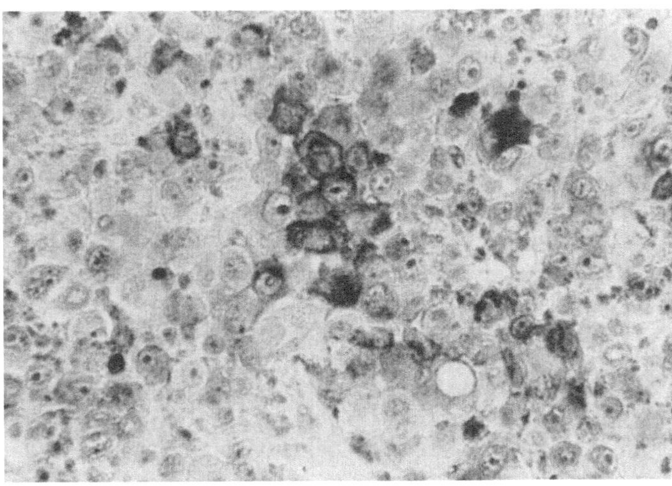

Fig. 1. Paraffin section of melanoma metastasis stained with MoAb NKI/C3. Note preferential staining in large epitheloid tumor cells. (x 400 with hematoxylin counterstaining).

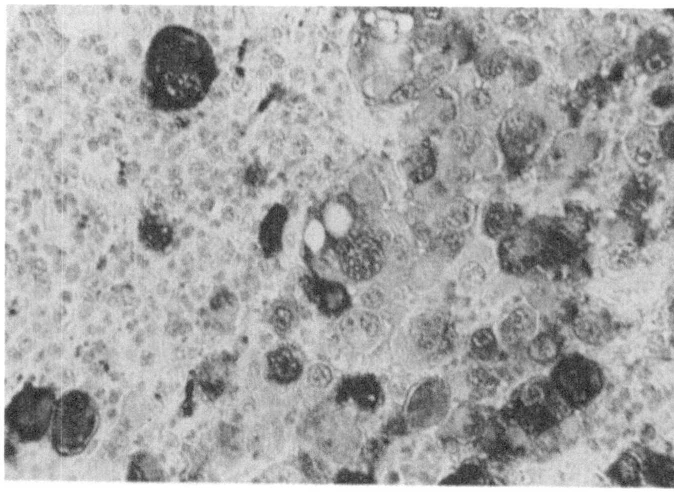

Fig. 2. Paraffin section of melanoma metastasis stained with anti-S100. Note staining of both nuclei and cytoplasm of the tumor cells (x 400, with hematoxylin counterstaining).

TABLE 2 A. Distribution of melanoma-associated antigen recognized by MoAb NKI/C3 in paraffin sections.

Lesions tested and staining results*					
NN	PCM	MM	Other APUD-omas	Other malignant tumors+	Reference
9/9 (100%)	17/23 (74%)	18/18 (100%)	11/23 (48%)	2/60 (3%)	Van Duinen et al. (8)
55/69 (80%)	18/18 (100%)	21/21 (100%)	0/2	4/44 (9%)	MacKie et al. (17)
22/26 (85%)	36/37 (97%)	60/61 (98%)	18/27 (67%)	12/187 (6%)	Vennegoor et al. (7)
NT	NT	44/47 (94%)	NT	NT	Palmer et al. (18)
NT	34/39 (87%)	20/21 (95%)	NT	NT	Hagen et al. (19)
NT	31/36 (86%)		NT	1/7 (14%)	Gatter et al. (20)

* number of lesions positive/number of lesions examined.

+ tumors relevant for differentrial diagnosis with MM

NT = not tested

NN = nevocellular nevus

PCM = primary cutaneous melanoma

MM = melanoma metastasis

TABLE 2B. Specification of non-melanocytic tumors reported to react with NKI/C3.

Lesions tested and staining results*	
Carcinoid	12/14
Medullary carcinoma of thyroid	2/2
Clear cell sarcoma	2/9
Neuroendocrine carcinoma	1/5
Undifferentiated large-cell carcinoma of the lung	2/5
Carcinoma of breast	3/46
Carcinoma of prostate	6/10
Carcinoma of ovary	4/30
Carcinoma of lung	4/31

* number of lesions positive/number of lesions examined after Van Duinen et al. (8), Gatter et al. (20), MacKie et al. (17) and Vennegoor et al. (7).

Interestingly, it is also expressed in clear cell sarcoma, which has recently been defined as melanoma of soft tissue (21). In other malignant tumors that histologically may mimic melanoma the antigen is infrequently expressed, i.e. in less than 10% of the lesions studied (7,8,17).
By use of an enzyme immunoassay it was shown that the gp 90-34 antigen recognized by NKI/C3 is a glycoprotein with a disulfide-dependent configuration (7). Its nature as differentiation marker is supported by its topological association with melanosomes, as demonstrated by immunoelectronmicroscopy (7), and the correlation between the degree of staining with NKI/C3 and the degree of pigmentation in melanoma lesions (19).
S-100 protein may also be found in other neuroendocrine tumors, but the frequency observed in the different series varies markedly (Table 3A,B) (9,22,23).

More consistently the presence of S-100 protein has been reported in benign tumors of the peripheral nervous tissue (data not shown) (23),and variably in their malignant counterparts (9,22). S-100 protein was first described as a nervous tissue-specific protein by Moore (25), and was named because of its solubility in 100% ammonium sulfate solution at neutral pH. It was further shown that S-100 protein consists of two similar subunits, S-100a (α,β subunits) and S-100b (α,β subunits), all with a molecular weight of 21 kD. The biological function of S-100 protein is unknown, although it has been considered as a member of the Ca-binding protein family (24).

TABLE 3A. Distribution of melanoma-associated antigen recognized by anti-S100 in paraffin sections

Lesions tested and staining results.

NN	PCM	MM	Other APUD-omas	Other malig-nant tumors	Reference
20/25 (80%)	20/23 (87%)	24/24 (100%)	17/64 (27%)	PNT 10/14 (71%)	Nakijima et al. (9)
				OT 4/67 (6%)	
0/4 (0%)	NT	8/10 (80%)	0/16 (0%)	PNT 0/4 (0%)	Stefansson et al. (22)
				OT 0/18 (0%)	
12/12 (100%	8/8 (100%)	13/13 (100%)	4/5 (80%)	5/55 (9%)	Kahn et al. (23)
22/23 (96%)	30/30 (100%)	30/30 (100%)	NT	0/27 (0%)	Kindblom et al. (24)
NT	39/39 (100%)	21/21 (100%)	NT	NT	Hagen et al. (19)
NT	31/36 (86%)		NT	4/7 (57%)	Gatter et al. (20)

NT = not tested

PNT = peripheral nervous tumor

OT = other tumors

NN = nevocellular nevus

PCM = primary cutaneous melanoma

MM = melanoma metastasis

TABLE 3B. Non-melanocytic malignant tumors reported to react with anti-S-100.

Lesions tested and staining results*	
Neurogenic sarcoma	10/14
Chondrosarcoma	2/2
Duct carcinoma (breast)	2/7
Medullary carcinoma (breast)	4/4
Neuroblastoma	4/4
Ganglioneuroblastoma	2/4

* number of lesions positive/number of lesions examined after Nakijima et al. (19) and Kahn et al. (23)

2.1.2. Antigens detectable in frozen sections.

Differentiation markers detectable in frozen sections only include high molecular weight proteoglycans (12, 26) as recognized by several MoAbs (e.g. 653.40S), p97 (27) recognized by the MoAb 96.5 and ganglioside GD3 (28) recognized by several MoAbs (e.g. R-24), and an unknown antigen recognized by the MoAb M-2-2-4 (see Table 1).

The antigens mentioned are expressed in a high percentage of melanocytic lesions tested and in a low percentage of other tumors. The antigen recognized by MoAb 653.40S was found only in 6/111 other tumors tested, i.e. in 4/6 basal cell carcinomas of skin and 2/5 squamous cell carcinomas of skin (11). The antigen recognized by MoAb 225.28S was found in 5/10 basal cell and squamous cell carcinomas tested (12). P97 was not found in 5 basal cell and squamous cell carcinomas tested (13).

In a large series of non-melanocytic tumors tested GD3 was demonstrated in two carcinoid tumors only by Dippold et al. (14). However, it was reported in 4/4 astrocytomas, 3/13 lung carcinomas, 2/8 breast carcinomas, 2/3 embryonal carcinomas and 7/15 sarcomas by Real et al. (15). The antigen recognized by M-2-2-4 was found in 1/2 lung carcinomas and 1/2 breast carcinomas tested (16).

2.2 Markers associated with stages of neoplastic progression.

Immunohistochemical analysis of a large number of melanocytic lesions in different stages of local and systemic neoplastic progression with a panel of monoclonal antibodies against melanoma-associated antigens and HLA antigens has clearly demonstrated phenotypic heterogeneity (3). Despite this heterogeneity, principles of antigen expression were found based on the relative frequency of antigens in various types and stages of melanocytic lesions (see Table 4).

Based on these data on the tissue distribution the melanoma-associated antigen K.1.2. (29) can be classified as "early" antigen, and A-1-43 and A-10-33 as "late" markers of tumor progression. HLA-A,B,C and HLA-DR antigens, gp75, p89 and the antigens recognized by MoAbs PAL-M1, PAL-M2, 2-139-1 and 6-26-3 in this respect can be classified as "intermediate" markers (3,30,31,32). Melanoma-associated antigens M.2.2.4 and H.2.8.10 (not mentioned in table 4) that are expressed over a wide range of local and dissemintated melanoma lesions can be depicted as "constitutive" markers of melanocytic cells (3) as was discussed earlier. It was found that the proportion of melanocytic cells stained for PAL-M1 and PAL-M2 was higher in primary melanomas than in dysplastic nevi and even higher in metastases (31). This supports the proposition that the antigens recognized by these antibodies may be markers for neoplastic progression of melanocytic proliferations. Little is known about the nature of these antigens. Mab 15.75 defines a 75kD glycoprotein expressed on the surface of human melanoma cell lines (30). MAb P3.58 immunoprecipitated

TABLE 4. Melanoma-associated antigens associated with certain stages of neoplastic progression.

Antigen	Monoclonal antibody	Tissue preparation	Distribution* NN	DN	PCM	MM	Reference
mw?	K-1-2	F	17/24	5/6	76/92	35/118	Suter et al. (29)
gp 75	15.75	F	1/19	0/2	9/12	3/3	Holzmann et al.(30)
p 89	P3.58	F	2/19	0/2	9/12	3/3	Holzmann et al.(30)
mw?	PAL-M1	F	2/26[+]	9/35	14/19	15/15	Ruiter et al.(31)
mw 95-100	PAL-M2	F	0/26	3/35	5/19	9/15	Ruiter et al.(31)
mw?	2-139-1 (human)	P	0/20	2/5	18/18	18/18	Imam et al.(32)
mw?	6-26-3 (human)	P	0/20	2/5	18/18	18/18	Imam et al.(32)
					II ≥III		
mw?	A.1.43	F	3/50	NT	1/10 53/160	67/155	Bröcker et al. (3)
mw?	A.10.33	F	0/56	NT	0/12 36/160	47/157	Bröcker et al. (3)

*number of lesions positive/number of lesions examined. [+] nevus cells were only sporadically positive.

NN = nevocellular nevus

DN = dysplastic nevus

PCM = primary cutaneous melanoma

MM = melanoma metastasis

mw? = molecular weight not known

NT = not tested

II = Clark Level II

≥III = Clark Level III and more.

proteins with an approximate molecular weight of 89kD under nonreducing conditions, and 93 kD under reducing conditions (30). Immunoblotting with PAL-M2 revealed two well-demarcated lines situated at 95 and 100 kD (31). Further characterization showed that PAL-M2 recognizes a molecule associated with adhesion of human melanoma cells to cultured endothelial cells (33).

2.3 Markers associated with cell function.

Antigens involved in immune regulation, i.e. Class I and Class II HLA antigens may be expressed on both cultured melanoma cells and in melanoma cells in tissue sections (33,4,5,34-36)). The distribution of these antigens in tissue sections points towards an association with the adjacent and intratumoral mononuclear cell inflammatory infiltrate (see Table 5) (5).

Therefore, these antigens may be involved in eliciting or mediating the immune response directed against the tumor (5). Because certain expression patterns of these antigens were found to have prognostic implications they are discussed under paragraph 3.5.

TABLE 5. Distribution of HLA antigens in melanocytic lesions and relationship with mononuclear inflammatory infiltrate.

	STAINING RESULTS*		
Type of lesions	HLA-A,B,C[1]	HLA-DR[2]	Inflammatory infiltrate
Nevocellular nevus	4/37	1/56	-
Dysplastic nevus	12/15	1/15	+/-
Primary melanoma			
Clark II-III	32/33	16/63	+
Clark IV-V	26/36	59/109	+/-
Melanoma metastasis			
Locoregional	49/76	39/85	-/+
Visceral	1/18	2/23	-/+

After Bröcker et al. (3) and Ruiter et al. (5, 36)

* number of lesions positive/number of lesions tested

\- = absent, -/+ = mostly absent, +/- = mostly present, + = present

1 = ≥ 50% positive melanocytic cells per section

2 = ≥ 10% positive melanocytic cells per section

The antigen p97, already mentioned under 2.1, has been shown to have a high degree of structural homology with the iron-binding protein transferrin (37). A novel molecule, MACAM-1, recognized by Moab AMF-7 (not mentioned in tables) was shown to be involved in the adhesion of human melanoma cells to cultured endothelial cells (33). This is a complex molecule that under non-reduced conditions consists of two components with a molecular weight of 150 kD and 95 kD. In a reduced state the molecular complex consists of 4 subunits with a molecular weight of 120 kD, 45 kD, 29 kD and 25kD (33).

3. APPLICATION OF MONOCLONAL ANTIBODIES IN THE PHENOTYPING OF MELANOCYTIC LESIONS.

Immunohistochemical phenotyping of melanoma lesions using monoclonal antibodies has contributed to: 1) assessment of the tumor cell type, 2) discrimination between benign and malignant lesions, 3) identification of early metastases, 4) assessment of the prognosis, and 5) improvement of insight into the pathogenesis and development of neoplasms.
Before a review will be given on the phenotyping of melanocytic lesions some technical aspects of the immunohistological techniques used will be discussed.

3.1. Technical aspects

Most monoclonal antibodies that recognize melanoma-associated antigens are applicable on frozen sections only. The degree of staining may vary with the affinity of the antibody used and with the staining procedure. Especially if the differences in expression of certain antigens between different lesions are quantitative it is mandatory to chose standardized staining conditions, such as dilution of antibodies and developing time of the chromogen. The specificity of an antibody as defined on buffered formalin fixed paraffin sections may be different from that in paraffin sections fixed otherwise or pretreated with digestive enzymes, and from that on frozen sections. This is the case for the MoAb NKI/C3, that should be used for diagnostic purposes on formalin fixed paraffin sections only (8,17). In order to avoid confusion with melanin we exclusively use 3-amino-9 ethylaminocarbazole as a chromogen, of which the red color contrasts well with the brown pigment. It should be noted, that the interpretation of immunohistochemical sections of tumorous lesions should be performed by experienced pathologists in order to avoid confusion of non-neoplastic cells with tumor cells.

3.2 Assessment of the tumor cell type.

In poorly differentiated malignant tumors the differential diagnosis based on conventional histological sections may include undifferentiated carcinoma, non-Hodgkin lymphoma, sarcoma and amelanotic malignant melanoma. Absolute proof for melanocytic differentiation are the demonstration of (pre-)melanosomes by transmission electron microscopy and/or of tyrosinase activity by enzyme histochemistry. However, these methods have a low sensitivity.Because MoAbs with absolute specificity for melanocytic differentiation are still lacking, a panel of monoclonal antibodies with different specificities can be applied. This panel and the step-wise diagnostic approach (38) are shown in Table 6 (part 1 and part 2) (see fig. 3).

The use of a panel of MAbs recognizing melanoma-associated antigens increases both sensitivity and specificity. For example, Hellström and Hellström (39) found 60%, 80% and 85% of 100 melanoma metastases reactive with anti-p97, anti-GD3 and anti-proteoglycan, respectively. All melanoma lesions had one of the antigens expressed, 96% two, and 50% all three. Only 15% of about 30 other malignant tumors expressed two of these antigens, in particular undifferentiated carcinoma (39).

3.3 Discrimination between benign and malignant melanocytic lesions.

MoAbs have been developed that preferentially stain malignant melanoma, and do not stain nevocellular nevi (30,31,32). These include anti-gp75, anti p89, PAL-M1, PAL-M2 and 2-139-1 and 6-26-3 (see Table 4). Only the human MoAbs 2-139-1 and 6-26-3 (32) were shown to react with paraffin tissue sections, which makes them suitable for

TABLE 6. Application of immunohistochemistry employing monoclonal antibodies in the diagnosis of amelanotic malignant melanoma.

Conventional histopathology: poorly differentiated malignant tumor

Step 1:	Monoclonal antibodies recognizing	Results obtained* 1	2	3	4
	cytokeratin	+	-	-	-
	vimentin	-	+	+	-
	desmin	-	-	-	+
	common leukocyte antigen	-	-	+	-

Interpretation of results

1) carcinoma
2) sarcoma, malignant melanoma
3) non- Hodgkin lymphoma
4) leiomyosarcoma, rhabdomyosarcoma

* co-expression of intermediate-sized filaments is not considered here.

Step 2: A second set of MoAbs that permits further differentiation can be applied, dependent on results of sept 1.
Suppose the tumor contains vimentin only. The following (monoclonal) antibodies are useful for the diagnosis of melanoma

Monoclonal antibodies	Specificity	Results obtained 1	2	3	4	5
M-2-2-4 (16)	Melanoma-associated antigen	+	+	-	-	-
HMW 653.40S (11)	detectable in frozen sections only	+	+	+	-	-
NKI/C3 (7)	Melanoma-associated antigen	+	-	-	-	-
anti-S100 (9)*	detectable in buffered formaldehyde fixed paraffin embedded tissues	+	+	+	+	-

* Anti-S-100 is a polyvalent antibody

Interpretation of results

1) strongly supports melanoma
2) supports melanoma
3) supports melanoma
4) compatible with melanoma

(2–4: other diagnoses should be considered)

5) no support for melanoma; does not exclude melanoma

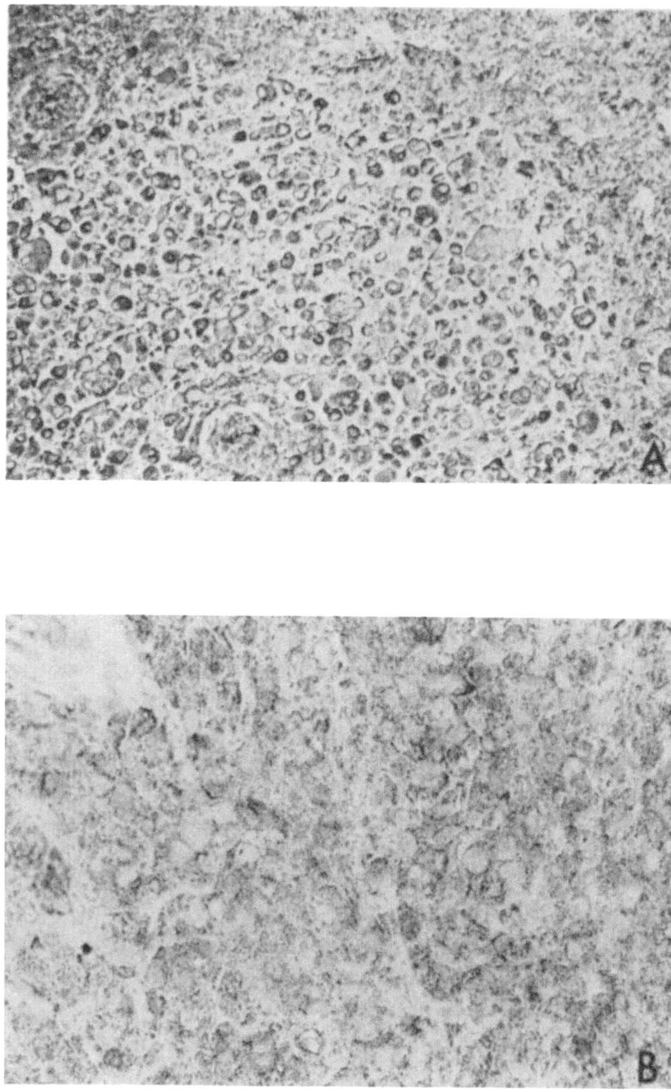

Fig. 3. Staining results of a poorly differentiated malignant tumor with MoAbs used in the panel indicated in Table 6. a) anti-vimentin: positive and b) anti-HMW 763.74T: positive). (a: x 160, b: x 400; frozen sections with hematoxylin counterstaining).

routine diagnostic application. However, these antibodies were shown also to react with a proportion of dysplastic nevi, which is interesting for the insight into the pathogenesis of melanoma, but a potential limitation for diagnostic application.
Because the problem of distinguishing cancer and noncancer is very complex (40) further studies testing the diagnostic value of combinations of these monoclonal antibodies using diagnostically difficult nevoid cases studied by a multivariate analysis should be awaited.
A marked expression of HLA class I and HLA class II antigens has been described in primary malignant melanomas and not in nevocellular nevi (see Table 5) (35, 36). However, in our experience the diagnostic role of MoAbs recognizing these antigens is limited because the differences in HLA class I expression are quantitative and the distribution pattern is complex. Furthermore, HLA class II expression in melanoma lesions is variable and mostly focal. However, the distribution of these antigens may give important information on the prognosis and pathogenesis, as will be discussed later.

3.4 Identification of early metastasis.

Identification of individual tumor cells in highly cellular tissues such as lymph nodes or bone marrow by conventional morphological examination is often difficult and time-consuming. Both monoclonal and polyvalent antibodies recognizing melanoma-associated antigens were shown to identify micrometastases in histological sections or individual melanoma cells in cytological preparations (41,42). Cochran et al. (42) detected occult melanoma metastases in 363/1273 lymph nodes by staining with anti-S100, and by conventional histology in only 128/1273 lymph nodes. This indicates that immunohistochemistry has a higher sensitivity than conventional histology in the identification of early metastasis.

3.5 Assessment of the prognosis of primary cutaneous melanoma and locoregional melanoma metastasis.

3.5.1 Primary cutaneous melanoma

In primary cutaneous melanoma expression of HLA-DR, A.1.43 or A.10.33 in 10% or more tumor cells was shown to have a relationship with early recurrence of disease (3, 43). This relationship was found especially in primary tumors below 3 mm thickness. In the whole group of 172 primary tumors the rate of metastasis was low when none of these "risk antigens" was expressed and increased in proportion to the number of these antigens expressed (3, Table 7) (see Fig. 4). Rode and Dhillon (44) reported that marked or moderate staining for neuron specific enolase and S-100 protein is associated with a relatively short time before metastases occur. However, Hagen et al. (19) could not demonstrate differences in staining with NKI/C3 or anti-S-100 between a group of primary cutaneous melanoma with metastases, and a group of primary cutaneous melanoma without metastases (minimal follow-up period of 5 years).

TABLE 7. Frequency of early metastasis from primary cutaneous melanoma according to number of risk antigens expressed.

Number of risk antigens expressed	Frequency of metastasis
0	6/77 (8%)
1	14/44 (32%)
2	19/38 (50%)
3	9/13 (69%)
(after Bröcker et al. (3)	

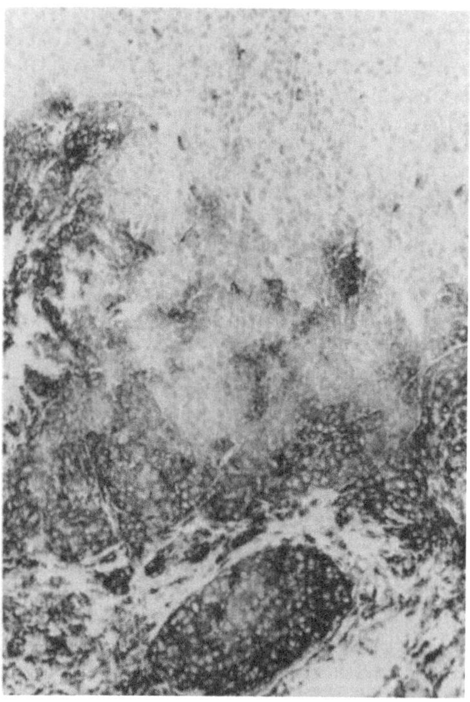

Fig. 4.

Frozen section of primary cutaneous melanoma stained with MoAb recognizing HLA-DR backbone determinant. Note the focal staining pattern. (x 160, with hematoxylin counterstaining).

3.5.2 Locoregional melanoma metastases.

In a series of 47 locoregional melanoma metastases certain patterns of HLA class I and HLA class II antigen expression have been described by our group (45). An U-shaped frequency distribution of the proportion of melanoma cells stained for HLA class I antigens in these lesions was found, with a break-point at 50% of melanoma cells stained. If the same breakpoint of 50% is used for HLA class II antigens, and the topological relation between melanoma cells expressing these antigens is accounted for, three different expression patterns can be discerned (45): pattern A: more than 50% of melanoma cells stain for HLA class I antigens and 50% or less for HLA class II antigens; pattern B: 50% or less of the melanoma cells stain for both HLA class I or II antigens; and pattern C: more than 50% melanoma cells stain for both HLA class I or II antigens. Pattern A was found in 55% of the locoregional metastases studied, pattern B in 35% and pattern C in 10%. The existence of expression patterns on individual melanoma cells derived from metastases was demonstrated by double-labeling immunofluorescence and double-labeling immunoelectronmicroscopy (46). A low expression of HLA class I antigens in melanoma lesions was further shown to correlate with a low level of m.RNA coding for HLA class I (47).

Cases with locoregional melanoma metastases showing pattern A had a statistically significant (p=0.02) longer survival than those showing pattern B or C (45,47). Survival analysis was performed in cases having either one metastasis only or more metastases if the same expression pattern was found in each metastasis. The same expression pattern between autologous locoregional metastases was found in 8 out of 9 cases. The data on the survival analysis are shown in Table 8.

TABLE 8. HLA expression patterns and survival in locoregional melanoma metastasis.

Expression pattern	Survival*
A	14/21 (67%)
B	5/13 (38%)
C	0/4 (0%)

* Survival calculated according to Kaplan and Meier (48).
The follow-up period of patients still alive ranged from 10 to 41 months, with an average of 30 months.

The relationship between the HLA expression patterns and survival was independent of other known prognostic factors for patients with locoregional metastasis, such as the interval between primary melanoma and the occurrence of metastasis, or the number of metastases. Patients that had primary tumors with a Breslow thickness of 1.5 mm or less tended to have expression pattern A more often than patients with thicker tumors (p=0.2).

3.6 Possible implications for the biology of melanoma.

The correlation of the immunohistochemical findings in locoregional melanoma metastases with the course of the disease indicate that a low expression of HLA class I antigens on melanoma cells (pattern B) is associated with a high grade of malignancy. Earlier immunohistochemical work on melanocytic tumors (35, 63) and other human tumors (49, 50) points into the same direction. A low content of H-2 antigens has been reported to be associated with increased tumorigenicity in mice (51). In an adenovirus transformed rat tumor cell line a low level of class I antigens also correlated with a high degree of tumorigenicity (52). Interestingly, the expression of class I antigens was switched off by a highly oncogenic adenovirus. A low or absent expression of HLA class I antigens would provide melanoma cells with a mechanism to evade cytotoxic T cells. Such a mechanism was indeed demonstrated in the adenovirus transformed rat tumor model mentioned earlier (53). The low expression of these antigens may represent a lack of susceptibility to modulation by lymphokines, such as immune interferon (54). Alternatively, it may reflect loss of tumor cell-tumor cell interactions associated with tumor progression or a recapitulation of an early stage of melanocytic differentiation.

The association between a high expression of HLA class II antigens (in combination with high expression of HLA class I antigens; pattern C) and an unfavorable outcome is more difficult to interpret as presentation of HLA class II antigens would sensitize T cells and HLA class I antigens would offer a recognition site for such sensitized T cells. Additional immunohistochemical analysis has shown that the staining distribution of HLA class II antigens in melanoma corresponds with that of HLA-DR; staining for HLA-DR mostly exceeds that for HLA-DQ or HLA-DP (55). Although an unbalanced expression of HLA class II locus products may have an adverse effect on the cellular immune response, other interpretations for the correlation between the high expression of HLA-DR and a high grade of malignancy seem more attractive. It has been shown that melanoma cells derived from metastases expressing HLA-DR were resistant to stimulation by autologous lymphocytes in vitro, whereas those derived from primary tumors were immunostimulatory (56, 57, 58). In case of metastatic melanoma this would give an explanation for the association of a high expression of HLA-DR on melanoma cells and an unfavorable outcome. However, the correlation between HLA-DR expression and increased risk for recurrence in primary melanomas (3,43,45) needs other explanations. An alternative, non-immunological interpretation is that HLA class II antigen expression on melanoma cells may represent an early stage of differentiation (59).

4. MONOCLONAL ANTIBODIES AGAINST MELANOMA ASSOCIATED ANTIGENS: SERUM TESTS, TUMOR DETECTION AND THERAPY.

In addition to the application of monoclonal antibodies against melanoma-associated antigens for tissue diagnosis such antibodies have been used for detection and quantification of antigens in sera from melanoma patients. Also these antibodies have been used for in vivo localization of melanoma metastases. Finally, efforts have been made to apply the antibodies for therapeutical purposes.

4.1 Serum detection of melanoma-associated antigens.

With monoclonal antibodies against the high molecular weight melanoma-associated proteoglycan antigen as well as with monoclonal antibodies against the 100 kD cytoplasmic antigen described by Galloway et al. (60) elevated antigen levels have been detected in sera from Stage III and Stage IV melanoma patients (61, 62, 63). The results of these studies are summarized in Table 9..
Unfortunately, the antigens have also been detected in sera from healthy donors and non-melanoma tumor-bearing patients (61, 62). Therefore, these antibodies can neither be used for early detection of melanoma, nor for tumor diagnosis. Measuring of the circulating antigen level, however, may be used to provide some information on the extent of the disease in melanoma patients.

4.2 In vivo tumor detection.

In vivo tumor localization studies require high affinity antibodies directed against surface antigens that will not disappear from the cell surface after binding to the antibody. For melanoma the studies have been focused on two melanoma-associated surface antigens, namely the p97 antigen and the Mr 250.000 glycoprotein-chondroitin sulfate proteoglycan complex.
For in vivo localization studies mainly radiolabeled monoclonal antibodies have been used, although localization by unlabeled antibody has also been described (64, 65; see also Table 10).
General problems in tumor localization studies have been the initial high radiolabel in the blood pool, the uptake in liver being most markedly of antibodies labeled with iodine or indium labeled antibodies, and uptake in spleen, kidney, bone marrow and/or gastrointestinal tract (66-71). With iodine labeling the iodine accumulation in the liver may be ascribed partially to loss of the radiolabel from the monoclonal antibody (71). The problems with indium labeled antibodies are being caused by the selective accumulation of the metal in the liver. With ^{111}In-conjugates loss of the

TABLE 9. Detection of melanoma-associated antigen in serum with monoclonal antibodies.

		Elevated antigen level			
Antigen	Monoclonal antibody	Normal donors	Melanoma patients	Other tumor patients	Reference
gp 250	763.74T (catcher)	2/49[1]	9/137	9/78	Giacomini
gp 250	225.28S (tracer)		0/7 Stage I		et al. (61)
			2/68 Stage II-III		
			3/14 Stage IV		
			0/18 NED[2]		
gp 250	ME 95-45 (catcher)	2/52[3]	40/203[4]	11/51	Ross et al.
gp 250	ME 31.3 (tracer)		0/3 none or trace[5]		(62)
			8/22 light		
			6/136 intermediate		
			26/35 heavy		
gp 100	250/165 (inhibitor)	1/15[1]	10/16	NT[6]	Morgan et al.
			0/4 Stage I		(63)
			0/1 Stage II		
			5/10 Stage III		
			7/17 Stage IV		
			3/16 NED		

1) As calculated from the figure in the reference. The data are compared with the antigen level in normal donors + 2 x S.D.

2) NED = no evidence of disease

3) Sera higher than 35 Units

4) Patients with a light, intermediate and heavy metastatic tumor burden

5) Tumor burden

6) NT = not tested

radiolabel from the antibody has been considerably less than with iodine conjugates (72). Application of radiolabeled Fab or F(ab')2 fragments instead of intact monoclonal antibodies reduces the background label in bone marrow, liver and spleen (66), probably because the blood and soft tissue clearance is more rapidly (67, 71). Radioactive uptake in liver has been especially high when ^{111}In-labeled monoclonal antibody 96.5 (IgG2a isotope) directed against the transferrin like p97 antigen was administered and in this situation no liver metastases could be localized (68, 79). With ^{123}I-Fab against p97 antigen, however, a liver metastasis has been visualized by using photo emission tomography (70) and with ^{131}I-Fab against the HMW-MAA using a gamma camera (67).

Tumor localization has appeared to be dependent on the absolute amount of antibody, and whether or not the antibody is radiolabeled (64,65,68,69,71). In vivo localization is influenced by reactions of the monoclonal antibody with normal tissue (64,65,66-68,71) . This holds particularly for the antibodies against p97. High antigen density on the tumor has a positive effect on the localization (66, 67,71),

TABLE 10. In vivo tumor localization studies with monoclonal antibodies against melanoma-associated antigens.

Antigen	Monoclonal antibody				Specific labeling of metastases		Number of	Reference
	Name	Subclass	Dose (mg)	Labeling	Known	Unknown	patients	
gp 250	9-2-27 whole	IgG_{2a}	200 or more	none	6/8[1]		8	Oldham et al. (64)
gp 250	225.28S whole	IgG_{2a}	0.014 - 0.750	^{131}I	1/6[2]	0	4	Buraggi et al.(66)
gp 250	225.28S $F(ab')_2$				9/12	0	8	
gp 250	48.7 Fab	IgG_1	2 - 10	^{131}I	17/23[3]	1	8	Larson et al. (67)
gp 97	96.5 whole	IgG_{2a}	1 - 20	^{111}In mixed with unlabeled MoAb	48/79[4]	8	21	Halpern et al.(68)
gp 97	96.5 whole	IgG_{2a}	0.5 - 20	^{111}In	50/100	2	31	Murray et al. (69)

1) Only skin lesions were examined

2) The negative lesions were about 1 cm in diameter

3) Patients with lesions greater than 1.5 cm in diameter

4) Found by an informed observer. Only lesions greater than 1.5 cm in diameter were examined

whereas large necrotic metastases don't image (69). The anatomical site of the tumor also plays a role in tumor visualization. The uptake of ^{131}I-labeled monoclonal antibody Fab fragments directed against p97 antigen has found to be greater in visceral lesions than in subcutaneous lesions (71). With ^{131}I-labeled antibodies against the HMW-MAA the uptake in brain metastases was less avid than in systemic sites (66). A more detailed study has been described by Murray et al. (69), who found that with ^{111}In-labeled monoclonal antibodies against p97 and using a longitudinal tomographic imager in thirty-one patients the most frequent metastases imaged were skin lesions (100%) and lymph nodes (89%). Metastases less likely to take up tracer were bone (75%), lung (67%) and brain (33%). In total 50% of the known lesions imaged in this study. In most cases, using a gamma camera, the tumors that have been localized were more than 1.5 cm in diameter (66,68,71). Because the sensitivity of tumor localization is dependent on antigen density, and the high molecular weight melanoma-associated proteoglycan antigen as well as the p97 antigen appear to have a heterogeneous distribution on melanomas, the patients subjected to scintigraphy have in some studies been selected for high antigen density on skin metastases. Therefore, the data on in vivo localization like 20/33 patients (71) 8/8 patients, 74% of the metastases (67), 6/10 patients (64) or 100% of the biopsy specimens when doses of 200 mg antibody or greater were used (65) are flattered.

4.3 Therapy of melanoma with monoclonal antibodies.

4.3.1. General aspects

The therapeutical effect of monoclonal antibodies against melanoma-associated antigens has been low (Table 11).

Using therapeutical doses of radiolabeled antibody or antibody fragments partial regression has been observed in 4 patients, namely one out of two patients who received ^{131}I-Fab (IgG1) against the high molecular weight melanoma-associated proteoglycan antigen (67) and three out of twelve patients who had previously been selected for high antigen density on the tumor and who recieved unlabeled intact mouse IgG3 against the GD3 antigen (73). In two other patients who were treated with monoclonal antibody against the GD3 antigen a mixed response has been observed (73).

The higher doses of antibody necessary for therapy usually evoked transient anti-mouse immunoglobulin responses in the patients (64,67,69,71,73). Allergic reactions have been skin rash, erythema, local urticaria and/or pruritis (64,67,69,71,73). In one patient infusion of monoclonal antibody had to be discontinued after administration of 15 mg of antibody because the patient developed severe allergy (69). In two patients treatment had to be abrogated because of the anti-mouse immunoglobulin responses (71,73). Another patient experienced serum sickness after intraveneous administration of mouse monoclonal antibody (64). The inflammatory reactions responded to benadryl and either epinephirine or hydrocortisone (69,71), whereas the patient

TABLE 11. Therapy of melanoma patients with monoclonal antibodies against melanoma-associated antigens.

Antigen	Monoclonal antibody					Regression in no. of patients	Reference
	Name	Subclass	Dose (mg)	Labeling	Cumulative dose (mCi)		
gp 250	48.7 Fab	IgG_1	10	^{131}I	142 - 374	1/2 1)	Larson et al. (67)
gp 97	8.2 Fab	IgG_1	5 - 10	^{131}I	132 - 529	0/7 2)	Larson et al. (71)
gp 97	96.5 Fab	IgG_{2a}					
GD_3	R_{24} whole	IgG_3	8 mg/m^2	none		5/12 3)	Houghton et al. (73)

1) Greater than 50% reduction in the size of pelvic and pericaval nodes; stabilization of the diseaseat the smaller nodal size for three months

2) All patients had advanced disease and a favorable ratio between tumor and potential target organs, liver and bone marrow. One patient, who recieved a cumulative dose of 529 mCi ^{131}I-anti-p97 Fab, has been stable for two months

3) Two patients had a mixed response; three other patients showed major tumor regression

with serum sickness responded to a high-dose of intravenous steroids (64). The toxic effects due to application of mouse monoclonal antibody were usually low, the most serious being temporal fall in blood lymphocytes and thrombocytes in patients receiving more than 500 mCi ^{131}I-Fab anti-p97 (71). In one patient further therapy with monoclonal Fab fragments against the high molecular weight melanoma-associated proteoglycan antigen had to be abrogated because of a drop in platelet count and the debilitated state of the patient (67). Other effects recorded are temperature elevation (73), flushing and transient hypotension (71), tachycardia (71), mild nausea and vomiting or anorexia (64, 73) and headache (64).

4.3.2. Mechanisms of therapeutic effects using unlabeled monoclonal antibodies against melanoma-associated antigens in experimental tumor systems.

Unlabeled monoclonal antibodies against melanoma have in some cases been shown to selectively inhibit tumor growth in vitro, as well as in vivo in nude mice carrying human melanoma inoculates (see Table 12, A and B).

Antibody dependent cellular cytotoxicity (ADCC) may be one of the mechanisms for in vivo inhibition of tumor growth by monoclonal antibodies. With antibodies (IgG3) against the melanoma-associated GD3 ganglioside antigen the outgrowth of human melanoma in nude mice was inhibited when an antibody giving an ADCC with mouse lymphocytes was injected (80). With a mouse monoclonal antibody 9.2.27 (IgG2a subclass) against the HMW-MAA antigen tumor regression was achieved only when simultaneously compatible mouse splenocytes were injected (78). In the latter study evidence has been given that cells with natural killer cell activity were responsible for the destruction of the melanoma cells. The results of Herlyn et al. (79) indicated that macrophages were responsible for in vivo tumor cell suppression. Only melanoma cells with a high surface antigen density (more than 1×10^6 MoAb binding sites per cell) appeared to be susceptible for in vitro antibody dependent cellular cytotoxicity and growth inhibition in the nude mouse by monoclonal antibodies. With human anti-OFA-1-2 (IgM subclass) no cellular cytotoxicity on melanoma cells was observed, but the cells were very susceptible for the monoclonal antibody in the presence of complement (81). Therefore, different monoclonal antibodies may induce tumor cell killing by different effector mechanisms.

4.3.3. Therapy with monoclonal antibody conjugates.

Immunotherapy with monoclonal antibodies might be improved by administration of antibodies conjugated to toxic substances. With conjugates of monoclonal antibodies and radionuclides like ^{125}I selective killing of melanoma cells in vitro has been observed in mixtures of melanoma and lung cancer cells (84). In vitro, in non-adherent SK-Mel 28 cells specific inhibition of protein synthesis by ricin A anti-p97

TABLE 12A. Efficacy and possible mechanism of therapy with unlabeled monoclonal antibodies against melanoma-associated antigens in experimental tumor models (part 1).

Antigen	Monoclonal antibody		In vitro effect			Tumor suppression in the nude mouse	Reference
	Name	Subclass	Cytostatic and cytoloytic	CMC[1)]	ADCC[2)]		
gp 250	225.28S	IgG_{2a}		-	+[3)]		Imai et al. (74)
gp 250	653.40S	IgG_1		-	±[3)]		
gp 250	9.2.27	IgG_{2a}	+				Harper et al.(75)
gp 250	9.2.27	IgG_{2a}		-	+[4)] ±[5)]	++ i.v.[4)] + i.v.[6)]	Schulz et al.(76)
gp 250	9.2.27	IgG_{2a}			±	+ i.p	Bumol et al. (77)
gp 250	9.2.27	IgG_{2a}			+[7)]	- i.v.[8)] + i.v.[7) 8)]	Schulz et al.(78)
gp 250	ME 126	IgG_{2a}			+[9)]	+ i.p.	Herlyn et al.(79)
gp 250	48.7	IgG_1			-		Hellströom et al.(80)

1) Human complement mediated cytotoxicity

2) Antibody dependent cellular cytotoxicity; unless indicated otherwise the effecter cells are human lymphocytes

3) Also positive with murine lymphocytes

4) Murine spleen cells armed with monoclonal antibody 9.2.27 by polyethylene glycol

5) Effector cells are murine spleen cells

6) With eigther antibody 9.2.27 alone or antibody 9.2.27 and murine spleen cells

7) Effector cells are murine natural killer cells

8) Therapy started 14 days after tumor inoculation

TABLE 12B. Efficacy and possible mechanism of therapy with unlabeled monoclonal antibodies against melanoma-associated antigens in experimental tumor models (part 2).

Antigen	Monoclonal antibody		In vitro effect			Tumor suppression in the nude mouse	Reference
	Name	Subclass	Cytostatic and cytolytic	CMC[1]	ADCC[2]		
gp 116, 95	MeNu4B	IgG_{2a}			-[3]	- i.p.	Herlyn et al.(79)
gp 97	96.5	IgG_{2a}			-	- i.v.	Hellström et al.(80)
gp 97	MED63	IgG_{2a}			-[3]	- i.p.	Herlyn et al.(79)
gp 97	MEC44	IgG_{2a}			-[3]	- i.p.	
GD_2	human anti-OFA-1-2	IgM		+	-	+ s.c. - i.p. ± i.l.	Katano et al. (81)
GD_3	R_{24}	IgG_3	+[4]				Dippold et al. (82)
GD_3	2B2	IgG_3		-	+[5]	+ i.v.	Hellström et al.(80)
GD_3	IF4	IgG_3		-	+[6]	- i.v.	
GD_3	MG-21	IgG_3		+	+[6]		
GD_3	MB3.6	IgG_3		+	+	+ i.p.[7] - i.l.[7]	Cheresh et al.(83)

1) Human complement mediated cytotoxicity
2) Antibody dependent cellular cytotoxicity; unless indicated otherwise the effector cells are human lymphocytes.
3) Effector cells are murine macrophages
4) Accompanied by change in morphology of the cells
5) Also positive with murine lymphocytes
6) Negative with murine lymphocytes.
7) Therapy started 8 days after tumor inoculation.

immunotoxin was at a consid[illegible]y lower concentration (CI 50 = 5×10^{-10} M) than by the ricin A - chain alone (CI 50 = 10^{-6} M) (85). In a similar way, in vitro colony formation was inhibited at a much lower concentration of ricin A-immunotoxin (2 x 10^{-9} M), than with the unlabeled ricin A-chain (10^{-6} M). These results were obtained only with target cells with a high antigen expression and after an incubation period of 60 hours. The slow action of the immunotoxin was probably the result of its slow internalization into the melanoma cells, as the same inhibition of colony formation was obtained after incubating the melanoma cells for only two hours with the immunotoxin in the presence of ammonium chloride (85).
Two reports have appeared on the application of immunotoxins in vivo in nude mice inoculated with rapidly growing melanoma cells. In one study the immunotoxin was prepared with diphteria toxin A, an inhibitor of protein synthesis, and monoclonal antibody 9.2.27 directed against the melanoma-associated proteoglycan antigen. The conjugate showed, however, no higher suppression of M21 tumor growth compared to the antibody alone (77). In the other study antibody 9.2.27 was bound to purothonin, a toxin that binds to the cell membrane and causes functional changes of the membrane and inhibition of sugar incorporation. This conjugate has shown significant increase of life span of nude mice inoculated with the ascitic form of human Colo 38 cells. With the subcutaneous solid form of these cells only inhibition of tumor growth, but no significant increase of life span was observed (86). Because of these results the authors suggested that immunotherapy with toxin conjucated to monoclonal antibodies against melanoma-associated antigens might be effective only in patients with a limited tumor burden.

5. CONCLUSIONS AND FUTURE DEVELOPMENTS.

The MoAb NKI/C3 and anti-S100 antiserum are useful tools for the diagnosis of amelanotic melanoma in paraffin sections and for the detection of micro-metastases. In frozen sections, the MoAbs recognizing ganglioside GD3, p97, a high molecular weight proteoglycan and M-2-2-4 are useful for this purpose. The sensitivity and specificity of the diagnostic test increases if panels of MoAbs with different specificites are used. Use of panels is strongly advocated because no MoAbs with absolute specificity for melanocytic differentiation have been produced. Although MoAbs have been produced that were selected to discriminate between nevocellular nevi and melanomas their contribution to the diagnosis of diagnostically difficult nevoid lesions still has to be established. For the assessment of prognosis of patients with primary cutaneous melanoma the MoAbs anti-HLA-DR, A.1.43 and A.10.33 are useful additional tools.

In patients with locoregional melanoma metastases, the number of lymph nodes involved (including those with micrometastases as identified by staining for S100 protein) has prognostic significance. Furthermore, certain patterns of expression of HLA-A,B,C and HLA-DR were shown to have prognostic significance in this group of patients.
Recently developed MoAbs were shown to recognize adhesion molecules on melanoma cells (33). These molecules may have relevance for the process of metastasis, because adhesion of tumor cells to endothelial cells or basal lamina is an important step in this process.
Metastasis of human melanoma cells have been obtained in the nude mouse model (87,88). We hope to develop MoAbs that can identify the antigenic phenotypes on human melanoma cells that are associated with the different steps of metastasis in this model. By doing so one may obtain more insight into this highly complex process. MoAbs related to this process may have relevance for the assessment of prognosis and may have great potential for immunotherapy of early metastases.
Until now no diagnostic serum test for melanoma patients exists. However, melanoma patients can already be followed for progression of the disease with serum markers that are more tumor-associated than lactate dehydrogenase, alkaline phosphatase and gamma glutamyl transpeptidase used at present. In vivo localization studies have shown that tumor targetting is possible. However, high antigen density on the tumor cells should be present. Because of the observed heterogeneity in melanomas, mixtures of monoclonal antibodies directed against several melanoma-associated antigens should be applied to detect a higher proportion of metastases. As regards to immunotherapy more experimentation in model systems is required on mechanisms of antibody mediated tumor cell destruction and selection of proper toxins or drugs for antibody conjugates.

ACKNOWLEDGEMENTS.

This work was in part supported by a grant of the Queen Wilhelmina Foundation, the Netherlands Organisation for the Fight against Cancer. The excellent technical assistance of Mrs. M.E. van Beveren-Hooijer and C.B. de Graaff-Reitsma, and the excellent secretarial assistance of Mrs. I.A. Bruinenberg-Kruyff is gratefully acknowledged.

ADDENDUM.

After the completion of this chapter a monoclonal antibody HMB-45, has been published* that showed absolute specificity and a very high sensitivity for melanocytic tumors in methacarn or formaldehyde fixed paraffin sections. This antibody therefore has great utility for the diagnosis of oligomelanotic and amelanotic melanoma.

*Gown Am, Vogel AM, Hoak D, Gough F, McNutt MA. Monoclonal antibodies specific for melanocytic tumors distinguish subpopulations of melanocytes. Am. J. Pathol. 1986; 123: 195-203.

REFERENCES

1. Mastrangelo MJ, Baker AR and Katz HR. Cutaneous melanoma. In De Vita VT, Hellman S and Rosenberg SA (eds.): Cancer, Principles and practice of oncology. 1985; pp. 1371-1442, Lippincott, Philadelphia.
2. Clark Jr. WH, Reimer RR, Greene M. Origin of familial melanoma from heriditable melanocytic lesions the BK mole syndrome. Arch. Dermatol. 1978; 114: 732-38.
3. Bröcker E-B, Suter L, Brüggen J, Ruiter DJ, Macher E, Sorg C. Phenotypic dynamics of tumor progression in human malignant melanoma. Int. J. Cancer 1985; 36: 29-35.
4. Natali PG, Cordiali- Fei P, Cavaliere R, Difilippo F, Quaranta V, Pellegrino MA and Ferrone S. Ia-like antigens on freshly explanted human malignant melanoma. Clin. Immunol. Immunopathol. 1981; 19: 250-9.
5. Ruiter DJ, Bhan AK, Harrist TJ, Sober AJ and Mihm Jr. MC. Major histocompatibility antigens and mononuclear inflammatory infiltrate in benign nevomelanocytic proliferations and malignant melanoma. J. Immunol. 1982; 129: 2808-15.
6. Damjanov J, Knowles BB. Biology of Disease. Monoclonal antibodies and tumor-associated antigens. Lab. Invest. 1983; 48: 510-25.
7. Vennegoor C, Calafat J, Hageman Ph. Van Buitenen F, Janssen H, Kolk A, Rümke Ph. Biochemical characterization and cellular localization of a formalin-resistant melanoma-associated antigen reacting with monoclonal antibody NKI/C3. Int. J. Cancer 1985; 35: 287-295.
8 Van Duinen SG, Ruiter DJ, Hageman Ph, Vennegoor C, Dickersin GR, Scheffer E, Rümke Ph. Immunohistochemical and histochemical tools in the diagnosis of amelanotic melanoma. Cancer 1984; 53: 1566-73.
9. Nakajima T, Watanabe S, Sato Y, Kameyo T, Shimosato Y, Ishihara K. Immunohistochemical demonstration of S100 protein in malignant melanoma and pigmented nevus, and its diagnostic application. Cancer 1981; 50: 912-8.
10. Atkinson B, Ernst CS, Ghrist BFD, Herly M, Blaszcyk M, Ross AH, Herlyn D, Steplewski Z, Koprowski H. Identification of melanoma-associated antigens using fixed tissue screening fo antibodies. Cancer Res. 1984; 44: 2577-81.
11. Natali PG, Imai K, Wilson BS, Bigotti A, Cavaliere R, Pellegrino MA, Ferrone S. Structural properties and tissue distribution of the antigen recognized by the monoclonal antibody 653.40S to human melanoma cells. J. Natl. Cancer Inst. 1981; 67: 591-5.
12. Wilson BS, Imai K, Natali PG, Ferrone S. Distribution and molecular characterization of a cell-surface and a cytoplasmic antigen detectable in human melanoma cells with monoclonal antibodies. Int.J. Cancer 1981; 28: 293-300.

13. Garrigues HJ, Tilgen W, Hellström I, Franke W, Hellström KE. Detection of a human melanoma-associated antigen, p97 in histological sections of primary human melanomas. Int. J. Cancer 1982; 29: 511-5.
14. Dippold WG, Dienes HP, Knuth A, Meijer zum Büschenfelde K-H. Immunohistochemical localization of ganglioside GD3 in human malignant melanoma, epithelial tumors and normal tissues. Cancer Res. 1985; 45: 3699-3706.
15. Real FX, Houghton AN, Albino AP, Cordon-Cardo C, Melamed MR, Oettgen HF, Old LJ. Surace antigens of melanomas and melanocytes defined by mouse monoclonal antibodies: specificty analysis and comparison of antigen expression in cultured cells and tissues. Cancer Res 1985; 45: 4401-11.
16. Suter L, Bröcker E-B, Brüggen J, Ruiter DJ, Sorg C. Heterogeneity of primary and metastatic human malignant melanoma as detected with monoclonal antibodies in cryostat sections of biopsies. Cancer Immunol. Immunother. 1983; 16: 53-8.
17. MacKie RM, Campbell J, Turbitt ML. Use of NKI/C3 monoclonal antibody in the assessment of benign and malignant melanocytic lesions. J. Clin. Pathol. 1984; 37: 367-72.
18. Palmer AA, Hall BE, Lew M. A comparison of some methods for identifying amelanotic and oligomelanotic melanoma metastases in paraffin sections. Pathology 1985; 17: 335-9.
19. Hagen EC, Vennegoor C, Schlingemann RO, Van der Velde EA, Ruiter DJ. Correlation of histopathological characteristics with staining patterns in human melanoma assessed by monoclonal antibodies reactive on paraffin sections. Histopathology 1986 (in press).
20. GatterKC, Ralfkiaer E, Skinner J. Brown D, Heryet A, Pulford KAF, Hou-Jensen K, Mason DY. An immunocytochemical study of malignant melanoma and its differntial diagnosis from other malignant tumours. J. Clin. Pathol. 1985; 38: 1353-7.
21. Chung EB, Enzinger FM. Malignant melanoma of soft parts. A reassessment of clear cell sarcoma. Am. J. Surg. Pathol. 1983; 7: 405-13.
22. Stefansson K, Wollmann R, Jerkovic M. S100 protein in soft-tissue tumors derived from Schwann cells and melanocytes. Am. J. Pathol. 1982; 106: 261-8.
23. Kahn HJ, Marks A, Thom H, Baumal R. Role of antibody to S100 protein in diagnostic pathology. Am. J. Pathol. 1983; 79: 341-7.
24. Kindblom L-G, Lodding P, Rosengren L, Bandier J, Haglid K. S100 protein in melanocytic tumors. Acta Pathol. Microbiol. Scand. Sect A. 1984; 92: 219-30.
25. Moore B. Chemistry and biology of the two proteins S100 and 14-3-2 specific to the nervous system. Int. Rev. Neurobiol. 1972; 15: 215-25.
26. Bumol TF and Reisfeld RA. Unique glyocprotein-proteoglycan complex defined by a monoclonal antibody on human melanoma cells. Proc. Natl. Acad. Sci. USA, 1982; 79: 1245-49.

27. Woodbury RG, Brown JP, Yeh MY, Hellström I, Hellström K-E. Identification of a cell surface protein, p97, in human melanomas and certain other neoplasms. Proc. Natl. Acad. Sci., USA, 1980; 77: 2183-87.
28. Pukel CS, Lloyd KO, Travassos LR, Dippold WG, Oettgen HF, Old LJ. GD3 - a prominent ganglioside of human melanoma: detection and characterization by mouse monoclonal antibody. J. Exp. Med. 1982; 155: 1133-47.
29. Suter L, Brüggen J, Bröcker E-B, Sorg C. A tumor-associated antigen expressed in melanoma cells with lower malignant potential. Int. J. Cancer 1985; 35: 787-91.
30. Holzmann B, Johnson JP, Kaudewitz P, Riethmüller G. In situ analysis of antigens on malignant and benign cells of the melanocyte lineage: differential expression of two surface molecules, gp75 and p89. J. Exp. Med. 1985; 161: 366-77.
31. Ruiter DJ, Dingjan M, Steijlen PM, Van Beveren-Hooijer M, De Graaff-Reitsma CB, Bergman W, Van Muyen GNP, Warnaar SO. Monoclonal antibodies selected to discriminate between malignant melanomas and nevocellular nevi. J. Invest. Dermatol. 1985; 85: 4-8.
32. Imam A, Mitchell MS, Modlin RL, Taylor CR, Kempf RA, Kan-Mitchell J. Human monoclonal antibodies that distinguish cutaneous malignant melanomas from benign nevi in fixed tissue sections. J. Invest. Dermatol. 1986; 86: 145-8.
33. De Vries JE, Keizer GD, Te Velde AA, Voordouw A, Ruiter DJ, Figdor CG. A melanoma-associated cellular adhesion molecular (MACAM-1) involved in the adhesion, motility and migration of melanoma cells. Int. J. Cancer 1986; in press.
34. Natali PG, Cordiali-Fei P, Cavaliere R, DiFilippo F, Quaranta V, Pellegrino MA, Ferrone S. Ia-like antigens on freshly explanted human malignant melanoma. Clin. Immunol. Immunopathol. 1981; 19: 250-9.
35. Wilson BS, Indiveri F, Pellegrino MA, Ferrone S. DR (Ia-like) antigens on human melanoma cells: Serological detection and immunological characterization. J. Exp. Med. 1979; 149: 658-68.
36. Ruiter DJ, Bergman W, Welvaart K, Scheffer E, Van Vloten WA, Russo C, Ferrone S. Immunohistochemical analysis of malignant melanomas and nevocellular nevi with monoclonal antibodies to distinct monomorphic determinants of HLA antigens. Cancer Res. 1984; 44: 3930-5.
37. Brown JP, Heurick RM, Hellström I, Hellström KE, Doolittle RF, Dreyer WJ. Human melanoma-associated antigen p97 is structurally and funtionally related to transferrin. Nature 1982; 296: 171-3.
38. Ruiter DJ, Van Muyen GNP, Warnaar SO. Monoclonal antibodies in diagnostic tumor pathology. In: Biotechnology in Diagnostics. H. Koprowski, S. Ferrone, A. Albertini (eds.). Elsevier Science Publ. BV, Amsterdam, 1985; pp. 31-43.

39. Hellström KE, Hellström I. Monoclonal anti-melanoma antibodies and their possible clinical use. In: Monoclonal antibodies for cancer detection and therapy. R.W. Baldwin, V.S. Byers (eds), Academic Press, London 1985; pp. 17-51.
40. Elder DE. Editorial: Distinguishing cancer and noncancer. J. Invest. Dermatol. 1985; 85: 1-3.
41. Dantas ME, Brown JP, Thomas MR, Robinson WA, Glode LM. Detection of melanoma cells in bone marrow using monoclonal antibodies. Cancer 1983; 52: 949-53.
42. Cochran AJ, Wen D-R, Herschman HR. Occult melanoma in lymph nodes detected by antiserum to S100 protein. Int. J. Cancer 1984; 34: 159-63.
43. Bröcker E-B, Suter L, Sorg C. HLA-DR antigen expression in primary melanomas of the skin. J. Invest. Dermatol. 1984; 82: 244-7.
44. Rode J, Dhillon AP. Neuron specific enolase and S100 protein as possible prognostic indicators in melanoma. Histopathology 1984; 8: 1041-52.
45. Van Duinen SG, Ruiter DJ, Bröcker E-B, Sorg C, Welvaart K, Ferrone S. Association of low level of HLA-ABC antigens or high level of Ia antigens in metastatic melanoma with a high grade of malignancy. J. Invest. Dermatol. 1984; 82: 558.
46. Van Duinen SG, Ruiter DJ, Ferrone S. Associated expression of HLA class I and class II antigens on melanoma cells in surgically removed metastases. J. Pathol. (in press)
47. Ruiter DJ, Van Duinen SG, Bröcker E-B, Schrier PI, Welvaart K, Ferrone S. Low level of class I or high level of class II Major Histocompatibility Complex antigens in metastatic melanoma is associated with a high grade of malignancy. Proc. Amer. Ass. Cancer Res. 1985; 26: 315.
48. Kaplan EL, Meier P. Non-parametric estimation from incomplete observations. J. Am. Statistic. Assoc. 1958; 53: 457-8.
49. Holden CA, Sanderson AR, MacDonald DM. Absence of human leukocyte antigen molecule in skin tumors and some cutaneous appendages: evidence using monoclonal antibodies. J. Am. Acad. Dermatol. 1983; 9: 867-71.
50. Kawabat SE, Bast Jr RC, Knapp RC; Bhan AK. Expression of major histocompatibility antigens and nature of inflammatory cellular infiltrate in ovarian neoplasms. Int. J. Cancer 1983; 32: 547-54.
51. Dennis JW, Donaghue TP, Carlow DA, Kerbel RS. Demonstration of a correlation between tumor cell H-2 antigen content, immunogenicity, and tumorigenicity using lectin-resistant tumor variants. Cancer Res. 1981; 41: 4010-9.
52. Schrier PI, Bernhards R, Vaessen RTMJ, Houweling A, Van der Eb AJ. Expression of class I major histocompatibility antigens switched off by highly oncogenic adenovirus 12 in transformed rat cells. Nature 1983; 305: 771-5.

53. Bernhards R, Schrier PI, Houweling A, Bos JL, Van der Eb AJ, Zijlstra M, Melief CJM. Tumorigenicity of cells transformed by adenovrius type 12 by evasion of T-cell immunity. Nature 1983; 305: 776-9.
54. Sanderson AR, Beverley PCL. Interferon, B2-microglobulin and immunoselection in the pathway to malignancy. Immunology Today 1983; 4: 211-3.
55. Ruiter DJ, Bröcker E-B, Jager M, Koning F, Schrier PI, Ferrone S. HLA-DR and HLA-DQ expression in cutaneous melanoma. J. Invest. Dermatol. 1985; 84: 442.
56. Fossati G, Taramelli D, Balsari A, Bogdanovich G, Andreola S, Parmiani G. Primary but not metastatic human melanomas expressing DR antigens stimulate autologous lymphocytes. Int. J. Cancer 1984; 33: 591-7.
57. Guerry IV D, Alexander MA, Herlyn MF, Zehngebot LM, Mitchell KF, Zmijewski CM. Lusk EJ. HLA-DR histocompatibility leukocyte antigens permit cultured human melanoma cells from early but not advanced disease to stimulate autologous lymphocytes. J. Clin. Invest. 1984; 73: 267-71.
58. Taramelli D, Fossati G, Balsari A, Marolda R, Parmiani G. The inhibition of lymphocyte stimulation by autologous human metatastic melanoma cells correlates with the expression of HLA-DR antigens on the tumor cells. Int. J. Cancer 1984; 34: 797-806.
59. Houghton AN, Eisinger M, Albino AP, Cairncross JG, Old LJ. Surface antigens of melanocytes and melanomas. J. Exp. Med. 1982; 156: 1755-66.
60. Galloway DR, McGabe RP, Pellegrino MA, Ferrone S, Reisfeld RA. Tumor associated antigens in spent medium of human melanoma cells: immunochemical characteristization with xenoantisera. J. Immunol. 1981; 126: 62-6.
61. Giacomini P, Veglia F, Fei PC, Rehle T, Natali PG, Ferrone S. Level of a membrane-bound high molecular weight melanoma-associated antigen and a cytoplasmic melanoma-associated antigen in surgically removed tissues and in sera from patients with melanoma. Cancer Res. 1984; 44: 1281-87.
62. Ross AH, Herlyn M, Ernst CS, Guerry D, Bennicelli J, Ghrist BFD, Atkinson B, Koprowsky H. Immuno-assay for melanoma-associated proteoglycan in the sera of patients using monoclonal and polyclonal antibodies. Cancer Res. 1984; 44: 4642-47.
63. Morgan AC, Crane MM, Rossen RD. Measurement of a monoclonal antibody-defined, melanoma-associated antigen in human sera: correlation of circulating antigen levels with tumor burden. J. Natl. Cancer Inst. 1984; 72: 243-48.
64. Oldham RK, Foon KA, Morgan AC, Woodhouse CS, Schroff RW, Abrams PG, Fer M, Schoenberger CS, Farral M, Kimball E, Sherwin SA. Monoclonal antibody therapy of malignant melanoma: in vivo localization in cutaneous metastasis after intravenous administration. J. Clin. Oncol. 1984; 2: 1235-44.

65. Schroff RW, Woodhouse CS, Foon KA, Oldham RK, Farrell MM, Klein RA, Morgan AC. Intratumor localization of monoclonal antibody in patients with melanoma treated with antibody to a 250,000-Dalton melanoma-associated antigen. J. Natl. Cancer Inst. 1985; 74: 299-306.
66. Buraggi GL, Callegar L, Mariani G, Cascinelli N, Attilli A, Bombardieri E, Terno G, Plassio G, Dovis M, Mazzuca N, Natali PG, Scassellati GA, Ferrone S. Imaging with ^{131}I-labeled monoclonal antibodies to a high-molecular-weight melanoma-associated antigen in patients with melanoma: efficacy of whole immunoglobulin and its F(ab')2 fragments. Cancer Res. 1985; 45: 3378-87.
67. Larson SM, Carrasquillo JA, McGuffin RW, Krohn KA, Ferens JM, Hill LO, Beaumier PL, Reynolds JC, Hellström K-E, Hellström I. Use of I-^{131}-labeled murine Fab against a high molecular weight antigen of human melanoma: preliminary experience. Radiol. 1985; 155: 487-92.
68. Halpern S, Dillman RO, Witztum KF, Shega JF, Hagan PL, Burrows WM, Dillman JB, Clutter ML, Sobol RE, Frinke JM, Bartholemew RM, David GS, Carlo DJ. Radio-immunodetection of melanoma utilizing ^{111}In 96,5 monoclonal antibody: a preliminary report. Radiol. 1985; 155: 493-99.
69. Murray JL, Rosenblum MG, Sobol RE, Bartholomew RM, Plager CE, Haynie TP, Jahns MF, Glenn HJ, Lamki L, Benjamin R, Papadopoulos N, Boddie AW, Frinke JM, David GS, Carlo DJ, Hersch EM. Radio-immuno-imaging in malignant melanoma with ^{111}In-labeled monoclonal antibody 96.5. Cancer Res. 1985; 45: 2376-81.
70. Larson SM, Carrasquillo JA, Krohn KA, McGuffin RW, Williams DL, Hellström I, Hellström K-E. Diagnostic imaging of malignant melanoma with radiolabeled antitumor antibodies. J. Amer. Med. Ass. (JAMA) 1983; 249: 811-12.
71. Larson SM, Carrasquillo JA, Krohn KA, Brown JP, McGuffin RW, Ferens JM, Graham MM, Hill LD, Beaumier PL, Hellström K-E, Hellström I. Localization of ^{131}I-labeled p97-specific Fab fragments in human melanoma as a basis for radiotherapy. J. Clin. Invest. 1983; 72: 2101-14.
72. Rosenblum MG, Murray JL, Haynie TP, Glenn HJ, Jahns MF, Benjamin RS, Frincke JM, Carlo DJ, Hersch EM. Pharmacokinetics of ^{111}IN-labeled anti p97 monoclona antibody in patients with metastatic malignant melanoma. Cancer Res. 1985; 45: 2382-86.
73. Houghton AN, Mintzer D, Cordon-Cardo C, Welt S, Fliegel B, Vadhan S, Carswell E, Melamed MR, Oettgen HF, Old LJ. Mouse monoclona IgG3 antibody detecting GD3 ganglioside: a phase I trial in patients with malignant melanoma. Proc. Natl. Acad. Sci. USA. 1985; 82: 1242-46.
74. Imai K, Pellegrino MA, Wilson BS, Ferrone S. Higher cytolytic efficiency of an IgG2a than of an IgG1 monoclonal antibody reacting with the same (or

spationally close) determinant on a human high-molecular-weight melanoma-associated antigen. Cell. Immunol. 1982; 72: 239-47.
75. Harper JR, Reisfeld RA. Inhibition of anchorage-independent growth of human melanoma cells by a monoclonalantibody to a chondroitin sulfate proteoglycan. J. Natl. Caner Inst. 1983; 71: 259-63.
76. Schulz G, Bumol TF, Reisfeld RA. Monoclonal antibody-directed effector cells selectively lyse human melanoma cells in vitro and in vivo. Proc. Natl. Acad. Sci. USA 1983; 80: 5407-11.
77. Bumol TF, Wang EQ, Reisfeld RA, Kaplan NO. Monoclonal antibody and an antibody-toxin conjugate to a cell surface proteoglycan of melanoma cells suppress in vivo tumor growth. Proc. Natl. Acad. Sci. USa, 1985; 80: 529-33.
78. Schulz G., Staffileno LK, Reisfeld RA, Dennert G. Eradication of established human melanoma tumors in nude mice by antibody-directed effects cells. J. Exp. Med. 1985; 161: 1315-25.
79. Herlyn D, Powe J, Ross AH, Herlyn M, Koprowski H. Inhibition of human tumor growth by IgG2a monoclonal antibodies correlates with antibody density on tumor cells. J. Immunol. 1985; 143: 1300-04.
80. Hellström I, Brankovan V, Hellström K-E. Strong antitumor activities of IgG3 antibodies to a human melanoma-associated ganglioside. Proc. Natl. Acad. Sci. USA, 1985; 82: 1499-02.
81. Katano M, Jien M, Irie RF. Human monoclonal antibody to ganglioside GD2-inhibited human melanoma xenograft. Eur. J. Cancer Clin. Oncol. 1984; 20: 1053-59.
82. Dippold WG, Knuth A, Meyer zum Buschenfelde K-H. Inhibition or human melanoma cell growth in vitro by monoclonal anti-GD3-ganglioside antibody. Cancer Res. 1984; 44: 806-10.
83. Cheresh DA, Honsik CJ, Staffileno LK, Jung G, Reisfeld RA. Disialoganglioside GD3 on human melanoma serves as a relevant target antigen for monoclonal antibody-mediated tumor cytolysis. Immunol. 1985; 82: 5155-59.
84. Lindmo T, Boven E, Mitchell JB, Morstyn G, Bunn PA. Specific killing of human melanoma cells by ^{125}I-labeled 9.2.27 monoclonal antibody. Cancer Res. 1985; 45: 5080-87.
85. Casellas P, Brown JP, Gros O, Gros P, Hellström I, Jansen FK, Poncelet P, Roncucci R, Vidal H, Hellström K-E. Human melanoma cells can be killed in vitro by an immunotoxin specific for melanoma-associated antigen p97. Int. J. Cancer 1982; 30: 437-43.
86. Matsui M, Nakanishi T, Noguchi T, Imai K, Yachi A, Ferrone S. Suppression of human melanoma growth in nude mice injected with anti high-molecular-weight melanoma-associated antigen monoclonal antibody 225.28S conjugated to purothionin. Jpn. J. Cancer Res. (Gann). 1985; 76: 119-23.

87. Kerbel RS, Man MS, Dexter D. A model of human cancer metastasis: extensive spontaneous and arteficial metastasis of a human pigmented melanoma and derived variant sublines in nude mice.J. Natl. Cancer Inst. 1984; 72: 93-101.
88. Lockshin A, Giovanella BS, de Ipolyi PD, Williams Jr. LJ, Mendoza JT, Ockyim S, Stehlin Jr. JS. Exceptional lethality for nude mice of cells derived from a primary human melanoma. Cancer Res. 1985; 45: 345-60.

9. MONOCLONAL ANTIBODIES IN BREAST TUMOR PATHOLOGY.

PH.C. HAGEMAN, J.L. PETERSE, J. HILKENS, J. HILGERS

1. INTRODUCTION

Several reviews have recently appeared on the use of monoclonal antibodies (MAbs) in breast cancer research and diagnosis (1, 2, 3, 4, 5). In particular the chapter written by Sloane (4) places immunohistochemistry of breast and breast tumors in the context of pathology and also underlines the continuing value of more conventional staining techniques. We will discuss the MAbs from a pathological/histological point of view, in respect to practical problems in diagnosis and as tools for fundamental research of structure and biology of the human mammary gland. Some but not all problems of unwanted cross-reactions have been solved since the introduction of monoclonal antibodies. Our preoccupation with routine diagnosis leads to an emphasis on the antibodies that detect antigens in formalin-fixed and paraffin-embedded tissues.

Special attention will be paid to some pitfalls that may lead to misinterpretation of immunohistochemical data.

2. TUMOR-ASSOCIATED ANTIGENS

2.1. Undefined immunogens

In recent years MAbs were generated against new and unknown antigens using as immunogens mammary tumor cells, cell membranes or human milk fat globule membranes (HMFGM) representing the mammary gland cells in their functional state. These antigens could be characterized after raising the corresponding antibodies. A list of the most important MAbs that were also used in immunohistochemical studies is given in Table 1. Although the starting material was an undefined immunogen, MAbs with the required reactivity have been obtained by careful selection procedures. Dairkee (6) used a breast tumor cell line as an immunogen and was able to select a MAb that was specific for myoepithelial cells.

The growing jungle of MAbs directed to HMFGM or tumor cell membranes will sort itself out in the next few years. Several of the antibodies appear to be directed to a family of high molecular weight mucus glycoproteins which are rather heterogeneous in size. Similar antigens were found irrespective of the chosen immunogen: HMFGM, fresh mammary tumor cells or cells of mammary tumor cell lines.

NCRC-11, HMFG-1, HMFG-2, M8 and anti-EMA (epithelial membrane antigen) (39) and probably also DF3 and 115D8 react with the same antigenic molecule which we have called MAM-6. We could not detect any difference in the tissue distribution of commercially available monoclonal anti-EMA (Dakopatts, Copenhagen) and 115D8. Reactions with the MAb to EMA are reported to have a distribution pattern identical to that of rabbit anti-EMA used by the same group of authors (40, 41, 42).

Most and probably all of these antibodies are directed to the carbohydrate moiety of the glycoprotein as was shown for EMA (42), HMFG-1 and HMFG-2, (9, 43) and 115D8 (44). The carbohydrate composition of these determinants has not been determined yet. Gooi et al. (12, 13) described the determinants of the antigen corresponding to antibody 67D11 and M18 as a combined Lewis^a-SSEA-1 carbohydrate sequence.

TABLE 1. Monoclonal antibodies raised to undefined immunogens reactive with formalin-fixed mammary tumors.

Immunogen	Antibody	Antigen	Reference
HMFGM	Mc5	high Mr glycoprotein	(7)
	HMFG-1	300-400 kD glycoprotein	(8, 9)
	HMFG-2	80-400 kD glycoprotein	(10)
	115D8	MAM-6, >400 kD glycoprotein	(11, 48)
	67D11, 115H10	MAM-3 high Mr glycoprotein	(11, 12, 13)
	M8	high Mr glycoprotein	(12, 13)
	M18	glycoprotein(I/MA epitope)	(14, 15, 16)
	M24	39-59 kD glycoprotein	(14, 15, 16)
	E29	EMA, 265-400 kD glycoprotein	(17, 18)
fresh mammary tumor cells or membranes	B 72.3	220-400 kD glycoprotein	(19, 20)
	NCRC-11	high Mr glycoprotein	(21, 22)
	DF3	290 kD glycoprotein	(23)
	3E 1.2	unidentified	(24)
mammary tumor in lymph node	MBE6[1]	cytoplasmic antigen	(25, 26)
	CF 29/34[1]	on poorly differentiated tumors	(27)
secondary breast tumor culture	312C-1	51 kD polypeptide in myoepithelium	(6)
mammary tumor cell lines:			
MCF-7	MBr1	high Mr glycolipid	(28, 29, 30
ZR-75-1	H59	glycoprotein in ER pos. tumors	(31, 32)
MCF-7 and SK-DR-3	F 36/22	glycoprotein	(33, 34)
MCF-7	24-17.2	100 kD molecule	(35)
MCF-7	AB/3	glycoprotein	(36)
MCF-7	3B18[2]	unidentified	(37)
	15A8[2]	unidentified	(37)
MCF-7	45-B/B3[2]	cytokeratin	(38)

[1] human monoclonal antibodies
[2] can not be used on formalin-fixed and embedded tissue

The work of Shimizu and Yamaughi contributed much to the knowledge of the molecules that carry the antigenic determinants for most of the MAbs raised against HMFGM (45). They isolated and characterized from HMFGM a high molecular weight glycoprotein called PAS-0. In amino acid, carbohydrate composition and in antigenic properties PAS-0 was similar to MAM-6 and also to EMA but was not identical (46). Recently Shimizu et al.

described an even more glycosylated glycoprotein (HMFG-A) isolated from human milk (47). PAS-0, EMA and MAM-6 have several antigenic determinants in common. 115D8 and M8 react with PAS-0 and MAM-6 (48), HMFG-1, HMFG-2 and M8 react both with PAS-0 and EMA. HMFG-A seems to be recognized by polyclonal anti-EMA only.

Several of the antibodies directed to the same or comparable glycoproteins exhibit a comparable reaction pattern on histological preparations: in normal mammary epithelium the reaction is predominantly apical, in mammary tumor cells the antigen is located in the cytoplasm, but can also be apical, depending on the differentiation of the tumor (46, for DF3; see for 115D8 Figure 1).

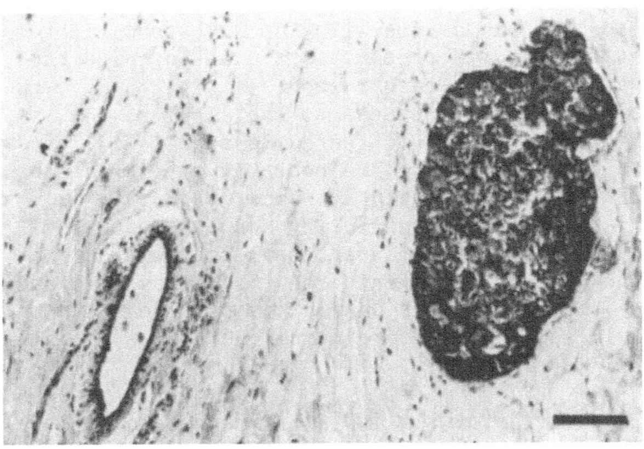

FIGURE 1. Apical staining of normal mammary duct and cytoplasmic reaction of tumor cells with antibody 115D8.
Bar: 100 µ

As a rule these MAbs react with epithelial cells of several organs and the tumors derived from them. For instance many react strongly with ovarian carcinomas: 115D8 (11, 49), F36/22 (34) and HMFG-1 and -2. Variations can be caused by slight differences in tissue sampling, fixation or differences in the immunoperoxidase procedure used. Some epitopes are represented more abundantly on certain tissues than others. HMFG-1 reacts preferentially with lactating mammary gland and normal breast, but is also positive on mammary tumors whereas HMFG-2 gives a stronger reaction on breast tumors, especially on metastatic carcinoma (9).

The distribution pattern of some MAbs has special characteristic features, of which a few will be discussed. Binding of antibody H59 is supposed to be correlated to the presence of estrogen and progesterone receptor in mammary carcinomas. The same phenomenon is reported for the MAbs that are discussed in paragraph 2.6 and 2.7.

3E 1-2 was different from most other antibodies because it was positive on all mammary tumors tested and did not react with mammary tumor cell lines (24).

Antibody 15A8 (37) recognizes a surface membrane antigen on frozen sections of mammary tumors and on normal mammary epithelium. 3B18 tested on the same group of tumors is reported to react with a cytoplasmic antigen in tumor cells with a more malignant appearance and to be absent from normal cells. The MAbs stain about 90% of the mammary tumors tested. Reaction of mammary tumors with DF3 (50) correlates with tumor differentiation, measured both as nuclear grade and histological grade and with the presence of ER.

2.2. Milk proteins

Casein and lactalbumin are rather unique constituents of milk and it was to be expected that these substances would be good markers to demonstrate the tissue origin of a breast tumor. More than sixty percent of mammary carcinomas and their metastases were reported to be positive for lactalbumin in immunoperoxidase tests using a polyclonal antiserum to lactalbumin (51, 52). Normal tissues other than breast and their tumors were negative. However, Bailey et al. (53) did not detect α-lactalbumin in breast tumors. This observation is in accordance with the results of Hall (54), who was not able to detect any messenger RNA for lactalbumin in breast carcinomas. The false positive reactions with the antiserum might be caused by the contamination of lactalbumin preparations used to raise the polyclonal antisera by a substance that co-electrophoreses with prelactalbumin and that cross-reacts with antisera to lactalbumin. The value of this molecule as a marker is as yet not established. It will be interesting to know the tissue distribution of the recently developed MAb to a cross-reacting determinant of α-lactalbumin and casein (55).

Tests for casein in mammary tumors gave conflicting results because casein preparations used for the production of polyclonal antisera can be contaminated with traces of the highly immunogenic EMA (56). MAbs to casein have been produced now (55, 57) but at present casein has been demonstrated in the normal mammary gland only, but not in carcinomas (58).

2.3. Contractile proteins

Antisera to the contractile proteins myosin and actin have been used to study myoepithelial cells, in which these proteins are highly expressed. In the majority of these studies (59, 60, 61) polyclonal sera have been used but recently MAbs to myosin and actin have become commercially available (Eurodiagnostics, Apeldoorn, The Netherlands). In contrast to several of the polyclonal sera the MAbs react on cryosections only.

2.4. Basal membrane components

Disruption of the basal membrane separating epithelial and myoepithelial cells in the normal breast from the surrounding stroma, is an important feature in tumor pathology. The basal membrane components, type IV collagen, laminin, heparan sulphate proteoglycan and fibronectin have been identified in sections of human breast tissue (59, 60, 61, 62, 63, 64) mainly using polyclonal sera. Several MAbs against these components are now available (for collagen IV, see Carter (65). Laminin binds much stronger to the receptors of breast carcinoma cells than to normal breast. Recently a MAb to the 67 kD laminin receptor protein has been developed (66, 67). Mammary carcinoma cells in formalin-fixed tissue showed more binding to this MAb than cells of normal breast tissue or benign lesions.

2.5. Oncofetal antigens

Work on the tissue distribution of carcinoembryonic antigen (CEA) has been hampered by the fact that this glycoprotein has many epitopes in common with other antigens such as the Non-Specific Cross-reacting Antigens I and II, present in splenic thymocytes and in pneumocytes of the lung and with the biliary protein in bile ducts. Methods to remove the cross-reactivity from polyclonal sera have been described (68, 69) and will be discussed in chapter 4. Many MAbs to CEA detect these cross-reacting molecules. Very promising seems Parlam-4 (Eurodiagnostics, Apeldoorn, The Netherlands) a MAb produced by Verstijnen et al. (70). In preliminary experiments on sections of formalin-fixed and embedded tissues we found no reaction on spleen or in granulocytes, bile canaliculi or lung tissue, whereas colon carcinomas were positive. On frozen sections granulocytes show some reaction with Parlam-4. Our results on paraffin sections are even more satisfactory than those reported by Verstijnen, probably because his pre-incubation of the tissue sections with trypsin uncovers some cross-reacting epitopes on bile ducts and lung tissue.

2.6. Estrogen receptors

The presence of functional estrogen receptor (ER) molecules is an important prognostic factor especially for the prediction of the response of mammary carcinoma patients to hormonal treatment. Several methods exist for the quantitative measurement of ER in cytosols of which the dextran-coated charcoal analysis is the most generally used. As some tissue samples are too small for biochemical detection methods and as the distribution of ER-positive and -negative cells in a tissue might give additional information, methods have been developed to detect ER in histological sections. Reviews on the use of fluorescein-labeled steroids to detect ER or the use of antibodies to detect estrogens bound to ER (71, 72, 73) show that these methods do not yield satisfactory results and can not replace biochemical detection of ER in cytosols. The labeled steroids bind as well to the high affinity ER as to other more abundant intracellular proteins that have a low affinity but a high capacity to bind estrogen.

More promising than the work with labeled steroids seem the MAbs to ER that detect the presence of the ER antigen. Green et al. (74) developed 5 rat MAbs to ER from the human mammary tumor cell line MCF-7. All antibodies detected ER in the nuclei of mammary carcinoma cells in cryosections (75) and not in the cytoplasm (Figure 2).

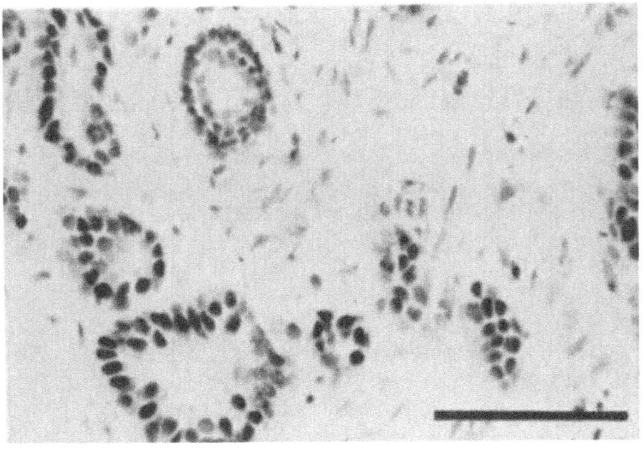

FIGURE 2. Nuclear staining of tumor cells in ER-positive breast tumor with a MAb to ER. Bar: 100 μ

The nuclear localization seemed remarkable because the bulk of functional ER was believed to be present in the cytosol, but later data suggest that free receptor resides in the nucleus and that localization in the cytosol is an artefact (76). A good correlation between the results obtained with these MAbs and the dextran coated charcoal detection of ER in cytosols is reported (77) but the more important correlation between immunohistochemical detection of ER and clinical response to hormone treatment remains to be proven. A recent studies (78, 79) indicate that in a small series of patients with metastatic breast cancer who received hormonal therapy a good correlation existed of positive reactions of the tumor with a MAb to ER and objective clinical response to the therapy.

Two MAbs of this set (Abbott, North Chicago, USA) (80, 81, 82) have been used to detect ER in formalin-fixed and embedded material. When the material was fixed in buffered formalin at 4° C the staining for ER correlated well with that on frozen sections or with the ER content in the respective tumor determined by the dextran-coated charcoal assay.

2.7. Estrogen-regulated proteins

MAbs to ER of myometrium react with a cytosol estradiol receptor associated antigen in human breast tumor tissue. The reaction product is found in the cytoplasm instead of the nucleus (83). The reacting antigen is not ER but a closely related antigen (84). The antigen can be detected in Carnoy- or methacarn-fixed and embedded tissue.

Search for ER-related proteins can be useful because they might be present in larger amounts than ER itself and they indicate that cells are responding to estrogen and that ER is functional. Several MAbs to ER-related proteins are listed in Table 2.

TABLE 2. Monoclonal antibodies to estrogen receptor-related proteins

Immunogen	Antigen	Reactive on frozen or embedded tissue	Tissue	Author
52 kD glycoprotein from MCF-7 cells	52 kD cytoplasmic glycoprotein	frozen	breast tumor not on normal breast	(85, 86)
24 kD protein from MCF-7 cells	24 kD cytoplasmic protein	embedded	breast tumor occasionally normal breast	(87, 88)
MCF-7 cells	54 kD cellular prot. 56 kD cellular prot. 52 kD extra-cellular protein	embedded	breast tumor	(89)
ER myometrium	29 kD ER-related cytoplasmic antigen	embedded	ER pos.tumor less in normal breast	(83, 84)
ZR 75-1 cell line	cell surface glycoprot. of 30kD peptides	frozen and embedded	ER pos.tumor	(32)

2.8 Miscellaneous antigens

Ectopic hormones such as β-human chorion gonadotrophin (90), pregnancy specific β-1-glycoprotein (91, 92, 93) and pregnancy-associated plasma protein A (94) have been immunohistochemically demonstrated in sections of formalin-fixed breast cancer tissue. Although these antigens have been identified by polyclonal antisera the antigens are mentioned because some of them might be useful markers for prognosis.

Transferrin receptor is a cell surface protein that has been found in breast tumor cells and that is related to cell proliferation (95). To our knowledge no antisera have been prepared yet to detect transferrin receptor in formalin-fixed material.

The production of MAbs to onc gene products and to cytoskeletal proteins and the tissue distribution of the corresponding antigens is described in chapters 16 and 5 of this volume.

3. APPLICATION OF MABS TO PATHOLOGICAL PROBLEMS

3.1. Identification of a tumor as metastasis of mammary carcinoma

To distinguish carcinoma from tumors of non-epithelial origina a panel of antibodies should be used, containing a MAb reacting with widely distributed keratin epitopes, that can be recognized on formalin-fixed material and a MAb directed to one of the EMA-like antigens. The MAb to keratin should recognize keratin 8, 18 and 19, as these are present in mammary tumors (96). Such an antibody is CAM 5.2 of Makin et al. (97).

Another 'pan-keratin' reagent consists of a mixture of the antibodies AE1 and AE3 recognizing most keratin classes (98). Tissues have to be pretreated with trypsin to obtain optimal reactivity with several antibodies to keratin (99). Many antibodies to keratins only react on frozen material. Several antigenic determinants seem to be preserved better after methacarn-fixation of the tissue than in formalin (60, 100). The MAb directed to the EMA-like antigen could be chosen from Table 1, for instance HMFG-2, 115D8 or E29 (101), since these antibodies react with a high percentage of mammary tumor cells in nearly all mammary tumors (Table 3).

Antibodies to EMA-like antigens generally have the advantage that they react with formalin-fixed tissue without needing pretreatment of the section with trypsin for optimal results. MBr1 would be another option but this antibody does not react with all mammary tumors (30, 102). Gatter and Mason used a panel of antibodies including HMFG-1 and HMFG-2 (103) or the anti-EMA E 29 (104) as a tool for diagnosis of cancer of unknown origin. One could argue whether MAbs directed to keratins are preferable to those reacting with EMA-like substances. In a study on the efficiency to recognize epithelial tumors Pinkus et al. (98) compared a mixture of the two anti-keratins AE1 and AE3 with polyclonal and monoclonal anti-EMA. In the majority of cases (including all breast cancer cases) both groups of markers yielded comparable results. In 33% of their cases keratins were superior to EMA as a tumor marker and in 9% anti-EMA detected the carcinoma cells, whereas the anti-keratins did not. It seems therefore advisable to use both types of antibodies in a diagnostic panel (Figure 3 and 4), that should contain in addition MAbs to other tissue types (anti-vimentin, antibodies directed to melanoma- and to lymphoma-associated antigens).

Most MAbs from Table 1 react in addition to mammary carcinomas also with carcinomas from other sites.

Anti-EMA, 115D8 and some other antibodies from Table 1 react occasionally with T cell lymphoma and anti-EMA also with histiocytic lymphomas and plasmacytoma (101). Occasional plasma cells in cases of Hodgkin's disease may exhibit staining with anti-EMA.

TABLE 3. Immunoreactivity for MAM-6 detected with MAb 115D8 on formalin-fixed and embedded tumor tissues of various sites

	Positive	Negative
tumors[1]		
mammary carcinomas	119	1
Paget's disease of the nipple	10	0
Paget's disease of the vulva	1	0
lung carcinomas, different types	34	6
colorectal carcinomas	70	2
gastric carcinomas	15	2
renal carcinomas	4	0
ovarian carcinomas (epithelial), different types	89	0
cervical carcinomas	7	2
endometrial carcinomas	9	0
bladder carcinomas	3	0
prostate carcinomas	1	3
seminomas	0	6
carcinoma of the thyroid (follicular or papillary)	5	0
medullary carcinoma of the thyroid	0	3
basal cell carcinomas	0	2
melanomas[2]	0	49
nevocellular nevi	0	7
clear cell sarcomas	0	2
neuroblastomas and ganglioneuroblastomas	0	8
astrocytomas	0	42
sarcomas[3]	2	8
synoviosarcomas	4	1
epitheloid sarcomas	2	0
lymphomas (B cell)	0	10
histiocytic tumors	3	0
carcinoids	5	6

[1] primary tumors or metastases
[2] small positive foci in some cells of melanoma
[3] slight reactivity in one lymphangiosarcoma

3.2. Recognition of metastatic tumor cells in peritoneal and ascites fluids, bone marrow and lymph nodes

As in most of these cases the tissue of origin of these metastases is already known, the tissue specificity of the MAb is less important. The MAb should not react with non-tumorous cells in fluids or bone marrow. Antibodies to EMA and EMA-related substances have been widely used for this purpose (105, 106, 107, 108, 109, 110, 111). Redding et al. (112) reported EMA-positive cells in the bone marrow of 30% of mammary carcinoma patients.

In such tests it is imperative that the morphology of the cells is well preserved, to allow the cytologist to check the nature of the antigen-positive cells, because several MAbs to mammary tumor antigens cross-react with plasma cells and other components of bone marrow (113, 114, 115, 116). We regularly find cross-reaction of 115D8 with plasma cells in bone marrow. Because the biological significance of single tumor cells in bone marrow is as yet uncertain, we have to await the value of these observations. In a few publications the number of tumor cells might be overestimated because in samples with poor morphology EMA-positive plasma cells might be mistaken for tumor cells.

The MAbs H59 and H72, reactive with breast cancer bind to sinus histiocytes and perivascular cells in uninvolved hyperplastic lymph nodes of breast cancer patients and in hyperplastic nodes of mastectomy specimens without tumor. Since these antibodies do not react with normal or reactive

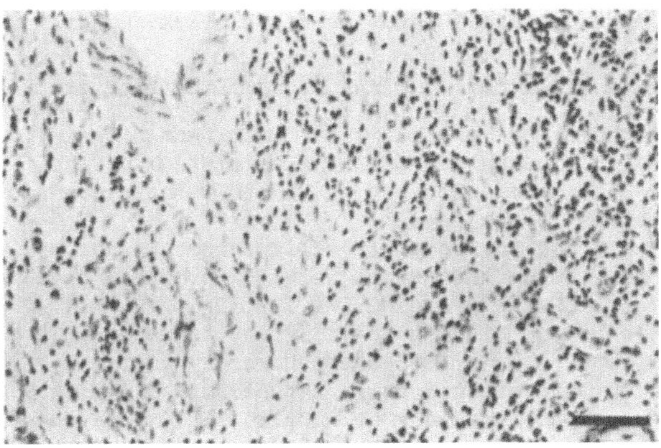

FIGURE 3. Polyclonal antikeratin stains only slightly carcinoma cells in a breast cancer mimicking lymphoma. Bar: 100 µ

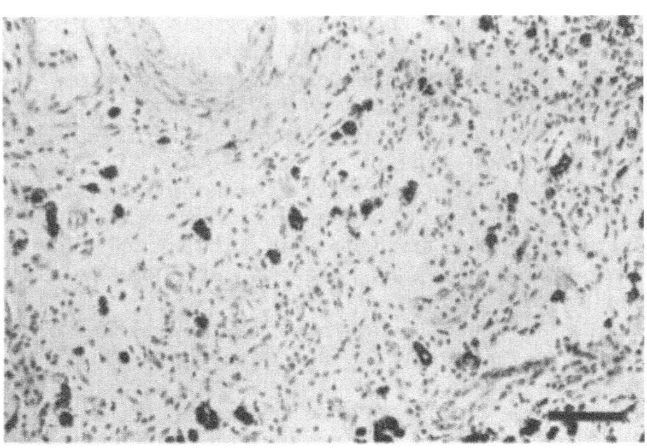

FIGURE 4. Carcinoma cells in the same preparation as in figure 3 can be distinguished easily with MAb 115D8. Bar: 100 µ

lymphoid cells Hendler and House (117) suggest that these lymph node cells are able to present breast antigens. The number of these cells in the uninvolved node correlated with the pathological stage. Moreover, Hendler and House observed single cells in the lymph node with a very strong binding of the antibody. These cells could not be identified morphologically as tumor cells.

The detection of mammary tumor cells in effusion fluids can be hampered by reactions of MAbs with reactive mesothelial cells. Mariani-Costantini reports that MBr1 does not show such cross-reactions, but immunocytology using MBr1 can miss tumor positive cases. Mènard (105) found MBr1-positive cells in 60% of pleural and peritoneal fluids that were considered positive for mammary carcinoma cells by conventional cytology. We have encountered the same dilemma when MAbs to MAM-6, for instance 115D8 or to MAM-3 (115H10) are used to detect tumor cells in effusion fluids. The MAb 115H10 does not react on reactive mesothelium but might miss several tumor cases since it reacts only with 60% of the breast tumors, whereas 115D8 seldom fails to react on tumor cells but can stain reactive mesothelium.

3.3. Use of MAbs in differential diagnosis of malignant and benign breast lesions

The value of MAbs in distinghuishing (pre)malignant from benign breast lesions has not been very great, illustrating that the assumption of the existence of a specific tumor antigen probably is a too simple approach to one of the major problems of breast pathology.

The CA1 antibody that was selected to recognize malignant cells has no specificity for malignant breast tissue and reacts as well on normal breast tissue (118, 119). The human MAbs CF 29/34 and MB E/6 (25, 26, 27) are reported to have strong preference for binding to malignant mammary cells as opposed to normal breast tissue. 3 B 18 (37) seems to be a tumor-specific MAb that can be used on cryosections only. Cytoplasmic staining with anti-CEA is a marker for malignant mammary cells (120, 121) but the value of this marker is limited because several mammary tumors are negative for CEA or contain only a small number of positive cells (see chapter 4 of this volume).

Reactions of MAbs to epithelial markers (keratin), myoepithelial cells (actin and myosin) and to components of the basement membrane (mainly laminin and collagen IV) can give information on the histogenesis of breast carcinoma and can be used as an aid for the differential diagnosis of proliferative and malignant breast lesions. Benign proliferative lesions (adenosis, epitheliosis and intraductal papilloma) normally consist both of myoepithelial and epithelial cells that are often arranged in bilayers. Carcinoma in situ and papillary carcinoma consist of epithelial cells only (60, 61, 122, 123). Papotti observed in cases of multiple ductal papillomas the presence of areas lacking myoepithelium. These areas contained CEA-positive cells that were arranged as ductal carcinoma in situ. This could be an example of a proliferative lesion developing into a carcinoma is a rare event in the breast according to Azzopardi (124).

Adenosis can be distinguished from tubular carcinoma by the absence of myoepithelial cells in the latter, revealed by absence of myoepithelial markers.

Destruction of basement membrane may be considered as marker to distinguish invasive from in situ carcinomas. Destruction of the basement membrane can be observed using antibody to type IV collagen. However, integrity of the basal lamina can not be considered as a reliable indicator for the absence of metastic tumor. Gusterson showed that basement membrane was present in highly differentiated infiltrating carcinoma (60). Using polyclonal and monoclonal antibodies to type IV collagen a redevelopment of the basal lamina could be demonstrated around invasive primary tumors and around tumor metastases in brain (125) and in lymph nodes (65) for melanoma and several types of carcinomas. The basement membrane around invasive tumors seems to be somewhat irregular as focal abnormalities in the appearance of the basement membrane, such as thickening and aggregation, are observed.

The fact that tumor cells show a diffuse cytoplasmic reaction with many MAbs from Table 1 as opposed to the apical staining in normal tissue and benign lesions has no application in diagnosis because more differentiated parts of malignancies can also show an apical reaction. The MAbs Ba16 and Ba17 produced to keratin 19 (126, 127) have an interesting heterogeneous reaction pattern on frozen sections of normal mammary tissue and react uniformly positive on breast tumors. However, as frequently normal breast tissue also reacts homogeneously positive, these MAbs are not useful as indicators of malignancy.

3.4. Use of MAbs in the assessment of prognosis in breast cancer

Numerous are the attempts to identify mammary tumor types that are different in respect to prognosis or respond differently to treatment. Until now immunohistochemistry has made only a small contribution compared with other already existing prognostic indicators such as tumor size, histological grade and lymph node status. In some studies a correlation has been sought between the reaction of an antigen with other prognostic indicators, or a correlation with survival or disease free interval. Only the latter two approaches can yield new independent prognostic indicators.

Presence of CEA in the tumor tissue was mentioned as indicator for tumor metastases and lower survival rate in breast cancer patients (128, 129). The study was performed with polyclonal anti-CEA and several other groups have not been able to reproduce the results (130, 131).

Loss of blood group isoantigens of the ABH group on mammary tumors had no correlation with tumor recurrence, recurrence-free interval or development/incidence of metastases (132). Even if quantitative differences in antigen expression would exist in different subtypes of tumors, immunohistochemistry is not the method of choice to detect it.

Other studies that failed to show a relation between marker expression and prognosis include antibodies to casein, α-lactalbumin, pregnancy specific β-1-glycoprotein, secretory component, placental lactogen, α-HCG, β-HCG and receptor for peanut agglutinin (131, 133). Unfortunately the use of polyclonal antibodies for the detection of these markers makes the outcome of some of these studies less reliable.

The absence of reactivity of the MAb HMFG-1 with breast carcinomas was associated with unfavorable prognosis and patients whose tumor showed staining, particularly extracellular staining (outside the cell in tube-like spaces) had a very long recurrence-free period (134). A comparable study (135) using the same MAbs did not confirm these data.

Ellis (136) reported a strong relationship between the intensity of staining of mammary tumor tissue with MAb NCRC-11, an antibody that follows the staining pattern of most other antibodies to HMFGM, and survival of the patients. This prognostic factor seemed to be independent of other factors such as lymph node status or presence of estrogen receptor in the tumor. An extention of this study by the same group did not yield consistent results.

Rasmussen et al. (137) observed a correlation between the presence of epitopes of the MAM-3 antigen and survival, but the presence of these epitopes was related to other prognostic factors such as estrogen receptor status and grade of anaplasia and could not add additional information to the clinical prognostic factors.

In a study on 30 patients with stage II breast carcinoma receiving the same chemotherapy treatment, presence in the tumor of pregnancy-associated plasma protein A strongly correlated with early recurrence ($p<0.0005$) and with overall recurrence (94). This promising result is observed in a small series of patients, and a larger number of mammary tumors will have to be tested with a well-defined antibody, preferentially a MAb, to confirm these results.

3.5 Histogenesis of special types of mammary carcinomas

3.5.1. Paget's disease of the nipple (MP). The origin of the tumor cells in MP is not certain, but some authors favor an intra-epidermal origin of the tumor cells while others suppose that malignant cells of an underlying mammary carcinoma invade the epidermis from below (124). MP cells proved to be positive with the MAbs HMFG-1 and HMFG-2 (138, 139) and with antikeratin LE612, that does not react with epidermal cells, but is positive on mammary tumors. The antikeratins K20 and K92 that were positive on epidermal keratinocytes were negative on mammary Paget cells. This confirms older work of Bussolati and Pick (140) who reported positive reactions both in mammary tumors and in MP with polyclonal anti-casein, probably containing antibodies to EMA-like substances (56). These combined data suggest that MP cells are derived from the underlying carcinoma. The same conclusion can be made form the work of Mariano-Costantini et al. (141) who reported positive reaction of MBr1,with cells in a high percentage of MP cases. The reaction of the Paget cells was often but not always concordant with the reaction of the underlying carcinoma with MBr1. We found positive reactions with 115D8 (positive on mammary carcinoma, negative on melanoma) on all MP cases we tested (Figure 5) and we did not find MP cells positive with NKI/C3, an antibody raised against membranes of a melanoma cell line and positive with 90% of formalin-fixed and paraplast embedded melanoma metastases (142).

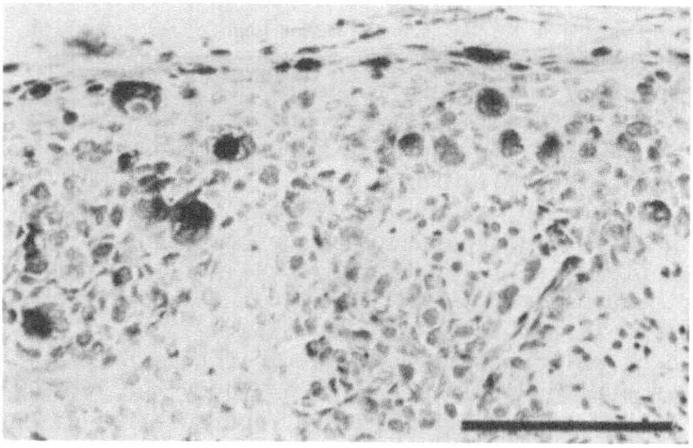

FIGURE 5. Reactivity of Paget cells with antibody 115D8. Bar: 100 μ

A different point of view is presented by Nagle et al. (143). They detected in normal nipple epithelium nests of clear cells that reacted with anticytokeratin KA4. This MAb was positive on MP, luminal cells of mammary ducti and lobuli but was negative on melanoma and intrafollicular stratified squamous epithelium. The authors propose that the KA4 positive clear cells in the normal nipple epithelium represent embryonal cell nests. This last finding supports the view of Azzopardi (124) that most evidence points to a migration of cells of the underlying carcinoma into the epidermis of the nipple, but that at least some Paget tumor cells might have an in situ origin. This would mean that some cases of Paget's disease of the nipple may have a different histogenesis.

3.5.2. Carcinosarcoma of the breast. Carcinosarcomas contain malignant cells of both epithelial and mesenchymal appearance. Most tumors presented as carcinosarcomas seem to be carcinomas with metaplasia (144). The epithelial elements in these tumors react with MAbs to epithelial elements of the breast (see positive reaction with 115D8 in Figure 6), the metaplastic dedifferentiated spindle-cell component reacts with anti-vimentin.

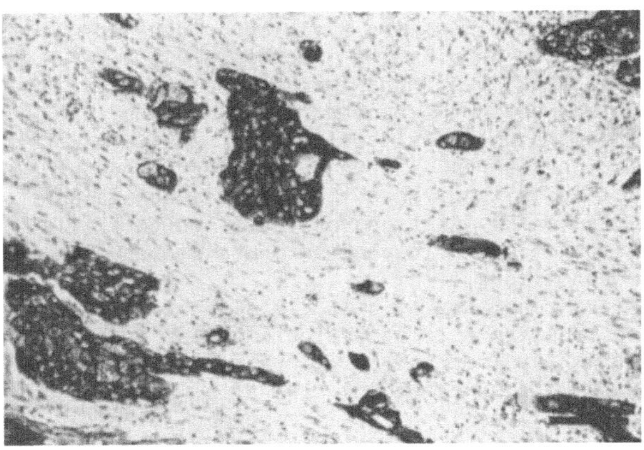

FIGURE 6. 115D8 stains epithelial cells in a metaplastic carcinoma of the breast. Bar: 100 µ

Some authors suggest (145) that the epithelial and mesenchymal components of carcinosarcoma are derived from different cell types. This point is difficult to prove because the mesenchymal marker vimentin is a rather unspecific tool to prove the origin of cells and because of the rare occurrence of the carcinosarcomas of the breast.

3.5.3. Endocrine mammary tumors. Cross et al. (146) studied cases of ductal carcinoma in situ of the breast, some of which had light-microscopical features that suggested an endocrine tumor. The tumors were positive for neuronspecific enolase and contained argyrophilic cells. Several of the tumors reacted positively with antisera to peptide hormones. Bussolati et al. (147) found in argyrophilic breast carcinomas but not in other breast carcinomas a positive reaction with the MAb LK2H10 directed against human chromogranin. This MAb reacts with most carcinoid tumors. In normal breast tissue rare chromogranin-positive cells were observed. These data support the view that some of the argyrophilic breast carcinomas are originating from cells belonging to the diffuse neuroendocrine (APUD) system (see chapter 4 of this volume).

4. FUTURE DEVELOPMENTS

In the near future the structure and the synthesis of the glycoproteins in HMFGM and breast cells will be elucidated. This will allow a better comparison between the numerous MAbs, directed to EMA-like substances and will give information on the occurrence and function of the epitopes detected by these MAbs. Reactions of these MAbs and of many antikeratins with well-defined specificity will improve the characterization of the cell types in the mammary gland. The ability of detection of the tissue origin of a tumor will be improved. For example, the MAbs of White et al. (37) seem to recognize rather breast tumor specific antigens.

More antibodies will be developed that recognize antigens in formalin-fixed and paraffin embedded tissue. On the other hand the choice of other fixation methods (60, 61) and the use of embedding methods that employ a lower temperature, such as replacing paraffin by polyester wax (148) will increase the number of MAbs that can be used on fixed material. It might be useful to go further into the possibilities of pregnancy-associated plasma protein A and other markers for prognosis, but it is of utmost importance to use better characterized antibodies.

As according to Baak et al. (149) mitotic activity is a good prognostic factor, antibodies reacting with cells that are dividing or that are at least not in G_0 phase could prove to be of great importance (150, 151, 152). In this respect the possibilities of MAbs against the transferrin receptor as prognostic indicators are not exhausted. The presence of transferrin receptor on cell membranes is related to cell proliferation and in lymphomas a strong correlation was found between transferrin receptor and malignancy grading (153). The drawback that the MAbs raised against transferrin receptor can be used on cryosections only will be partially overcome because a growing number of pathology departments store at least a part of their specimen as frozen tissue.

MAbs that react with substances related to cell division will allow the study of the expression of antigens related to the cell cycle. We may even expect that the lack of quantitative immunohistologic data will be overcome in the future. New developments in flow cytometry will allow simultaneous quantitation of different antigens even in paraffin-embedded pathology material, thus opening the possibility of objective measurements of the expression of antigens in tumor cell populations (154).

5. REFERENCES

1. Schlom J, Colcher D, Horan Hand P, Greiner J, Wunderlich D, Weeks M, Fisher PB, Noguchi P, Pestka S, Kufe D. Monoclonal antibodies reactive with breast tumor-associated antigens. Adv Cancer Res 1985; 43: 143-173.
2. Neville AM, Foster C, Redding H, Coombes RC. Monoclonal antibodies as probes in human breast disorders. In: Oncodevelopmental Biology and Medicine. Ann NY Ac Sci 1983; 417: 251-261.
3. Ceriani RL(ed): Monoclonal antibodies and breast cancer. Martinus Nijhoff Publ Boston/Dordrecht/Lancaster. 1984.
4. Sloane JP(ed): Biopsy pathology of the breast. London, Chapman and Hall 1985; 284.
5. Hageman Ph, Peterse JL. New approaches to the pathology of breast cancer; can immunohistochemistry add new information? In: Breast Cancer: Origins, detection and treatment. Rich MA, Hager J, Taylor-Papadimitriou J (eds). Martinus Nijhoff, Boston. 1986, pp. 94-111.
6. Dairkee SH, Blayney C, Smith HS, Hackett A. Monoclonal antibody that defines human myoepithelium. Proc Natl Acad Sci 1985; 82: 7409-7413.
7. Ceriani RL, Peterson JA, Lee JY, Moncada R, Blank EW. Characterization of cell surface antigens of normal human mammary epithelial cells with monoclonal antibodies. Somat Cell Genet 1983; 9: 415-427.
8. Arklie J, Taylor-Papadimitriou J, Bodmer W, Egan M, Millis R. Differentiation antigens expressed by epithelial cells in the lactating breast are also detectable in breast cancers. Int J Cancer 1981; 28: 23-30.
9. Burchell J, Durbin H, Taylor-Papadimitriou J. Complexity of expression of antigenic determinants recognized by monoclonal antibodies HMFG-1 and HMFG-2 in normal and malignant human mammary epithelial cells. J Immunol 1983; 131: 508-513.
10. Taylor-Papadimitriou J, Peterson JA, Arklie J, Burchell J, Ceriani RL, Bodmer WF. Monoclonal antibodies to epithelium-specific components of the human milk fat globule membrane: production and reaction with cells in culture. Int J Cancer 1981; 28: 17-21.
11. Hilkens J, Buys F, Hilgers J, Hageman Ph, Calafat J, Sonnenberg A, Van der Valk M. Monoclonal antibodies against human milk fat globule membranes detecting differentiation antigens of the mammary gland and its tumors. Int J Cancer 1984; 34: 197-206.
12. Gooi HC, Jones NJ, Hounsell EF, Scudden P, Hilkens J, Hilgers J, Feizi T. Novel antigenic specificity involving the blood group antigen Le^a, in combination with oncodevelopmental antigen SSEA-1, recognized by two monoclonal antibodies to human milk fat globule membranes. Biochem Biophys Res Comm 1985; 131: 543-550.
13. Gooi HC, Jones NJ, Hilkens J, Hilgers J, Feizi T. Lewis blood group-related specificities of monoclonal antibodies designated Mam-3a, b and c against human milk fat globule membranes. Glycoconjugate J 1985; 2: 409.
14. Foster CS, Edwards PAW, Dinsdale EA, Neville AM. Monoclonal antibodies to the human mammary gland. 1. Distribution of determinants in non-neoplastic mammary and extra mammary tissues. Virchows Arch (Pathol Anat) 1982; 394: 279-293.
15. Foster CS, Dinsdale EA, Edwards PAW, Neville AM. Monoclonal antibodies to the human mammary gland. 2. Distribution of determinants in breast carcinomas. Virchows Arch (Pathol Anat) 1982; 394: 295-305.
16. Foster CS, Neville AM. Monoclonal antibodies to the human mammary gland. III. Monoclonal antibody LICR-LON-M16 identifies impaired

expression and excess sialylation of the I (Ma) cell surface antigen by primary breast carcinoma cells. Hum Pathol 1984; 15: 502-513.
17. Cordell J, Richardson TC, Pulford KAF, Ghosh AK, Gatter KC, Heyderman E, Mason DY. Production of monoclonal antibodies against human epithelial membrane antigen for use in diagnostic immunocytochemistry. Br J Cancer 1985; 52: 347-354.
18. Heyderman E, Strudley I, Powell G, Richardson TC, Cordell JL, Mason DY. A new monoclonal antibody to epithelial membrane antigen (EMA)-E29. A comparison of its immunocytochemical reactivity with polyclonal anti-EMA and with another monoclonal antibody, HMFG-2. Br J Cancer 1985; 52: 355-361.
19. Colcher D, Hand PH, Nuti M, Schlom J. A spectrum of monoclonal antibodies reactive with human mammary tumor cells. Proc Natl Acad Sci 1981; 78: 3199-3203.
20. Nuti M, Teramoto YA, Mariani-Costantini R, Horan Hand P, Colcher D, Schlom J. A monoclonal antibody (B 72.3) defines patterns of distribution of a novel tumor-associated antigen in human mammary carcinoma cell-populations. Int J Cancer 1982; 29: 539-545.
21. Ellis IO, Robbins RA, Elston CW, Blamey RW, Ferry B, Baldwin RW. A monoclonal antibody NCRC-11 raised to human breast carcinoma: Production and immunohistological characterization. Histopathology 1984; 8: 501-516.
22. Price MR, Edwards S, Owainati O, Bullock JE, Ferry B, Robbins RA, Baldwin RW. Multiple epitopes on a human breast carcinoma-associated antigen. Int J Cancer 1985; 36: 567-574.
23. Kufe D, Inghirami G, Abe M, Hayes D, Justi-Wheeler H, Schlom J. Differential reactivity of a novel monoclonal antibody (DF3) with human malignant versus benign breast tumors. Hybridoma 1984; 3: 223-232.
24. Stacker SA, Thompson C, Riglar C, McKenzie IFC. A new breast carcinoma antigen defined by a monoclonal antibody. J Natl Cancer Inst 1985; 75: 801-811.
25. Schlom J, Wunderlich D, Teramoto YA. Generation of human monoclonal antibodies reactive with human mammary carcinoma cells. Proc Natl Acad Sci 1980; 77: 6841-6845.
26. Teramoto YA, Mariani R, Wunderlich D, Schlom J. The immunohistochemical reactivity of a human monoclonal antibody with tissue sections of human mammary tumors. Cancer 1982; 50: 241-249.
27. Imam A, Drushella MM, Taylor CR, Tökès ZA. Generation and immunohistological characterization of human monoclonal antibodies to mammary carcinoma cells. Cancer Res 1985; 45: 263-271.
28. Mènard S, Tagliabue E, Canevari S, Fossati G, Colnaghi MI.Generation of monoclonal antibodies reacting with normal and cancer cells of human breast. Cancer Res 1983; 43: 1295-1300.
29. Canevari S, Fossati G, Balsari A, Sonnino S, Colnaghi MI. Immunochemical analysis of the determinant recognized by a monoclonal antibody (MBr1) which specifically binds to human mammary epithelial cells. Cancer Res 1983; 43: 1301-1305.
30. Mariani-Costantini R, Colnaghi MI, Leoni F, Mènard S, Cerasoli S, Rilke F. Immunohistochemical reactivity of a monoclonal antibody prepared against human breast carcinoma. Virchows Arch (Pathol Anat) 1984; 402: 389-404.
31. Yuan D, Hendler FJ, Vitetta ES. Characterization of a monoclonal antibody reactive with a subset of human breast tumors. J Natl Cancer Inst 1982; 68: 719-728.

32. Hendler FJ, Yuan D. Relationship of monoclonal antibody binding to estrogen en progesterone receptor content in breast cancer. Cancer Res 1985; 45: 421-429.
33. Papsidero LD, Croghan GA, O'Connell MH, Valenzuela LA, Nemoto T, Ming Chu T. Monoclonal antibodies (F36/22 and M7/105) to human breast carcinoma. Cancer Res 1983; 43: 1741-1747.
34. Croghan GA, Papsidero LD, Valenzuela LA, Nemoto T, Penetrante R, Ming Chu, T. Tissue distribution of an epithelial and tumor-associated antigen recognized by monoclonal antibody F36/22. Cancer Res 1983; 43: 4980-4988.
35. Thompson LH, Jones SL, Whitehead RH, McKenzie IFC. A human breast tissue-associated antigen detected by a monoclonal antibody. J Natl Cancer Inst 1983; 70: 409-420.
36. Iacobelli S, Natoli V, Scambia G, Santeusiano G, Negrini R, Natoli C. A monoclonal antibody (AB/3) reactive with human breast cancer. Cancer Res 1985; 45: 4334-4338.
37. White CA, Dulbecco R, Allen R, Bowman M, Armstrong B. Two monoclonal antibodies selective for human mammary carcinoma. Cancer Res 1985; 45: 1337-1343.
38. Karsten U, Widmaier R, Kunde D. Monoclonal antibodies against antigens of the human mammary carcinoma cell line MCF-7. Arch Geschwulstforsch. 1983; 53: 529-536.
39. Price MR, Edwards S, Robins RA, Hilgers J, Hilkens J, Baldwin RW. Epitopes with diagnostic and prognostic significance co-expressed on a human breast carcinoma-associated antigen. Eur J Cancer Clin Oncol 1986; 22: 115-117.
40. Heyderman E, Steele K, Ormerod MG. A new antigen in the epithelial membrane: Its immunoperoxidase localisation in normal and neoplastic tissue. J Clin Pathol 1979; 32: 35-39.
41. Sloane JP, Ormerod MG. Distribution of epithelial membrane antigen in normal and neoplastic tissues and its value in diagnostic tumor pathology. Cancer 1981; 47: 1786-1795.
42. Ormerod MG, Steele K, Westwood JH, Mazzini MN. Epithelial membrane antigen: partial purification, assay and properties. Br J Cancer 1983; 48: 533-541.
43. McIlhinney RAJ, Patel S, Gore ME. Monoclonal antibodies recognizing epitopes carried on both glycolipids and glycoproteins of the human milk fat globule membrane. Biochem J 1985; 227: 155-162.
44. Hilkens J. Unpublished observations. 1986.
45. Shimizu M, Yamauchi K. Isolation and characterization of mucin-like glycoprotein in human milk fat globule membrane. J Biochem 1982; 91: 515-524.
46. Ormerod MG, McIlhinney J, Steele K, Shimizu M. Glycoprotein PAS-O from the milk fat globule membrane carries antigenic determinants for epithelial membrane antigen. Molec Immunol 1985; 22: 265-269.
47. Shimizu M, Yamauchi K, Miyanchi Y, Sakurai T, Tokugawa K, McIlhinney RAJ. High Mr glycoprotein profiles in human milk serum and fat-globule membrane. Biochem J 1986; 233: 725-730.
48. Hilkens J, Kroezen V, Buys F, Hilgers J, Van Vliet M, De Voogd W, Bonfrèr J, Bruning PF. MAM-6, a carcinoma-associated marker; preliminary characterization and detection in sera of breast cancer patients. In: Monoclonal antibodies and breast cancer. Ceriani RL(ed). Martinus Nijhoff, Publ. Boston, pp 28-42, 1984.
49. Zotter S, Lossnitzer A, Kunze KD, Müller M, Hilkens J, Hilgers J, Hageman Ph. Epithelial markers for paraffin-embedded human tissues.

Immunohistochemistry with monoclonal antibodies against milk fat globule antigens. Virchows Arch (Pathol Anat) 1985; 406: 237-251.
50. Lundy J, Thor A, Maenza R, Schlom J, Forouhar F, Testa M, Kufe D. Monoclonal antibody DF3 correlates with tumor differentiation and hormone receptor status in breast cancer patients. Breast Cancer Res Treatm 1985; 5: 269-275.
51. Clayton F, Nelson GO, Hanssen GM. Immunoperoxidase localization of lactalbumin in malignant breast neoplasms. Arch Pathol Lab Med 1982; 106: 268-270.
52. Lee AK, Dellelis RA, Rosen PP, Herbert-Stanton T, Tallberg K, Garcia C, Wolfe HJ. Alpha-lactalbumin as an immunohistochemical marker for metastatic breast carcinomas. Am J Surg Pathol 1984; 8: 93-100.
53. Baily AJ, Sloane JP, Trickey BS, Ormerod MG. An immunocytochemical study of α-lactalbumin in human breast tissue. J Pathol 1982; 137:13-23.
54. Hall L, Craig RK, Campbell PN. mRNA species directing synthesis of milk proteins in normal and tumor tissue from human mammary gland. Nature 1978; 277: 54-56.
55. Burchell J, Bartek J, Taylor-Papadimitriou J. Production and characterization of monoclonal antibodies to human casein. A monoclonal antibody that cross-reacts with casein and α-lactalbumin. Hybridoma 1985; 4: 341-350.
56. Ormerod MG, Bussolati G, Sloane JP, Steele K, Gugliotta P. Similarities of antisera to casein and epithelial membrane antigen. Virchows Archiv (Pathol Anat) 1982; 397: 327-333.
57. Earl HM, McIlhinney RAJ. Monoclonal antibodies to human casein. Molecular Immunol 1985; 22: 981-991.
58. Earl HM. Markers of human breast differentiation and breast carcinomas and characterization of monoclonal antibodies to human casein. Ph.D. Thesis, London University, Sloane l.c., 1985.
59. Bussolati G, Botta G, Gugliotta P. Actin-rich (myoepithelial) cells in ductal carcinoma in situ of the breast. Virchows Archiv B (Cell Pathology) 1980; 34: 251-259.
60. Gusterson BA, Warburton MJ, Mitchell D, Ellison ML, Neville AM, Rudland PS. Distribution of myoepithelial cells and basement membrane proteins in the normal breast and in benign and malignant breast disease. Cancer Res 1982; 42: 4763-4770
61. Gusterson BA, Warburton MJ, Monaghan P, Foster C, Edwards P, Kraft N, Smith C, Mitchell D, Rudland PS, Neville AM, Hancock W. The use of immunohistochemical probes in the study of benign and malignant breast disease. Behring Inst Mitt 1984; 74: 39-48.
62. Siegal GP, Barsky SH, Terranova VP, Liotta LA. Stages of neoplastic transformation of human breast tissue as monitored by dissolution of basement membrane components: an immunoperoxidase study. Invest Metast 1981; 1: 54-70.
63. Demartino L, Bigotti A, Natali PG. Immunohistochemical localization of contractile proteins, basement membrane, laminin, type V collagen and fibronectin in the normal human breast and its disorders. J submicr cytol 1984; 16: 163-165.
64. Birembaut P, Caron Y, Adnet JJ, Foidart JM. Usefulness of basement membrane markers in tumoural pathology. J Pathol 1985; 145: 283-296.
65. Carter RL, Burman JF, Barr L, Gusterson BA. Immunohistochemical localization of basement membrane type IV collagen in invasive and metastatic squamous carcinomas of the head and neck. J Pathol 1985; 147: 159-164.

66. Liotta LA, Horan Hand P, Rao CN, Bryant G, Barsky SH, Schlom J. Monoclonal antibodies to the human laminin receptor recognize structurally distinct sites. Exp Cell Res 1985; 156: 117-126.
67. Horan Hand P, Thor A, Schlom J, Rao CN, Liotta L. Expression of laminin receptor in normal and carcinomatous human tissues as defined by a monoclonal antibody. Cancer Res 1985; 45: 2713-2719.
68. Nap M, Ter Hoor KA, Fleuren GJ. Cross-reactivity with normal antigens in commercial anti-CEA sera, used for immunohistology. The need for tissue controls and absorptions. Am J Clin Pathol 1983; 79: 25-31.
69. Walker RA. Demonstration of carcinoembryonic antigen in human breast carcinomas by the immunoperoxidase technique. J Clin Pathol 1980; 33: 356-360.
70. Verstijnen CPHJ, Arends JW, Moerkerk PTM, Warnaar S, Hilgers J, Bosman FT. CEA-specificity of CEA-reactive monoclonal antibodies. Immunochemical and immunocytochemical studies. Anticancer Res 1986; 6: 97-104.
71. Van Bogaert LJ. Present status of estrogen-receptor immunohistochemistry and its application in breast cancer research. Acta Histochem 1985; 76: 29-35.
72. McCarty KS, Reintgen DS, Seigler HF, McCarty KS. Cytochemistry of sex steroid receptors: a critique. Breast Cancer Res Treat 1981; 1: 315-325.
73. Janssens, JPh, Pylyser K, Bekaert J, Roelens J, Stuyck J, Dekeyser LJ, Lauwerijns JM, De Loecker W. Biochemical and histochemical analysis of steroid hormone binding sites in human primary breast cancer. Cancer 1985; 55: 2600-2611.
74. Greene GL, Nolan C, Engler JP, Jensen EV. Monoclonal antibodies to human estrogen receptor. Proc Natl Acad Sci 1980; 77: 5115-5119.
75. King WJ, Greene GL. Monoclonal antibodies localize oestrogen receptor in the nuclei of target cells. Nature 1984; 307: 745-747.
76. Welshons WV, Lieberman ME, Gorski J. Nuclear localization of unoccupied oestrogen receptors. Nature 1984; 307: 747-749.
77. King WJ, DeSombre ER, Jensen EV, Greene GL. Comparison of immunocyto-chemical and steroid-binding assays for estrogen receptor in human breast tumors. Cancer Res 1985; 45: 293-304.
78. Jonat W, Stegner HE, Maass H. Immunohistochemical determination of estrogen receptors in breast carcinoma using monoclonal antibodies. Geburtshilfe Frauenheilkd 1985: 473-476.
79. McCarthy Jr KS, Miller LS, Cox EB, Konrath J, McCarthy Sr KS. Estrogen receptor analyses, correlation of biochemical and immunohistochemical methods using monoclonal antireceptor antibodies. Arch Pathol Lab Med 1985; 109: 716-721.
80. Greene GL, Sobel NB, King WJ, Jensen EV. Immunochemical studies of estrogen receptors. J Steroid Chem 1984; 20: 51-56.
81. Skovgaard Poulsen H, Ozello L, King WJ, Greene GL. The use of monoclonal antibodies to estrogen receptors (ER) for immunoperoxidase detection of ER in paraffin sections of human breast cancer tissue. J Histochem Cytochem 1985; 33: 87-92.
82. Shimada A, Kimura S, Abe K, Nagasaki K, Adachi I, Yamaguchi K, Suzuki M, Nakajima T, Miller LS. Immunocytochemical staining of estrogen receptor in paraffin sections of human breast cancer by use of monoclonal antibody: comparison with that in frozen sections. Proc Natl Acad Sci 1985; 82: 4803-4807.
83. King RJB, Coffer AI, Gilbert J, Lewis K, Nash R, Millis R, Raju S, Taylor RW. Histochemical studies with a monoclonal antibody raised

against a partially purified soluble estradiol receptor preparation form human myometrium. Cancer Res 1985; 45: 5728-5733.

84. Coffer AI, Lewis KM, Brockas AJ, King RJB. Monoclonal antibodies against a component related to soluble estrogen receptor. Cancer Res 1985; 45: 3686-3693.
85. Garcia M, Salazar-Retana G, Richer G, Domergue J, Capony F, Pujol H, Laffargue F, Pau B, Rochefort H. Immunohistochemical detection of the estrogen-regulated 52,000 mol wt protein in primary breast carcinomas but not in normal breast and uterus.J Clin Endocrinol Metab 1984; 59: 564-566.
86. Garcia M, Capony F, Derocq D, Simon D, Pau B, Rochefort H. Characterization of monoclonal antibodies to the estrogen-regulated Mr 52,000 glycoprotein and their use in MCF7 cells. Cancer Res 1985; 45: 709-716.
87. Adams DJ, Hajj H, Edwards DP, Bjercke RJ, McGuire WL. Detection of a Mr 24,000 estrogen-regulated protein in human breast cancer by monoclonal antibodies. Cancer Res 1983; 43: 4297-4301.
88. Ciocca DR, Adams DJ, Bjercke RJ, Edwards DP, McGuire WL. Immunohistochemical detection of an estrogen regulated protein by monoclonal antibodies. Cancer Res 1982; 42: 4256-4258.
89. Brabon AC, Williams JF, Cardiff RD. A monoclonal antibody to a human breast tumor protein released in response to estrogen. Cancer Res 1984; 44: 2704-2710.
90. Wachner R, Wittekind Chr, Von Kleist S. Immunohistological localization of β-HCG in breast carcinoma. Europ J Cancer Clin Oncol 1984; 20: 679-684.
91. Horne CHW, Reid N, Milne GD. Prognostic significance of inappropriate production of pregnancy proteins by breast cancers. Lancet 1976, i: 279-282.
92. Kuhajda FP, Bohn H, Mendelsohn G. Pregnancy specific β-1 glycoprotein (SP-1) in breast carcinoma: pathologic and clinical considerations. Cancer 1984; 54: 1392-1396.
93. Sorenson S, Anderson J, Norgaard T. Pregnancy-specific B1-glycoprotein (SP-1) in serum and tissue from patients with benign and malignant breast tumours. Br J Cancer 1984; 49: 663-668.
94. Kuhajda FP, Abeloff MD, Eggleston JC. Pregnancy-associated plasmna protein A: A clinically significant predictor of early recurrence in stage II breast carcinoma. Hum Pathol 1985; 16: 228-235.
95. Shindelman JE, Ortmeyer AE, Sussman HH. Demonstration of the transferrin receptor in human breast cancer tissue. Potential markers for identifying dividing cells. Int J Cancer 1981; 27: 329-334.
96. Moll R, Franke WW, Schiller DL, Geiger B, Krepler R. The catalog of human cytokeratins: patterns of expression in normal epithelia, tumors and cultured cells. Cell 1982; 31: 11-24.
97. Makin CA, Bobrow LG, Bodmer WF. Monoclonal antibody to cytokeratin for use in routine histopathology. J Clin Pathol 1984; 37: 975-983.
98. Pinkus GS, Etheridge CL, O'Connor EM. Are keratin proteins a better tumor marker than epithelial membrane antigen? Am J Clin Pathol 1986; 85: 269-277.
99. Pinkus GS, O'Connor EM, Etheridge CL, Corson JM. Optimal immunoreactivity of keratin proteins in formalin-fixed, paraffin-embedded tissue requires preliminary trypsinisation. J Histochem Cytochem 1985; 33: 465-473.

100. Gown AM, Vogel AM. Monoclonal antibodies to human intermediate filament proteins. III. Analysis of tumors. Am J Clin Pathol 1985; 84: 413-424.
101. Pinkus GS, Kurtin PJ. Epithelial membrane antigen - a diagnostic discriminant in surgical pathology: Immunohistochemical profile in epithelial, mesenchymal and hematopoietic neoplasms using paraffin sections and monoclonal antibodies. Hum Pathol 1985; 16: 929-940.
102. Mariani-Costantini R, Barbanti P, Colnaghi MI, Mènard S, Clemente C, Rilke F. Reactivity of a monoclonal antibody with tissues and tumors from the human breast. Immunohistochemical localization of a new antigen and clinic pathological correlations. Am J Pathol 1984; 115: 47-56.
103. Gatter KC, Mason DY. The use of monoclonal antibodies for histopathologic diagnosis of human malignancy. Seminars in Oncology 1982; 9: 517-525.
104. Gatter KC, Alcock C, Heryet A, Mason DY. Clinical importance of analysing malignant tumours of uncertain origin with immunohistological techniques. Lancet 1985; i: 1302-1305.
105. Mènard S, Rilke F, Della Torre G, Mariani-Costantini R, Regazzoni M, Tagliabue E, Alasio L, Colnaghi MI. Sensitivity enhancement of the cytologic detection of cancer cells in effusions by monoclonal antibodies. Am J Clin Pathol 1985; 83: 571-576.
106. Johnston WW, Szpak CA, Lottich SC, Thor A, Schlom J. Use of a monoclonal antibody (B 72.3) as an immunocytochemical adjunct to diagnosis of adenocarcinoma in human effusions. Cancer Res 1985; 45: 1894-1900.
107. Sloane JP, Ormerod MG, Imrie S, Coombes RC. The use of antisera to epithelial membrane antigen in detecting micrometastases in histological sections. Br J Cancer 1980; 42: 392-398.
108. Epenetos AA, Canti G, Taylor-Papadimitriou J, Curling M, Bodmer WF. Use of two epithelium-specific monoclonal antibodies for diagnosis of malignancy in serous effusions. Lancet 1982; ii: 1004-1006.
109. Dearnaley, DP, Sloane JP, Ormerod MG, Steele K, Coombes RC, Clink HMcD, Powles TJ, Ford HT, Gazet JC, Neville AM. Increased detection of mammary carcinoma cells in marrow smears using antisera to epithelial membrane antigen. Br J Cancer 1981; 44: 85-90.
110. Gugliotta P, Botta G, Bussolati G. Immunocytochemical detection of tumour markers in bone metastases from carcinoma of the breast. Histochem J 1981; 13: 953-959.
111. Wells CA, Heryet A, Brochier J, Gatter KC, Mason DY. The immunocytochemical detection of axillary micro metastases in breast cancer. Br J Cancer 1984; 50: 193-197.
112. Redding WH, Monaghar P, Imrie SF, Ormerod MG, Gazet JC, Coombes RC, Clink HM, Dearnaley DP, Sloane JP, Powles TJ, Neville AM. Detection of micrometastases in patients with primary breast cancer. Lancet 1983; ii: 1271-1274.
113. Taylor-Papadimitriou J, Burchell J, Moss F, Beverley P. Monoclonal antibodies to epithelial membrane antigen and human milk fat globule mucin define epitopes expressed on other molecules. Lancet 1985; i: 458-459.
114. Heyderman E, Macartney JC. Epithelial membrane antigen and lymphoid cells. Lancet 1985, i: 109-110.
115. Delsol G, Gatter KC, Stein H, Erber WN, Pulford KAF, Zinne K, Mason DY. Human lymphoid cells express epithelial membrane antigen. Lancet 1984; ii: 1124-1129.
116. Sloane JP, Dearnaley DP, Ormerod MG. Letter. Lancet 1985; i: 109-110.

117. Hendler F, House D. Presence of breast cancer antigens in uninvolved axillary lymph nodes. Cancer Res 1985; 45: 3364-3373.
118. Simpson HW, Candlish W, Liddle C, McGregor M, Mutch F, Tinkler B. A critical investigation of the Oxford tumour marker Ca1 in the histological diagnosis of breast cancer and pre-cancer. Histopathology 1984; 8: 481-499.
119. Woodhouse CS, Seller C, Morgan AC, Oldham RK. Immunohistochemical detection of the Ca antigen in normal and tumor tissues of humans by the use of Ca1 monoclonal antibody. J Natl Cancer Inst 1985; 74: 383-389.
120. Papotti M, Gugliotta P, Eusebi V, Bussolati G. Immunohistochemical analysis of benign and malignant papillary lesions of the breast. Am J Surg Pathol 1983; 7: 457-461.
121. Nap M, Keuning H, Burtin P, Oosterhuis JW, Fleuren GJ. CEA and NCA in benign and malignant breast tumors. Am J Clin Pathol 1984; 82: 526-534.
122. Bussolati G, Gugliotta P, Papotti M. Detection and significance of epithelial and myo-epithelial cell markers in carcinoma of the breast.in: New Frontiers in mamma pathology, Vol 2. Hollman KM, Verley JM (ed) Plenum Press New York 1983; 249-264.
123. Papotti M, Gugliotta P, Ghiringhello B, Bussolati G. Association of breast carcinoma and multiple intraductal papillomas: an histological and immunohistochemical investigation. Histopathology 1984; 8: 963-975.
124. Azzopardi JG. Problems in breast pathology. W.B. Saunders, London, Philadelphia, Toronto, 1979.
125. McArdle JP, Müller HK, Roff BT, Murphy WH. Basal lamina redevelopment in tumours metastatic to brain: an immunoperoxidase study using an antibody to type-IV collagen. Int J Cancer 1984; 34: 633-638.
126. Bartek J, Taylor-Papadimitriou J, Miller N, Millis R. Patterns of expression of keratin 19 as detected with monoclonal antibodies in human breast tissues and tumours. Int J Cancer 1985; 36: 229-306.
127. Bartek J, Durban EM, Hallowes RC, Taylor-Papadimitriou J. A subclass of luminal epithelial cells in the human mammary gland defined by antibodies to cytokeratins. J Cell Science 1985; 75: 17-34.
128. Shousha S, Lyssiotis T. Correlation of carcinoembryonic antigen in tissue sections with spread of mammary carcinoma. Histopathology 1978; 2: 433-447.
129. Shousha S, Lyssiotis T, Godfrey VM, Scheuer PJ. Carcinoembryonic antigen in breast-cancer tissue; a useful prognostic indicator. Br Med J 1979; 1: 777-779.
130. Gilchrist KW, Kalish L, Gould VE, Hirschl S, Imbriglia JE, Levy WM, Patchewsky AS, Pickren J, Roth HA, Schinella RA, Schwartz IS, Wheeler JE, Tormey DC. Immunostaining for carcinoembryonic antigen does not discriminate for early recurrence in breast cancer. Cancer 1985; 56: 351-355.
131. Barry JD, Koch TJ, Cohen C, Brigati DJ, Sharkey FE. Correlation of immunohistochemical markers with patient prognosis in breast carcinoma: a quantitative study, Am J Clin Pathol 1984; 82: 582-585.
132. Lee AK, Delellis RA, Rosen PP, Saigo PE, Gangi MD, Bagin R, Grosken S, Wolfe HJ. ABH Blood group isoantigen expression in breast carcinomas. An immunohistochemical evaluation using monoclonal antibodies. Am J Clin Pathol 1985; 183: 308-319.
133. Lee AK, Rosen PP, Delellis RA, Saigo PE, Gangi MD, Grosher S, Bagin R, Wolfe HJ. Tumor marker expression in breast carcinoma and relationship

to prognosis. An immunohistochemical study. Am J Clin Pathol 1985; 84: 687-696.
134. Wilkinson MJS, Howell A, Harris M, Taylor-Papadimitriou J, Swindell R. The prognostic significance of two epithelial membrane antigens expressed by human mammary carcinomas. Int J Cancer 1984; 33: 299-304.
135. Berry N, Jones DB, Smallwood J, Taylor I, Kirkham N, Taylor-Papadimitriou J. The prognostic value of the monoclonal antibodies HMFG1 and HMFG2 in breast cancer. Br J Cancer 1985; 51: 179-186.
136. Ellis IO, Hinton CP, McNay J, Elston CW, Robins A, Owainati AARS, Blamey RW, Baldwin RW, Ferry B. Immunocytochemical staining of breast carcinoma with the monoclonal antibody NCRC 11: a new prognostic indicator. Br Med J 1985; 290: 881-883.
137. Bruun Rasmussen B, Pedersen BV, Thorpe SM, Hilkens J, Hilgers J, Rose C. Prognostic value of surface antigens in primary human breast carcinomas, detected by monoclonal antibodies. Cancer Res 1985; 45: 1424-1427.
138. Van Stapel MJ, Gatter KC, De Wolf-Peeters C, Millard PR, Desmet VJ, Mason DY. Immunohistochemical study of mammary and extra-mammary Paget's disease. Histopathology 1984; 8: 1013-1023.
139. Kirkham N, Berry N, Jones DB, Taylor-Papadimitriou J. Paget's disease of the nipple. Immunohistochemical localization of milk fat globule membrane antigens. Cancer 1985; 55: 1510-1512.
140. Bussolati G, Pick A. Mammary and extra-mammary Paget disease. An immunohistochemical study. Am J Pathol 1975; 80: 117-128.
141. Mariani-Costantini R, Andreola S, Rilke F. Tumour-associated antigens in mammary and extramammary Paget's disease. Virchows Arch (Pathol Anat) 1985; 405: 333-340.
142. Vennegoor C, Calafat J, Hageman Ph, Van Buitenen F, Janssen H, Kolk A, Rümke Ph. Biochemical characterization and cellular localization of a formalin-resistant melanoma-associated antigen reacting with monoclonal antibody NKI/C-3. Int J Cancer 1985; 35: 287-295.
143. Nagle RB, Lucas DO, McDaniel KM, Clark VA, Schmalzel GM. Paget's cells. New evidence linking mammary and extramammary Paget cells to a common cell phenotype. Am J Clin Pathol 1985; 83: 431-438.
144. Millis RR. Atlas of breast Pathology. Part of: Current histopathology, Vol 7, G Austin Gresham (ed), MTP Press Ltd, Lancaster, 1984.
145. Huszar M, Herczeg E, Lieberman Y, Geiger B. Distinctive immunofluorescent labeling of epithelial and mesenchymal elements of carcinosarcoma with antibodies specific for different intermediate filaments. Hum Pathol 1984; 15: 532-538.
146. Cross AS, Azzopardi JG, Krausz T, Van Noorden S, Polak JM. A morphological and immunocytochemical study of a distinctive variant of ductal carcinoma in-situ of the breast. Histopathology 1985; 9: 21-37.
147. Bussolati G, Gugliotta P, Sapino A, Eusebi V, Lloyd R. Chromogranin-reactive endocrine cells in argyrophilic carcinomas ('carcinoids') and normal tissue of the breast. Am J Pathol 1985; 120: 186-192.
148. Steedman HF. Polyester wax. A new ribboning embedding medium for histology. Nature 1957; 179: 1345.
149. Baak JP, Van Dop H, Kurver PH, Hermans J. The value of morphometry to classic prognosticators in breast cancer. Cancer 1985; 56: 374-382.
150. Gerdes J, Schwab U, Lemke H, Stein H. Production of a mouse monoclonal antibody reactive with a human nuclear antigen associated with cell proliferation. Int J Cancer 1983; 31: 13-20.

151. Gerdes J. An immunohistological method for estimating cell growth fractions in rapid histopathological diagnosis during surgery. Int J Cancer 1985; 35: 169-171.
152. Lloyd RV, Wilson BS, Varani J, Gaur PK, Moline S, Makari JG. Immunocytochemical characterization of a monoclonal antibody that recognizes mitosing cells. Am J Pathol 1985; 121: 275-283.
153. Oudemans PB, Brutel de la Riviere G, Hart AAM, Van Heerde P, Scholte G, Vroom Th M. Determination of transferrin receptors on frozen sections of malignant B cell lymphomas by immunofluorescence with a monoclonal antibody. Cancer 1986; in press.
154. Bauer KD, Clevenger CV, Endow RK, Murad T, Epstein AL, Scarpelli DG. Simultaneous nuclear antigen and DNA content quantitation using paraffin-embedded colonic tissue and multiparameter flow cytometry. Cancer Res 1986; 46: 2428-2434.

10. MONOCLONAL ANTIBODIES IN CLINICAL AND EXPERIMENTAL PATHOLOGY OF LUNG CANCER

L. DE LEIJ, J. BROERS, F. RAMAEKERS, H. BERENDSEN, SJ. SC. WAGENAAR

1. INTRODUCTION

Lung cancer is a major problem in oncology, since it is responsible for the highest amount of cancer deaths in western societies and shows a still rising incidence, especially among women and in developing countries (1,2). The best opportunity for curative treatment is in the first stage of disease, when cancer is limited to the lung and surgical intervention is the treatment of choice. The number of patients presenting with really limited disease is small, however, and epidemiological studies have given some indication that the overall survival will not ameliorate by screening programs set up to find such early cases (3).

Lung cancer can be histopathologically typed according to a revised version of the WHO classification published in 1982 (4). In this scheme, five major lung cancer types, comprising 95% of all lung tumors, are recognized on light-microscopically evaluable, histological criteria: squamous cell carcinoma, small cell carcinoma (SCLC), adenocarcinoma, large cell carcinoma and adenosquamous cell carcinoma. Within these types, further subtyping can be performed. In 1985, the pathology panel of the IASLC proposed to use for subtypes of SCLC the classification SCLC (classic type), SCLC (mixed small/large cell) and SCLC (combined). The last subtype comprises cases showing substantial squamous or adenocarcinoma component or both (5). The recently introduced plastic embedding technique has, as compared to the results obtained with conventional paraffin embedding techniques, resulted in a further refinement of morphological evaluation possibilities (6). As a result, it has become apparent that more lung cancer cases show combined histologies and, that the percentage of so called "undifferentiated" large cell carcinoma is much smaller than orginally thought. Implications of these findings are indicated below.

A clinically relevant histopathological subdivision in lung cancer is that between SCLC and non-SCLC (7), since SCLC generally shows earlier and more extensive metastatic spread, more rapid tumor cell proliferation and greater sensitivity to chemo- and radiotherapy. However, despite the fact that SCLC is initially highly sensitive to therapy, untreatable recurrences often occur within a year and, also for this type of lung cancer, overall five year survival is disappointingly low.

A histopathological classification of lung cancer can provide information on the nature and possible clinical behaviour of a tumor case. Nevertheless, a purely histologically based subdivision appears not completely satisfying. As indicated above, the application of new histological techniques has shown that a considerable number of cases shows admixtures of areas with different histology. These data have confirmed earlier electronmicroscopical studies indicating that, ultrastructurally, combinations of varying degrees of squamous-, adeno- and neuroendocrine differentiation are often present within one biopsy. This heterogeneity in tumor cell composition is also reflected in tissue culture studies in which profound heterogeneity can be observed within one cell line (8). In addition to a heterogeneous histological composition, changes in histological appearance have also been reported to occur in time, both in vivo (9) and in vitro (10). These observations have led to the idea that lung cancer comprises in fact a continuum of cancer types in which the different histologically recognizable groups represent preferentially expressed, non-fixed differentiation pathways (11). The implications of such an idea for treatment and diagnostic modalities are still unclear. However, the apparent present lack of further advance in therapeutical options demands intensive fundamental and clinical research to seek new treatment avenues. In addition, new methods in the diagnostic approach have to be developed in order to select lung cancer cases with a good prognosis for treatment.

It has been shown that lung cancer can be subtyped not only by histological criteria, but also by immunohistological procedures using poly- or, more recently, monoclonal antibodies. Since monoclonal antibodies define lung cancer on basis of the occurrence of specific antigenic features, that need not to parallel histologically based subdivisions, it can be anticipated that new classifications might eventually emerge from the application of monoclonal antibody based immunohistopathology. The clinical relevance of such a new classification should be established by careful clinical studies and comparison with the established morphological criteria of lung cancer typing. In the following, the occurrence of specific monoclonal antibody defined antigens in lung cancer will be discussed (section 2).

Major attention is paid to two groups of antigens: Firstly, the proteins that form the intermediate-sized filaments, and which can be considered as cell lineage associated antigens (section 2.2) and, secondly, a group of lung cancer associated antigens that can be classified as cell differentiation associated antigens (section 2.3). The application of monoclonal antibodies for pathological and cell biological purposes is dealt with in section 3 and 4 respectively. Because of its clinical relevance special emphasis is given to differences between SCLC and non-SCLC.

2. LUNG CANCER ASSOCIATED ANTIGENS

2.1. General overview

A considerable amount of biochemically (12-15) and immunologically (16-18) detectable differences between SCLC and non-SCLC have been reported. It is conceivable that these differences are translatable into differences detectable by monoclonal antibodies. Thus, after immunization of mice with different lung cancer derived cell lines, monoclonal antibodies have been isolated, that appear to be directed against various SCLC (19-26) and non-SCLC (27-34) associated antigens. These antigens are of (glyco)protein or glycolipid nature. It is still too early to judge the value of all these different monoclonal antibodies for a really specific detection of lung cancer (sub)groups, but at least some (19,21,25,26) appear promising for such an application.

In addition to monoclonal antibodies obtained after immunization with lung tumor cells, a number of other monoclonal antibodies have attracted a lot of interest because of their coreactivity with lung cancer.

Firstly, monoclonal antibodies directed against differentiation antigens, originally defined as leucocyte-associated, have been reported to be also reactive with (subsets of) lung cancer. Examples of these are OKM1 and HNK-1 (35-37). A possible clinical relevance of the occurrence of these antigens on lung cancer is unclear for the moment, however. Secondly, a number of monoclonal antibodies raised against neural or neuroendocrine components appear useful as markers of SCLC. Examples of these are antibodies directed against neuron specific enolase (38,39), chromogranin A (40), synaptophysin (41) and fetal brain antigens (42). These antibodies probably match with the antibodies directed against SCLC differentiation antigens as discussed in section 2.3.

2.2. Cell lineage antigens

Antisera to intermediate filament proteins (IFP) have proven to be powerful tools in the detection of cell lineages of both normal and neoplastic tissues. Intermediate filaments are cytoskeletal structures with diameters of about 10 nanometers, and occur in nearly all vertebrate cells. Their protein constituents have been shown to vary in a strongly tissue-type associated way. As described in chapter 4 this tissue-type associated expression of IFP is retained in most cases after malignant conversion. For instance, both normal epithelial cells and their malignant counterparts contain IFP of the cytokeratin type, whereas neural cells and some neuronal tumors contain neurofilaments. Since the derivation of certain types of lung cancer is still unclear, some investigators (43-45) have attempted to determine their origin using antisera to IFP. These investigations have led to contradictory results in the literature. For instance either cytokeratins or neurofilaments have been shown to be present in small cell lung cancer (SCLC), a lung tumor with neuroendocrine properties, and suggested to be the malignant counterpart of normal neuroendocrine (NE) cells of the lung (46). When tested with antibodies to cytokeratins and neurofilament proteins it turned out, however, that these NE cells express cytokeratin(s) and not neurofilament proteins (fig. 1). This finding indicates that these cells, like many other neuroendocrine cells (such as for example Merkel cells (47)) are of epithelial origin and nature.

For the detection of certain types of IFP special attention should be given to the specificity of the antibodies used, since for instance the family of cytokeratin IFP consists of about 20 different polypeptides, which show a nonrandom, tissue-specific distribution throughout epithelia. Lack of cross-reactivity of cytokeratin antibodies with one or more of these cytokeratin polypeptides may result in false-negative results in certain subtypes of epithelia or epithelial tumors, such as lung tumors. Also fixation artefacts can lead to false-negative results, as has become evident from the literature. Therefore we have employed well-characterized monoclonal and polyclonal antibodies for the detection of IFP in lung tumors, whereas frozen tissue sections were used as a substrate. Figure 2 shows some examples of reactivity of antibody preparations with different lung carcinomas.

All lung carcinomas can be stained by generally cross-reacting cytokeratin antibodies, such as the polyclonal rabbit antiserum pKer or the monoclonal antibody RCK 102 (fig. 2a). Chain-specific monoclonal antibodies reacting with only one cytokeratin polypeptide can recognize certain directions of epithelial differentiation, i.e. adenocarcinomatous differentiation as detected by a monoclonal antibody to cytokeratin 18 (RGE 53), or (keratinizing) squamous cell differentiation as detected by a monoclonal antibody to cytokeratin 10 (RKSE 60). In the normal lung RKSE 60 is unreactive with epithelial cells, whereas RGE 53 reacts with bronchial columnar epithelial cells and type 2 pneumocytes, but not with basal cells of the bronchus.

In epidermoid lung cancers, especially poorly differentiated squamous cell carcinomas, a profound heterogeneity was observed with these chain-specific antibody preparations. With respect to the presence of cytokeratin 18, staining with RGE 53 revealed that this could range from a nearly complete absence in well-differentiated carcinomas to an abundant presence in poorly differentiated squamous cell carcinomas. Figure 2b shows a case with an intermediate RGE 53 staining pattern. With respect to the presence of cytokeratin 10, it appeared that staining with RKSE 60 occurred only in keratinizing areas of well-differentiated squamous cell carcinomas (not shown). Interestingly, some (about 10%, see table 2) of the poorly differentiated squamous cell carcinomas proved to contain neuroendocrine components and even cells with neural characteristics, as indicated by a reactivity with antibodies to neuroendocrine (MOC-1, fig. 2c), and neural marker proteins (neurofilament proteins, fig. 2d).

Adenocarcinomas of the lung were always positive with antibodies broadly reacting with cytokeratins as well as with the monoclonal antibody to cytokeratin 18 (RGE 53). Our results furthermore show that all SCLCs and lung carcinoids also express cytokeratins (fig. 2e,g). These results are in accord with several reports in the literature (45,48,49). Carcinoids exhibit a characteristic staining pattern, with dot-like concentrations of cytokeratin-positive reactions close to the nucleus (fig. 2g). We have found some SCLCs (fig. 2f), and two carcinoids (fig. 2h), which expressed neurofilaments next to cytokeratins. Although both cytokeratins and neurofilaments could be demonstrated in the same SCLC case, double-immunofluorescence studies showed no overlap in expression of cytokeratins and neurofilaments. Therefore, we cannot sustain results described by Lehto et al. (43), who found extensive staining with an anti-neurofilament antibody in all SCLC tumors examined, but no reactivity with an anti-cytokeratin antibody. In double-immunofluorescence studies of the two lung carcinoids reacting with anti-neurofilament antibodies a co-expression of cytokeratins and neurofilaments in all tumor cells could be clearly observed (fig. 2g,h). These last results are in accord with those of Lehto et al. (50).

2.3. Cell differentiation antigens

It can be anticipated that many features of specific antigenic patterns of different lung tumor subgroups originate from differences in cellular differentiation status. The expression of such antigens could partly parellel morphologically based subdivisions and, in addition, such "differentiation antigens" are likely to be also present in the putative normal counterparts of these tumor subgroups. In agreement with this, neuroendocrine related antigens have been detected in normal pulmonary neuroendocrine (NE) cells, SCLC and carcinoids. Such antigens are absent from the normal lung epithelium and are also not present in non-SCLC lung tumors. Neuron-specific enolase is a well-known example of such a neuroendocrine marker (38), whereas the antigen defined by MOC-1 (19) also belongs to this category. There is a considerable amount of evidence indicating that pulmonary NE cells, like the other lung epithelial cells, are endodermally derived. Concordantly, the antigenic make-up of SCLC and carcinoid consists of neuroendocrine as well as epithelial related antigens. Thus, the endocrine tumors of the lung can be differentiated from neural derived tumors by their expression of epithelial antigens like MOC-31 (see table 1) or cytokeratin (see previous section). In addition to the neuroendocrine related antigens that NE cells, carcinoids and SCLC share, we have also

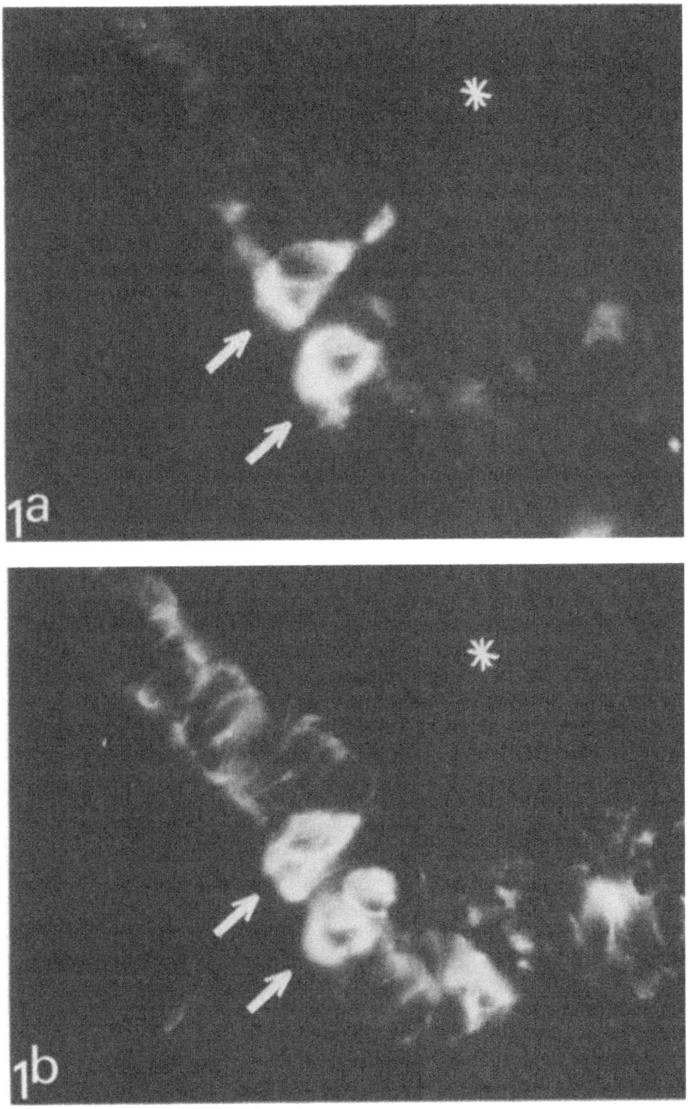

Figure 1: Double immunofluorescence staining with monoclonal antibodies leu 7 (a) and RGE 53 (b) on a developing bronchiolus in a human embryonic lung. The asterix indicates the lumen, whereas the arrows show the location of neuroendocrine cells inside the bronchial epithelium.

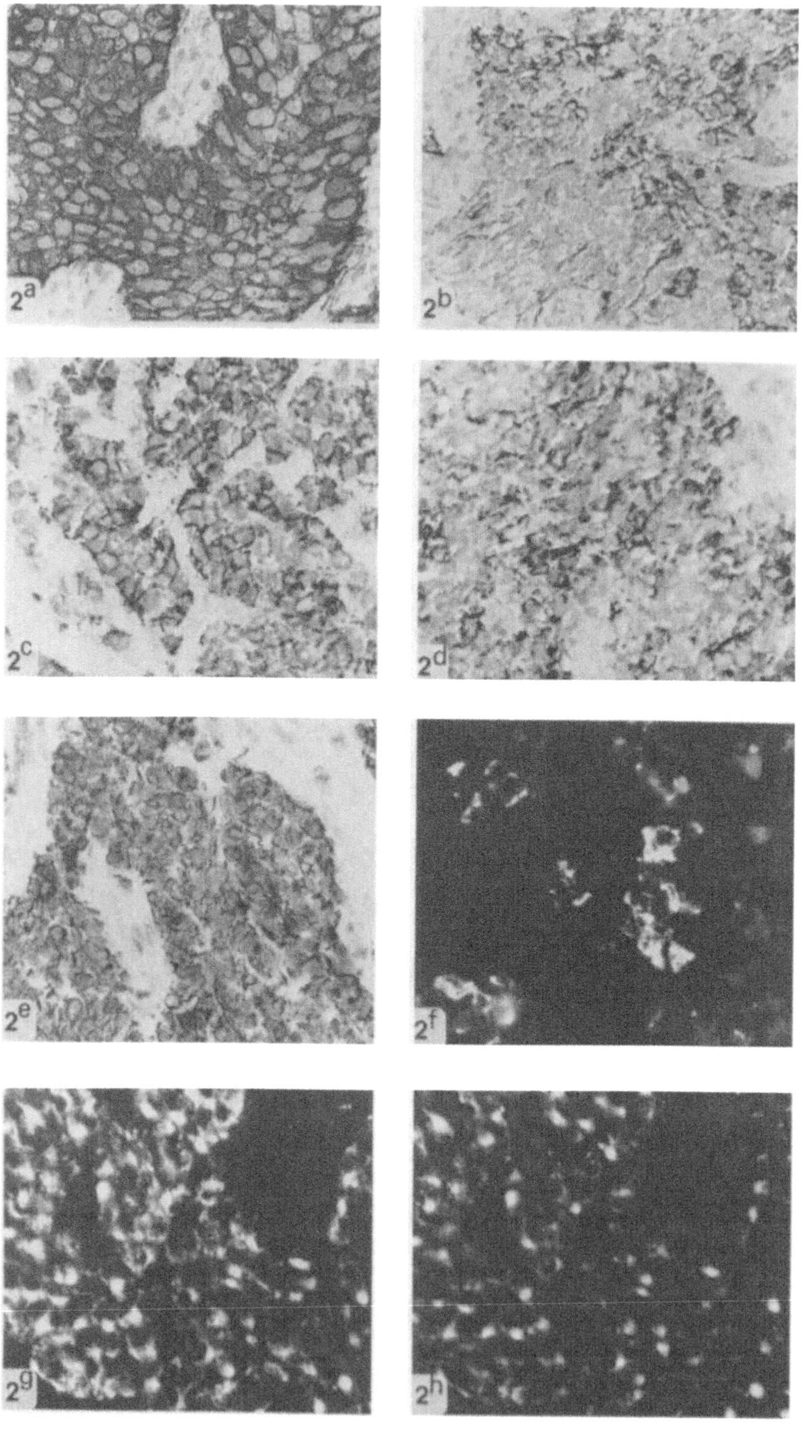
2a
2b
2c
2d
2e
2f
2g
2h

Figure 2: Pulmonary squamous cell carcinoma (a,b,c,d), small cell lung carcinoma (e,f) and a lung carcinoid (g,h) incubated with various antibody preparations directed against cytokeratins (a,b,e,g), neurofilaments (d,f,h) and the neuroendocrine marker MOC-1 (c). Antibody reactions are visualized by indirect immunoperoxidase (a,b,c,d,e) or immunofluorescence (f,g,h) staining techniques. Squamous cell carcinomas stain strongly with the generally cross-reacting antibody RCK 102 (a), while the antibody to cytokeratin 18 (RGE 53) stains variable amounts of cells within such tumors (b). Antibodies directed against neuroendocrine related antigens such as MOC-1 (c) and MNF (d) are unreactive with squamous cell carcinomas, but in a few cases can stain scattered cells or small tumor areas as shown here for two cases of poorly differentiated squamous cell carcinoma (c,d). In general, SCLC reacts strongly with RGE 53 (e) and is unreactive with MNF. The SCLC section shown in (f), however, contains cells reactive with a polyclonal rabbit antiserum to the 160 kDa neurofilament polypeptide in areas wich are unreactive with antibodies directed against cytokeratin. Co-expression of cytokeratin 18 (g, detected by RGE 53) and neurofilaments (h, detected by the rabbit antiserum to neurofilaments) occurs in lung carcinoid as shown here by an indirect double label immunofluorescence technique. Note the typical, dot-like staining pattern of both antibody preparations.

identified recently (51) some other neuroendocrine related antigens on SCLC and carcinoids that are absent in normal NE cells. These antigens are defined by the monoclonal antibodies MOC-21, MOC-32 and MOC-52 (table 1). They are pan-SCLC/carcinoid antigens and have a more restricted neuroendocrine distribution than for instance MOC-1. To study the nature of these neuroendocrine antigens, we have analysed their possible occurrence in fetal lungs of different gestational ages (L. de Leij, manuscript in preparation). Only in very young fetal lungs (first trimester), epithelial cells of some developing airways appear to express the MOC-21, MOC-32 and MOC-52 defined antigens. These same cells also express the MOC-1 (fig. 3), but not the HNK-1 defined antigen. They lack the typical morphology of pulmonary NE cells and have, in addition, a different localisation than putative NE cells present in first trimester fetal lungs (52). Therefore these fetal lung epithelium cells appear to be a distinct population. Thus, MOC-21, MOC-32 and MOC-52 apparently identify neuroendocrine related differentiation antigens, that are present only in very early fetal lung cells. These antigens are reexpressed during the malignant conversion of lung epithelium into carcinoid or SCLC later in life.
In conclusion, the "endocrine" (SCLC and carcinoid) and the non-"endocrine" (adenocarcinoma, squamous cell carcinoma, large cell carcinoma and adenosquamous cell carcinoma) tumors of the lung share epithelium-related differentiation antigens as a result of their common endodermal origin. They can be discriminated from each other by the fact that the "endocrine" tumors express (neuro)endocrine differentiation antigens. These neuroendocrine differentiation antigens are partly shared with normal pulmonary NE cells and appear to be reexpressed fetal (neuro)endocrine antigens.

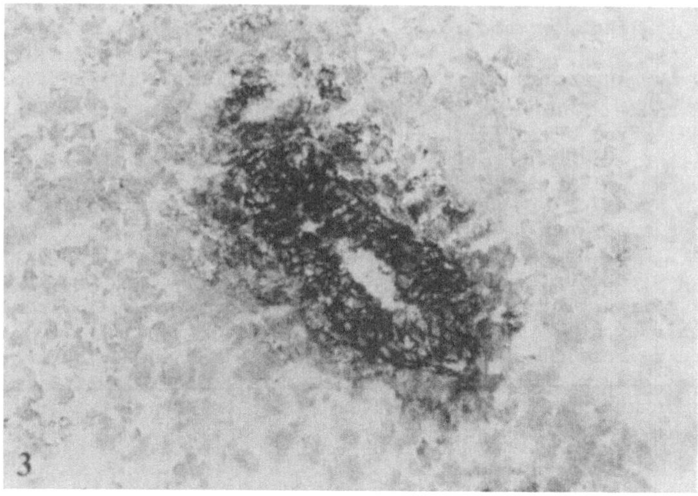

Figure 3: All fetal lung epithelium cells in a ten week old fetus react with the neuroendocrine marker MOC-1, as detected by an indirect immunoperoxidase technique. These fetal cells also react with MOC-21, MOC-32 and MOC-52, whereas normal adult bronchial epithelium cells are unreactive with these markers.

3. APPLICATION OF MONOCLONAL ANTIBODIES FOR ROUTINE PATHOLOGY

3.1. Materials and methods

Reactivity of poly- and monoclonal antibodies on frozen tissue sections of snap-frozen tumor biopsies and surgically resected tumor specimens was assessed according to described procedures using either an indirect immunofluorescence or immunoperoxidase method (53,54). The following antibodies have been used: pKer[1)] (a polyclonal rabbit antiserum to human skin keratins (55), RGE 53[1)] (monoclonal antibody directed against cytokeratin 18 (56), RKSE 60[1)] (monoclonal antibody directed against cytokeratin 10 (57), RCK 102[1)]), (a generally cross-reacting monoclonal antibody directed against at least cytokeratins 5 and 8 and reactive with all epithelia), anti-CEA[1)] (monoclonal antibody directed against the carcinoembryonal antigen), OKT9[2)] (directed against the transferrin receptor), VIM[1)] (directed against vimentin), MNF[1)] (directed against the 210 and 68 kDa components of neurofilaments (58)), 123 C3 (directed against a neuroendocrine related antigen), MOC-31[3)] (directed against an epithelium subset specific antigen, see table 1), MOC-1[3)] (directed against a neuroendocrine related antigen (19), see table 1), MOC-21[3] (directed against a neuroendocrine related antigen, see table 1), MOC-32[3] (directed against a neuroendocrine related antigen, see table 1), MOC-51 (directed against a neuroendocrine related antigen, see table 1) and MOC 52[3] (directed against a neuroendocrine related antigen, see table 1).

1) available from Eurodiagnostics, Apeldoorn, The Netherlands.
2) available from Ortho, USA.
3) available from Biotest.

Table 1. Reactivity of MOC antibodies with normal tissues

	MOC-31[a,b]	MOC-1[b]	MOC-21[b]	MOC-32[a]	MOC-52[a,b]	MOC-51[a]
skin	glands (+) hairshaft (+)	-	-	-	-	-
tonsil	-	-	-	-	-	-
spleen	-	-	-	-	-	-
bone marrow	-	-	-		-	-
respir. tract	epithelia (+) (incl. sero-mucous glands)	-	-		-	-
digest. tract	epithelia (+)	-	-		-	-
kidney	tubuli(+)	-	-		-	-
liver	parenchym (+)	-	-		-	-
pancreas						
exocrine	+	-	-	-	-	-
endocrine	+	+	+	+	±	-
thyroid	+	+	part.(+)		-	-
adrenal						
cortex	-	part.(+)	part.(+)	part.(+)	part.(+)	-
medulla	-	+	+	+	+	-
ovary	-	stromal cells(+) theca cells(+)	stromal cells(+)	stromal cells(+)	stromal cells(+)	-
brain	-	+	+	+	+	fibers(+)
peripheral nerves	-	+	+	+	+	+
ganglion cells	-	+	+	+	+	+

a) detecting an intracellular antigen
b) detecting a membrane antigen

3.2. Major lung tumor subgroups

In order to assess the potential value of immunohistochemistry for establishing a pathological diagnosis, the reactivity of a panel of monoclonal antibodies has been examined on frozen tissue sections of a large number of lung tumors. In almost all cases assessed a strongly positive reaction was obtained with antibodies directed against epithelial antigens like MOC-31 and the broadly reactive polyclonal anti-cytokeratin (tables 2-4). Thus these antibody preparations appear useful as general (lung) carcinoma

Table 2. Reactivity of specific antibodies with major "non-endocrine" lung tumors

	Histological diagnosis			
	squamous cell carcinoma		adenocarcinoma	
	completely positive	focally positive	completely positive	focally positive
polyclonal anti-cytokeratin	83/85	0/85	37/45	7/45
RGE 53	36/151	55/151	45/46	0/46
RKSE 60	3/151	21/151*	0/46	0/46
VIM	0/77	9/77	0/37	2/37
MNF	0/112	8/112**	0/29	0/29
anti-CEA	48/151	71/151	38/46	5/46
OKT9	138/151	9/151	33/46	7/46
123 C3	6/151**	13/151**	0/46	1/46
MOC-31	35/35	0/35	28/28	0/28
MOC-1	4/144**	22/144**	2/72	5/72
MOC-21	0/31	0/31	2/27	2/27
MOC-32	1/32**	0/32	2/28	3/28
MOC-51	0/27	0/27	2/27	1/27
MOC-52	0/27	0/27	1/27	1/27

*only keratinizing areas show a positive reaction
**reactivity only in poorly differentiated tumors

markers. No discrimination can be made with these antibodies between primary lung carcinoma and metastatic lesions originating from carcinomas that also express these markers.
MOC-31 recognizes an intracellularly located protein, which does not belong to the cytokeratin family. Interestingly, MOC-31 appears to be unreactive with normal mesothelium cells as well as mesotheliomas and can be used therefore for a differential diagnosis of mesothelioma versus lung carcinoma.
The monoclonal antibodies directed against chain-specific cytokeratins showed a preferential reactivity pattern in the different lung carcinomas. Thus the monoclonal antibody preparation directed against cytokeratin 18 (RGE 53) reacted preferentially with adenocarcinoma, SCLC and carcinoid, whereas the monoclonal antibody preparation directed against cytokeratin 10 (RKSE 60) reacted only with keratinizing areas present in well-differentiated squamous cell carcinoma (tables 2 and 3).
Concerning the expression of other intermediate filament proteins, it appeared that vimentin is coexpressed in a few carcinomas, whereas neurofilament is present in some poorly differentiated squamous cell carcinomas, some SCLCs and carcinoids. With respect to coexpression of vimentin and cytokeratin in the different types of lung cancer it should be noted that

Table 3. Reactivity of specific antibodies with major "endocrine" lung tumors

	Histological diagnosis			
	SCLC		carcinoid	
	completely positive	focally positive	completely positive	focally positive
polyclonal anti-cytokeratin	19/22	0/22	6/11	2/11
RGE 53	24/28	2/28	12/12	0/12
RKSE 60	1/22	0/22	0/12	0/12
VIM	0/21	2/21	0/7	0/7
MNF	0/20	4/20	3/10	1/10
anti-CEA	5/22	6/22	2/12	2/12
OKT9	18/22	4/22	0/12	0/12
123 C3	28/28	0/28	12/12	0/12
MOC-31	43/43	0/43	3/3	0/3
MOC-1	79/81	0/81	3/3	0/3
MOC-21	49/53	0/3	3/4	0/3
MOC-32	37/52	0/52	3/3	0/3
MOC-51	25/52	0/52	0/3	0/3
MOC-52	52/52	0/52	3/4	1/4

Jasani et al. (66) have found vimentin IF in 46% of all adenocarcinoma examined. Gatter et al. (67) reported coexpression of different IF in 40% of cases of lung cancer studied. There is no preferential reactivity of any lung cancer subtype with the antibody preparation directed against CEA, which appears, therefore, to be of no value as a support for a histopathological typing of lung cancer. Nevertheless, it has been claimed that the expression of CEA in SCLC could correlate with longer survival of the patient (59). The antibody directed against the transferrin receptor (OKT 9) proves to be unreactive with carcinoid but clearly reactive with SCLC and appears useful therefore for a differential diagnosis between these tumors. The expression of OKT9 in atypical carcinoids has still to be determined, however.

The monoclonal antibodies directed against neuroendocrine differentiation antigens (MOC-1, MOC-21, MOC-32, MOC-52 and 123C3) generally reacted with SCLC and carcinoids and not with the other non-SCLC tumors, in agreement with a general "endocrine" versus "non-endocrine" discrimination between these groups. Although such a reaction was a rule, exceptions were observed.

Firstly, non-SCLC cases (a few adenocarcinomas and a number of poorly differentiated squamous or large cell carcinomas) could be (partly) positive

Table 4. Reactivity of specific antibodies with other bronchial lung tumors

	Histological diagnosis							
	adenocystic carcinoma		carcino sarcoma		mucoepidermal carcinoma		pleomorphic adenoma	
	completely positive	focally positive	E*	M**	completely positive	focally positive	E*	M*
anti-cyto keratin	6/6	0/6	2/2	0/2	1/1	0/1	1/1	0/1
RGE 53	6/6	0/6	2/2	0/2	1/1	0/1	1/1	0/1
RKSE 60	0/6	0/6	1/2	0/2	0/1	0/1	0/1	0/1
VIM	0/5	4/5	0/2	2/2	0/1	0/1	0/1	1/1
MNF	0/5	0/5	0/2	0/2	0/1	0/1	0/1	0/1
anti-CEA	4/5	1/5	-	-	1/1	0/1	0/1	0/1
OKT9	4/5	1/5	1/1	1/1	1/1***	0/1	0/1	0/1
123 C3	4/5	0/5	0/1	0/1	1/1	0/1	0/1	0/1
MOC-31	5/5	0/5	1/1	0/1	1/1	0/1	1/1	0/1
MOC-1	2/5	1/5	2/2	0/2	1/1	0/1	0/1	0/1
MOC-21	0/5	0/5	0/1	0/1	0/1	1/1***	0/1	0/1
MOC-32	1/5	0/5	0/1	0/1	0/1	0/1	0/1	0/1
MOC-51	0/5	2/5	0/1	0/1	1/1	0/1	0/1	0/1
MOC-52	1/5	0/5	0/1	0/1	1/1	0/1	0/1	0/1

*epithelial part
**mesenchymal part
***only weakly positive

with these antibodies, indicating the presence of a neuroendocrine component in these cases, which was not apparent from the morphology. These observations could be of clinical relevance. In a recent electronmicroscopic study (60) it has been indicated that histologically undifferentiated large cell tumors, showing neuroendocrine differentiation features, have a clinical behaviour similar to SCLC. Although a similar clinical study with tumors having immunohistochemically detectable neuroendocrine features has to be done yet, the same could apply to this group. If so, we should like to suggest, in parallel with treatment schedules already applied to combined SCLC, that these tumors should be treated as combined SCLC, using irradiation and combination chemotherapy after surgery.
Secondly, not all neuroendocrine related antigens proved to be present on all SCLC cases assessed. Therefore these antigens could define subsets of SCLC. A possible clinical relevance of such a subtyping should be established, however, only after carefull clinical studies.

3.3. Bronchial gland tumors

Tumors originating from cells in the sero-mucous glands of the large airways are rare, representing less than 0.5% of all lung cancer cases. In table 4 the immunohistochemical staining results obtained with one muco-epidermoid, one pleomorphic adenoma, two carcinosarcomas and six adenoid cystic carcinomas are given.
Coexpression of epithelial (cytokeratins, MOC-31) and a number of neuro-endocrine (123 C3, MOC-1, MOC-51 and MOC-52) markers is seen in the muco-epidermoid case. Interestingly this case lacks vimentin expression, which contrasts to the results normally obtained in muco-epidermoid tumors derived from the major salivary glands. In the pleomorphic adenoma and the two carcinosarcomas assessed cytokeratin and vimentin are found in the epithelial and mesenchymal structures respectively. These tumors do not express neuroendocrine markers. In the six adenoid cystic carcinomas assessed epithelial markers (MOC-31, cytokeratins) were always present, whereas the different neuroendocrine markers were variably expressed.
Although the number of bronchial gland tumors presented is too small yet to draw definite conclusions, it is apparent that immunohistochemistry may be helpful to differentiate these tumors from other lung cancer types and between each other, if other morphological aspects fail to do so.

4. CELL CULTURES OF LUNG TUMORS

The high heterogeneity of lung tumors is reflected in established cell lines derived from patients with these cancers. Cell lines with characteristics of each subtype (squamous cell carcinomas, adenocarcinomas, large cell and small cell lung carcinoma) have been obtained and characterized. Investigations on these cell lines have led to the conclusion that they represent indeed certain (sub-)types of lung tumor and can be used therefore as model systems to study the cell biology of the different pathways of lung cancer differentiation. For instance "classic" SCLC cell lines have retained biological and biochemical features typical for the classic subtype of in vivo SCLC, while the "variant" SCLC cell lines represent the large cell component of the mixed small cell/large cell subtype of SCLC (61,62).

Applying antisera to cell differentiation and cell-lineage markers has shown that, also in vitro, such probes can discriminate between SCLC and non-SCLC, and even between "classic" and "variant" SCLC. Thus, using antibody preparations against IFP, all classic SCLC cell lines tested were shown to contain cytokeratins (7/7, fig. 4a), while the variant cell lines did not contain these cytokeratin IFP (0/6). Some of the latter cell lines, however, contained neurofilaments (3/6, fig. 4b), whereas the others (3/6) did not contain cytokeratins nor neurofilaments. These data were obtained after immunocytochemical studies using a large panel of polyclonal and monoclonal antibodies directed against cytokeratins and neurofilaments, and were confirmed by gelelectrophoretic and immunoblotting assays (55).

Cell lines derived from squamous cell carcinomas and adenocarcinomas contained cytokeratin (55) and did not react with anti-neurofilament antibodies. One cell line (GLC-3) showed a heterogeneous staining pattern when incubated with several monoclonal anti-cytokeratin antibodies (8), indicating that this cell line, which was derived from a patient with SCLC, had adapted both an adenocarcinomatous (RGE 53 positive, presence of microvilli at an electronmicroscopic level), as well as a squamous (RKSE 60 positive) differentiation pathway. The expression of the epithelial differentiation antigen defined by MOC-31 parallelled in all cell lines

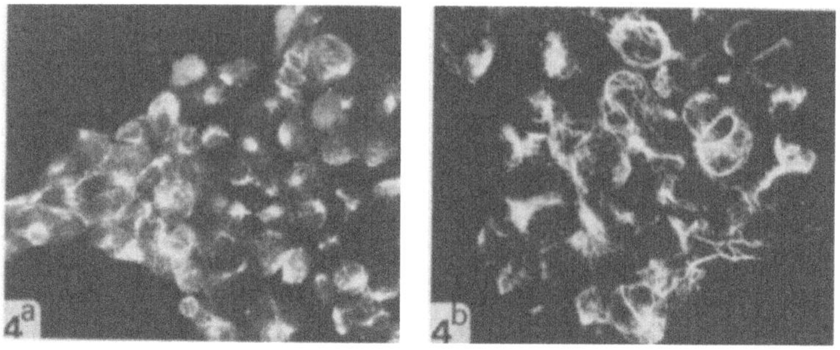

Figure 4: Immunofluorescence staining pattern of a classic (a) and a variant (b) SCLC cell line using different antibodies to IFP. Note the filamentous staining reaction of the classic line with the cytokeratin reactive antibody RGE 53 (a) and the reaction of the variant line with the rabbit antiserum to the 160 kDa neurofilament polypeptide (b).

assessed the presence or absence of cytokeratins. In contrast to the findings indicated above with neurofilaments, the neuroendocrine antigens defined by MOC-1, MOC-21, MOC-32, and MOC-52 could be demonstrated in both variant-and classic-type SCLC cell lines. MOC-51 was present only in a minority of classic-type cell lines.

In conclusion, our results concerning the cell lineage (IF) as well as cell differentiation protein phenotype of SCLC derived cell lines suggest different lineages of (de-)differentiation within SCLC, with classic cells having more epithelial characteristics and variant cells having lost these epithelial characteristics but having acquired some neuronal characteristics. Since a distinction of the variant type of SCLC from the classic type may be of clinical importance (63), it is of special interest to obtain a better understanding of the carcinogenesis of these two different types of SCLC. At this moment it is not clear whether "in situ" the variant cells differentiate spontaneously from a classic cell type or from a common neuroendocrine progenitor cell.

Expression of cytokeratins and neurofilament proteins within one tumor seems to be restricted to a limited number of neuroendocrine tumors. Neurofilaments have been found next to cytokeratins in neuroendocrine skin carcinomas (Merkel cell tumors; 64) and in some pancreatic islet tumors (65). The possible cell of origin for these tumors (Merkel cells in skin and pancreatic islet cell, respectively) express only cytokeratins and do not contain neurofilaments. Therefore it was of interest to study the intermediate filament expression in normal neuroendocrine cells of the lung. The finding that these cells contain only cytokeratins and not neurofilaments (fig. 1) supports the hypothesis that pulmonary neuroendocrine cells are of epithelial origin. However, apparently, neuroendocrine cells do have the potential to express neurofilaments as a result of malignant transformation and growth as shown both by in vitro and in vivo findings with SCLC. A possible clinical relevance of this has to be established yet.

5. CONCLUSION

Monoclonal antibody based immunohistochemistry is a very powerful tool for the establishment of a pathological diagnosis of lung tumor. With the advent of a growing number of different, well-defined monoclonal antibodies, it can be anticipated that this technique will become increasingly sophisticated and important. For the moment, however, the application of immunohistochemistry for diagnosis needs the preparation of two separate samples: one for immunohistochemistry (snap-frozen tissue specimen; the tissue antigens are not denaturated and stay optimally reactive with the different monoclonal antibodies) and one for normal histology (fixed and plastic embedded tissue specimen; optimal morphology can be obtained in the prepared sections). New fixation and embedding procedures that combine good morphology and preservation of tissue antigen reactivity are being developed now and will surely encourage the futher use of immunohistochemistry on a routine basis in the near future.

Summarizing the results presented in this chapter, it can be stated that immunohistochemistry can be helpfull in solving the following problems:

1. a differential diagnosis between epithelial and non-epithelial tumors in the lung by the application of antibodies directed against epithelial antigens (MOC-31 and the different cytokeratins).
2. a differential diagnosis between neuroendocrine and non-neuroendocrine lung tumors by the application of the monoclonal antibodies directed against neuroendocrine antigens.
3. a differential diagnosis between SCLC and carcinoid by the application of the monoclonal antibody directed against the transferrin receptor.
4. a better recognition of lung tumor heterogeneity within the established histologies. Examples of this phenomenon are:
   a. the presence of neuroendocrine components within non-neuroendocrine tumors. Possible clinical implications hereof are discussed in section 5.1.
   b. the presence of squamous cell or adenocarcinomatous differentiation in non-SCLC as detected by chain specific anti-cytokeratin antibodies.
   c. the degree of neuroendocrine differentiation within SCLC as detected by monoclonal antibodies directed against different neuroendocrine antigens or by the monoclonal antibody directed against neurofilaments.
5. a specific antigenic fingerprint of the bronchial gland tumors.

The application of monoclonal antibodies directed against specific cell lineage or cell-differentiation antigens will surely add to a better understanding of the histogenesis and cell biology of lung cancer. Future studies will have to show whether the application of these antibodies for a pathological diagnosis will also add to a better therapeutical approach.

6. ACKNOWLEDGEMENTS
The authors thank Ella Vaarkamp, Felie Schmitz du Moulin, Edwin Schwander, Anita ter Haar, Geert Mesander, Mirjam Klein Rot, Tineke Oostendorp, Gert Schaart and Anita Huijsmans for their excellent technical assistance, as well as Dr. Desmond Carney, Dr. Jo Hilgers and Dr. Y. Nakazato for providing cell lines and antisera. We appreciate the interest and helpfull discussions of Prof. Sibrand Poppema and Prof. Hauw The and thank Kiki Bugter for typing the manuscript.

7. REFERENCES

1. Parkin DM, Stjernswärd J, Muir CS: Estimates of the worldwide frequence of twelve major cancers. Bull World Health Organ 62: 163-182, 1984.
2. Stolley D: Lung cancer in women - five years later, situation worse. New Engl J Med 309: 428-429, 1983.
3. Early lung cancer cooperative study: Early lung cancer detection: summary and conclusions. Am Rev Respir Dis 130: 565-570, 1984.
4. World Health Organization: The world health organization histological typing of lung tumors, 2nd ed. Am J Clin Pathol 77: 123-136, 1982.
5. Yesner R: Classification of lung-cancer histology. New Engl J Med 312: 652-653, 1985.
6. Elema JD, de Leij L, Postmus P, Poppema S, The TH: Critical evaluation of new techniques in the morphological diagnosis of lung cancer. In: Clinical and experimental pathology of lung cancer. McVie JG, Bakker W, Wagenaar SjSc, Carney D (eds). The Hague, Martinus Nijhoff, pp 91-103, 1986.
7. Greco FA, Oldham RK: Current concepts in cancer. Small-cell lung cancer. New Engl J Med 301: 355-358, 1979.
8. de Leij L, Postmus PE, Buys Ch, Elema JD, Poppema S, Brouwer M, Ramaekers F, van der Veen A, Mesander G, The TH: Characterization of three new "variant type" SCLC derived cell lines. Cancer Res 45: 6024-6034, 1985.
9. Baylin SB, Mendelsohn G: Time dependent changes in human tumors: Implications for diagnosis and clinical behaviour. Semin Oncol 9: 504-512, 1982.
10. Carney DN, Mitchell JB, Kinsella TJ: In vitro radiation and chemotherapy sensitivity of established cell lines of human small cell lung cancer and its large cell morphological variants. Cancer Res 43: 2806-2811, 1983.
11. Gazdar A, Carney DN, Guccion J, Baylin S: Small cell carcinoma of the lung: cellular origin and relationship to other pulmonary tumors. In: Small cell lung cancer. Greco F, Oldham R, Bunn P (eds). New York, Grune and Stratton, pp 145-176, 1981.
12. Baylin SB, Gazdar AF, Minna JD, Bernal SD, Shaper JH: A unique cell-surface protein phenotype distinguishes human small cell from non small cell lung cancer. Proc Natl Acad Sci USA 79: 4650-4654, 1982.
13. Goodwin G, Shaper JH, Abeloff MD, Mendelsohn G, Baylin SB: Analysis of cell surface proteins delineates a differentiation pathway linking endocrine and nonendocrine human lung cancers. Proc Natl Acad Sci USA 80: 3807-3811, 1983.
14. Bergh J, Nilsson K, Cate CC, Pettengill O, Sorenson GD: Cell surface glycoprotein patterns of cell lines derived from human small cell carcinoma of the lung. Acta Path Microbiol Scand Sect A 91: 9-15, 1983.

15. Bernal SD, Baylin SB, Shaper JH, Gazdar AF, Chen LB: Cytoskeleton-associated proteins of human lung cancer cells. Cancer Res 43: 1798-1808, 1983.
16. De Schrijver-Kecskemeti K, Kyriakos M, Bell CE, Seetharam S: Pulmonary oat cell carcinoma. Expression of plasma membrane antigen correlated with presence of cytoplasmic neurosecretory granules. Lab Invest 41: 432-436, 1979.
17. Bell CE, Seetharam S, McDaniel RC: Endodermally derived and neural crest derived differentiation antigens expressed by a human lung tumor. J Immunol 116: 1236-1243, 1976.
18. Bell CE, Seetharam S: Identification of the Schwann cell as a peripheral nervous system cell possessing a differentiation antigen expressed by a human lung tumor. J Immunol 118: 826-831, 1977.
19. De Leij L, Poppema S, Klein Nulend J, ter Haar A, Schwander E, Ebbens F, Postmus PE, The TH: Neuroendocrine differentiation antigen on human lung carcinoma and Kulchitski cells. Cancer Res 45: 2192-2200, 1985.
20. Stahel RA, Speak JA, Bernal SD: Murine monoclonal antibody LAM2 defines cell membrane determinant with preferential expression on human lung small cell carcinoma and squamous cell carcinomas. Int J Cancer 35: 11-17, 1985.
21. Tong AW, Lee J, Stone MJ: Characterization of two human small cell lung carcinoma-reactive monoclonal antibodies generated by a novel immunization approach. Cancer Res 44: 4987-4992, 1984.
22. Okaba T, Kaizu T, Fujisawa M, Watanaba J, Koyoko K, Yamashita T, Takaku F: Monoclonal antibodies to surface antigens of small cell carcinoma of the lung. Cancer Res 44: 5273-5278, 1984.
23. Rosen ST, Mulshine JL, Cuttitta F, Fedorko J, Carney DN, Gazdar AF, Minna JD: Analysis of human small cell lung cancer differentiation antigens using a panel of rat monoclonal antibodies. Cancer Res 44: 2052-2061, 1984.
24. Ball HD, Graziano RF, Pettengill OS, Sorenson GD, Fanger MW: Monoclonal antibodies reactive with small cell carcinoma of the lung. J Natl Cancer Inst 72: 593-598, 1984.
25. Bernal SD, Speak JA: Membrane antigen in small cell carcinoma of the lung defined by monoclonal antibody. Cancer Res 44: 265-270, 1984.
26. Stahel RA, O'Hara CJ, Mabry M, Waibel R, Sabbath K, Speak JA, Bernal SD: Cytotoxic murine monoclonal antibody LAM8 with specificity for human small cell carcinoma of the lung. Cancer Res 46: 2077-2084, 1986.
27. Brenner BG, Jothy S, Shuster J, Fuks A: Monoclonal antibodies to human lung tumor antigens demonstrated by immunofluorescence and immunoprecipitation. Cancer Res 42: 3187-3192, 1982.
28. Kyoizumi S, Akiyama M, Kouno N, Kobuka K, Hakado M, Jones SK, Yamakido M: Monoclonal antibodies to human squamous cell carcinoma of the lung and their application to tumor diagnosis. Cancer Res 45: 3274-3281, 1985.
29. Brown DT, Moore M: Monoclonal antibodies against two human lung carcinoma cell lines. Br J Cancer 46: 794-801, 1982.
30. Varki NM, Reisfeld RH, Walker LE: Antigens associated with a human lung adenocarcinoma defined by monoclonal antibodies. Cancer Res 44: 681-687, 1984.
31. Mulshine JL, Cuttitta F, Bibro M, Fedorko J, Fargion S, Little C, Carney DN, Gazdar AF, Minna JD: Monoclonal antibodies that distinguish non-small cell from small cell lung cancer. J Immunol 131: 497-502, 1983.

32. Mazauric T, Mitchell KF, Letchworth GJ, Koprowski H, Steplewski Z: Monoclonal antibody defined human lung cell surface protein antigens. Cancer Res 42: 150-154, 1982.
33. Radosevich JA, Ma Y, Lee I, Salwen HR, Gould VE, Rosen ST: Monoclonal antibody 44-3A6 as a probe for a novel antigen found on human lung carcinomas with glandular differentiation. Cancer Res 45: 5808-5812, 1985.
34. Sobol RE, Astarita RW, Cook-Hinds T, Burton D, Falco M, Masui H, Handley HH, Royston I: A monoclonal antibody reactive with a subset of human lung carcinomas. Clinical Res 31: 412A, 1983.
35. Bunn PA, Linnoila I, Minna JD, Carney D, Gazdar AF: Small cell lung cancer, endocrine cells of the fetal bronchus and other neuroendocrine cells express the leu-7 antigenic determinant present on natural killer cells. Blood 65: 764-768, 1985.
36. Ball ED, Sorenson GD, Pettengill OS: Expression of myeloid and major histocompatibility antigens on small cell carcinoma of the lung cell lines analyzed by cytofluorography: modulation by -interferon. Cancer Res 46: 2335-2339, 1986.
37. Cole SPC, Mirski S, McGarry RC, Cheng R, Campling BG, Roder JC: Differential expression of the leu-7 antigen on human lung tumor cells. Cancer Res 45: 4285-4290, 1985.
38. Marangos PJ, Carney DN, Polak JM, Pearse AGE: Neuron specific enolase and small cell cancer of the lung. In: The endocrine lung in health and disease. Becker KL, Gazdar AF (eds), WB Saunders Company, Philadelphia pp 509-515, 1984.
39. Thomas P, Battifore H, Manderino G: Is neuron-specific enolase specific? An immunohistochemical comparison of a monoclonal and a polyclonal antibody against neuron-specific enolase. Lab Invest 54: 63A, 1984.
40. Kumar NB, Cookingham CL, Lloyd RV, Appelman HD: Detection of human chromogranin with a monoclonal antibody in carcinoid secretory granules and its comparison with the generic silver stains and with serotonin. Lab Invest 50: 33A, 1984.
41. Wiedemann B, Franke WW, Kuhn C, Moll R, Gould VE: Synaptophysin: a marker protein for neuroendocrine cells and neoplasms. Proc Natl Acad Sci USA 83: 3500-3504, 1986.
42. Allan PM, Garson JA, Harper EI, Asser U, Coakham HB, Brownell B, Kemshead JT: Biological characterization and clinical applications of a monoclonal antibody recognizing an antigen restricted to neuroectodermal tissues. Int J Cancer 31: 591-598, 1983.
43. Lehto V-P, Stenman S, Miettinen M, Dahl D, Virtanen I: Expression of a neural type of intermediate filament as a distinguishing feature between oat cell carcinoma and other lung cancers. Am J Pathol 110: 113-118, 1983.
44. Broers J, Huijsmans A, Moesker O, Vooijs P, Ramaekers F, Wagenaar S: Small cell lung cancers contain intermediate filaments of the cytokeratin type. Lab Invest 52: 113-115, 1985.
45. Blobel G, Gould VE, Moll R, Lee I, Huszar M, Geiger B, Franke WW: Coexpression of neuroendocrine markers and epithelial cytoskeletal proteins in bronchopulmonary neuroendocrine neoplasms. Lab Invest 52: 39-51, 1985.
46. Bensch KG, Corrin B, Pariente R, Spencer H: Oat-cell carcinoma of the lung: its origin and relationship to bronchial carcinoid. Cancer 22: 1163-1172; 1968.
47. Moll R, Moll I, Franke WW: Identification of Merkel cells in human skin by specific cytokeratin antibodies: changes of cell density and distri-

bution in fetal and adult plantar epidermis. Differentiation 28: 136-154, 1984.

48. van Muyen GNP, Ruiter DJ, van Leeuwen C, Prins FA, Rietsema K, Warnaar SO: Cytokeratin and neurofilament in lung carcinomas. Am J Pathol 116: 363-369, 1984.
49. Kahn HJ, Garrido A, Huang SN, Baumal R: Intermediate filaments and tumor diagnosis. Lab Invest 49: 509-510, 1983.
50. Lehto V-P, Miettinen M, Virtanen I: A dual expression of cytokeratin and neurofilaments in bronchial carcinoid cells. Int J Cancer 35: 421-425, 1985.
51. de Leij L, Postmus PE, Poppema S, Elema JD, The TH: The use of monoclonal antibodies for the pathological diagnosis of lung cancer. In: Lung cancer: basic and clinical aspects. Hansen HH (ed). The Hague, Martinus Nijhoff, pp 31-48, 1986.
52. Stahlman MT, Gray ME: Ontogeny of neuroendocrine cells in human fetal lung. I. An electron microscopic study. Lab Invest 51: 449-463, 1984.
53. Broers J, Carney D, de Leij L, Vooys G, Ramaekers F: Differential expression of intermediate filament proteins distinguishes classic from variant small cell lung cancer cell lines. Proc Natl Acad Sci USA 82: 4409-4413, 1985.
54. de Leij L, Poppema S, Klein Nulend J, ter Haar JG, Schwander E, The TH: Immunoperoxidase staining on frozen tissue sections as a first screening assay in the preparation of monoclonal antibodies directed against small cell carcinoma of the lung. Eur J Cancer Clin Oncol 20: 123-128, 1984.
55. Broers JLV, Carney DN, Klein Rot M, Schaart G, Lane EB, Vooijs GP, Ramaekers FCS: Intermediate filament proteins in classic- and variant-type small cell lung carcinoma cell lines. A biochemical and immunochemical analysis using a panel of monoclonal and polyclonal antibodies. J Cell Sc 1986, in press.
56. Ramaekers F, Huijsmans A, Moesker O, Kant A, Jap P, Herman C, Vooijs P: Monoclonal antibodies to keratin filaments, specific for glandular epithelia and their tumors. Use in surgical pathology. Lab Invest 49: 353-361, 1983.
57. Ramaekers F, Puts J, Moesker O, Kant A, Huijsmans A, Haag D, Jap P, Herman C, Vooijs G: Antibodies to intermediate filament proteins in immunohistochemical identification of human tumors: an overview. Histochem J 15: 691-713, 1983.
58. Klük P, van Muyen GNP, van der Kamp AWM, Tibboel D, van Hoorn WA, Warnaar SO, Molenaar JC: Hirschsprung's disease studied with monoclonal antineurofilament antibodies on tissue sections. Lancet i: 652-654, 1984.
59. Sehested M, Hirsch FR, Hou-Jensen K: Immunoperoxidase staining for carcinoembryonic antigen in small cell carcinoma of the lung. Eur J Cancer Clin Oncol 17: 1125-1131, 1981.
60. Hammond ME, Sause WT: Large cell neuroendocrine tumors of the lung. Clinical significance and histopathologic definition. Cancer 56: 1624-1629, 1985.
61. Carney DN, Gazdar AF, Bepler G, Guccion JG, Marangos PJ, Moody TW, Zweig MH, Minna JD: Establishment and identification of small cell lung cancer cell lines having classic and variant features. Cancer Res 45: 2913-2923, 1985.
62. Gazdar AF, Carney DN, Nau MM, Minna JD: Characterization of variant subclasses of cell lines derived from small cell lung cancer having

distinctive biochemical, morphological, and growth properties. Cancer Res 45: 2924-2930, 1985.

63. Hirsch FR, Osterlind K, Hansen HH: The prognostic significance of histopathological subtyping of small cell carcinoma of the lung according to the World Health Organization. Cancer 52: 2144-2150, 1983.
64. Gould VE, Moll R, Moll I, Lee I, Franke WW: Neuroendocrine (Merkel) cells of the skin: hyperplasias, dysplasias, and neoplasias. Lab Invest 52: 334-353, 1985.
65. Miettinen M, Lehto V-P, Dahl D, Virtanen I: Varying expression of cytokeratin and neurofilaments in neuroendocrine tumors of human gastrointestinal tract. Lab Invest 52: 429-436, 1985.
66. Jasani B, Edwards RE, Thomas ND, Gibbs AR: The use of vimentin-antibodies in the diagnosis of malignant mesotheliomas. Virch Arch [Pathol Anat] 406: 441-448, 1985.
67. Gatter KC, Dunnhill MS, Muyen GNP van, Mason DY: Human lung tumours may co-express different classes of intermediate filaments. J Clin Pathol, in press, 1986.

11. MONOCLONAL ANTIBODIES IN DIAGNOSIS AND PROGNOSIS OF COLORECTAL CANCER.

J.W. ARENDS, T. WIGGERS, C.P.H.J. VERSTIJNEN, F.T. BOSMAN.

1. INTRODUCTION.

In 1979 Koprowski et al, (1) described the first series of monoclonal antibodies (MoAbs) recognizing antigens associated with colorectal cancer. Since in incidence large bowel carcinoma ranks amongst the major cancers in the Western world, it is not surprising that numerous MoAbs have been generated against this tumor.
Most of these MoAbs, however, have not yet been sufficiently characterized with regard to the specificity and/or to the biochemical nature of their target antigens (2). Therefore, the role of MoAbs in diagnosis and prognosis of colorectal cancer so far is limited. In this chapter a review of antigens associated with large bowel carcinoma will be given. Also, the problems and pitfalls as well as the achievements of the application of MoAbs will be discussed highlighting MoAbs reactive with two well studied antigens, CEA and the Ca 19-9 antigen, for illustrative purposes.

2. ANTIGENS ASSOCIATED WITH COLORECTAL CANCER.

Antigens associated with colorectal cancer can be classified in different ways. Little is known of the biochemical structure of most antigens involved and of their function. We prefer to classify the antigens associated with colorectal cancer according to the cell and tissue distribution. In table 1 an example of such a classification is given. The antigens with an * have been studied with MoAbs.

TABLE 1. Antigens present in normal colonic epithelium and in colorectal carcinoma.

1. All cell types	oncogene products, like ras p21* (3) intermediate filaments, villin, CEA* (4,5,6,7)
	blood group antigens*
	ABH system
	Lewis
	HLA-A,B,C antigens*
	epithelial membrane antigen
	EMA
	HMFG series* (8)
	mam series* (9)
2. Cell type associated	
- stemcell	?
- goblet cell	mucins
	sialo/sulfomucins
	mucus associated gastro-intestinal antigen, M3

- columnar cells	secretory component (SC) adenosine deaminase - complexing protein (ADCP)
- endocrine cells	neuron - specific enolase (NSE) chromogranin serotonin other hormone products
(-Paneth cells	lysozyme)

In table 2 a further specification is given of MoAbs recognizing antigens associated with colorectal carcinoma. Only those MoAb reactive with colorectal carcinoma that have been intensively studied in the litterature are mentioned. It should be noted that many MoAbs claimed to be colorectal cancer specific have not been tested on tissue sections and therefore their specificity remains questionable.

3. SPECIFICITY PROBLEMS

Specificity problems should be distinghuished in two types:

1. specificity of the antigen for colorectal (cancer) tissue.
2. specificity of MoAbs for single antigens.

3.1. Specificity of an antigen for colorectal (cancer) tissue relates to the exclusive occurrence of this antigen in colonic epithelium and colorectal cancer.
Although some new MoAbs initially were claimed to detect large bowel cancer specific antigens, these claims often had to be withdrawn after more extensive and rigorous study of their immunoreactivity on a larger panel of different tissues. Both CEA and Ca 19-9 may serve as excellent examples to illustrate the gradual alteration of the designation "colorectal cancer specific" into the more non-committal term "colorectal cancer associated".
CEA after its isolation from hepatic metastases of colonic carcinoma in 1965 by Gold and Freeman (17) has been found to occur in colonic carcinoma tissue as well as in other cancers, such as those of respiratory and genitourinary tract origin. The antigen has also been demonstrated in normal colonic mucosa.
Ca 19-9 shows a similar fate. The Ca 19-9 antigen initially has been hailed as being a non CEA related antigen of oncofetal nature restricted to some gastrointestinal tumors (18). More detailed immunocytochemical studies demonstrated the antigen in carcinomas of other than gastrointestinal derivation as well as in various normal adult tissues (19, 20).

3.2 Another pressing problem relates to the specificity of antigen detection by MoAbs. The lack of specificity of CEA detection has been partly attributed to the existence of many cross-reactive antigens detected by conventional antisera and the occurrence of various molecular varieties

not identifiable with most of these antisera. It was hoped that with the help of MoAbs more exact immunological characterization of the CEA molecule would become possible and that recognition of epitopes specific for CEA and molecular subtypes would enable the detection of CEA varieties specific for particular tissue types or conditions of disease (21). This hope so far has not materialized.
Although CEA-reactive MoAbs recognizing CEA specific epitopes have been described (4, 5), most of these MoAbs after scrutinous biochemical as well as immunocytochemical tests reveal at least a trace of reactivity with other substances (6), perhaps due to epitope-cross reactivity (fig. 1) (7).
The epitope crossreactivity problem in the detection of antigens by MoAbs is also demonstrated in studies on Ca 19-9. The antigen binding site originally was shown to occur on glycolipids of the monosialoganglioside complex (10). Subsequently, however, the same epitope was demonstrated to occur also on glycoproteins of mucin nature (22).

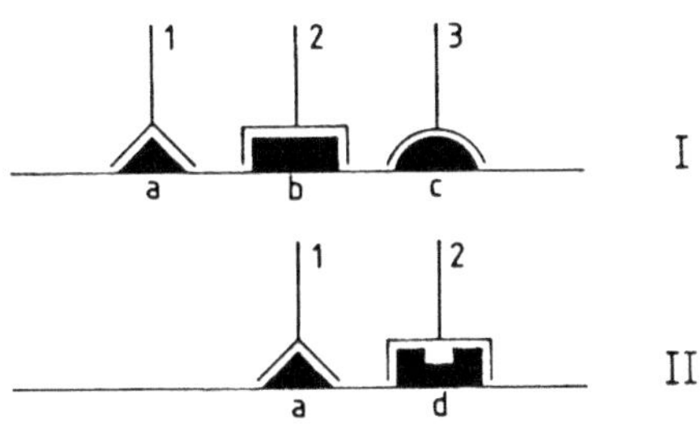

Fig. 1. MoAbs 1, 2 and 3 recognize the epitopes a, b, and c, respectively that are present on antigen I. The antigen II shares the epitope a with antigen I and in addition contains an epitope d having sufficient similarity to epitope b to react with MoAb 2, although the affinity of MoAb 2 for b may be reduced.
The epitope c is specific for antigen I.

4. APPLICATIONS OF MONOCLONAL ANTIBODIES
Some of the antigens listed in Table 2 like SC (23) ADCP (24) and serotonin (25) have been shown to be of prognostic value in large bowel carcinomas. These antigens have however been studied with polyclonal antisera. Studies with MoAbs have been of more limited value due to the circumstance that their and its tissue distribution are often incompletely characterized.

4.1 Diagnosis.
MoAbs useful for diagnosis of large bowel cancer are not available due to the specificity problems outlined above. Therefore, metastatic adenocarcinoma of unknown origin can not be unambiguously identified as of colorectal origin. In the diagnosis of primary, metastatic and recurrent lesions by immunoscintigraphic procedures, however, MoAbs may play a role. Especially CEA-reactive MoAbs have been used for this purppose and the first experiences with this procedure vary from encouraging (26) to cumbersome in certain technical and theoretical aspects (27, 28).

4.2 Tumor biology.
Phenotypic heterogeneity of tumors in regard of several features such as DNA-content, metastatic potential, clonogenicity, growth rate and also antigen composition has become one of the major topics of tumor research. Heterogeneity of antigen expression has been amply reported in large bowel carcinomas. Heterogeneity may exist between different large bowel carcinomas (intertumor heterogeneity) and between different clones in one tumor (intratumor heterogeneity. Both types of heterogeneity can be studied by means of differences in antigen profile. Here the application of MoAbs can be helpful. Especially study of intertumor heterogeneity is of importance, as this may allow the identification and classification of subsets of colorectal tumors on the basis of their cell of origin.
It is conceivable that such a classification will enable the identification of subsets of large bowel carcinomas with distinct biological behaviour and prognosis, as has been shown for malignant lymphomas.
Intratumor heterogeneity may complicate the assessment of prognosis based on antigen expression. Clones with a potentially different biological behaviour may have different antigen expression profiles. It is not well known what clone(s) determine the final outcome of a malignant proces. In addition, the interaction and interrelation of different clones may be important. Therefore, there is a certain inconsistency in characterizing tumors with respect to biological behaviour according to a feature heterogeneously expressed. Unfortunately, antigens expressed in the majority of clones of intestinal tumors appear to be scarce.Ca 19-9 for example was shown to be uniformly expressed in only 10.% of these carcinomas (29). Fig. 2 illustrates the expression patterns observed for Ca 19-9 in colorectal carcinomas.
CEA, in contrast, is one of the few antigens commonly present in most tumor cells (30).

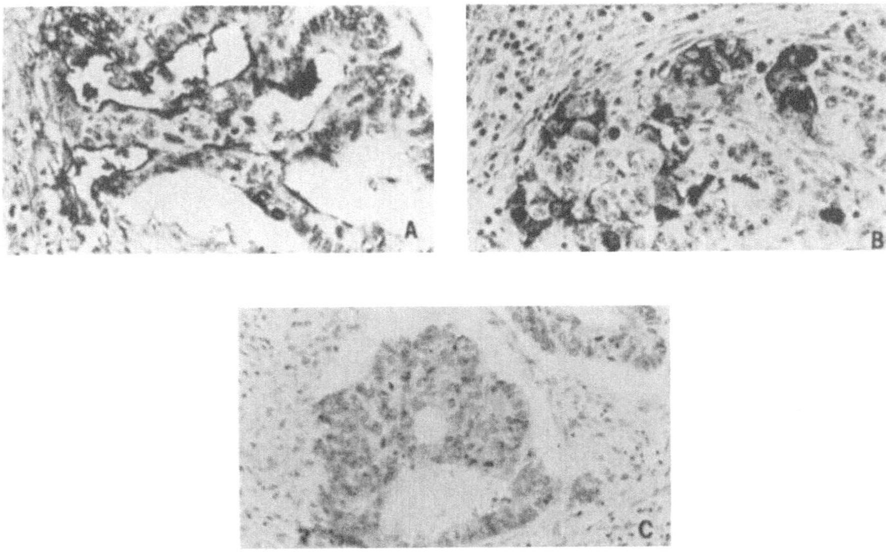

Fig. 2. Ca 19-9 expression patterns in colonic carcinoma. A. uniformly positive expression. B Focally positive expression. C. No expression (IP x 150).

4.3 Prognosis.
Despite the theoretical objections raised in paragraph 3.3 some encouraging results have been obtained in the assessment of prognosis of colorectal tumors using monoclonal antibodies. These are based on a few studies with large numbers of patients with adequate clinical pathological and follow-up data. Results of our group suggest that CEA and Ca 19-9 may be useful for the identification of subgroups of colorectal cancer patients with a poor prognosis. Patients with uniformly Ca 19-9 positive tumors and patients with CEA negative tumors or carcinomas demonstrating a membranous CEA expression pattern show a poor survival compared with Ca 19-9 negative or focally positive carcinomas and tumors displaying an apical/ cytoplasmic CEA immunoreactivity pattern respectively (fig. 3, 4 and 6) (29, 31).
These data encourage further studies.

5. FUTURE PERSPECTIVES
So far the impact of MoAbs in diagnosis and prognosis of colorectal cancer has been limited. This has been largely due to the rather crude preparations used for immunization. Therefore, selection of cell types or individual antigens of

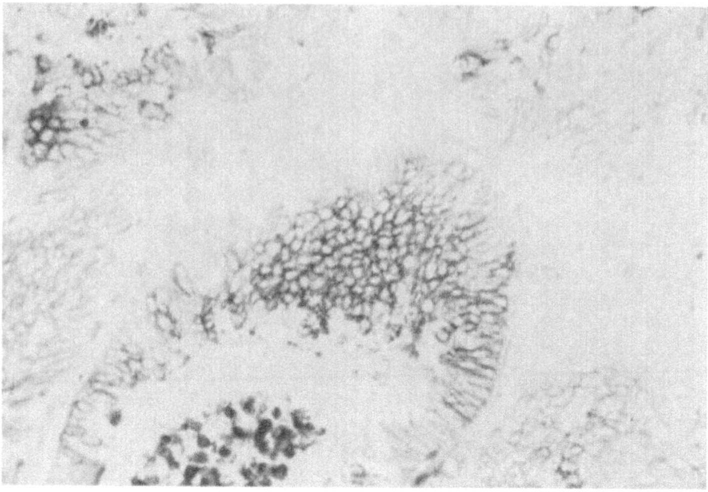

Fig. 3a. A colonic carcinoma with membranous CEA expression pattern (IP x 150).

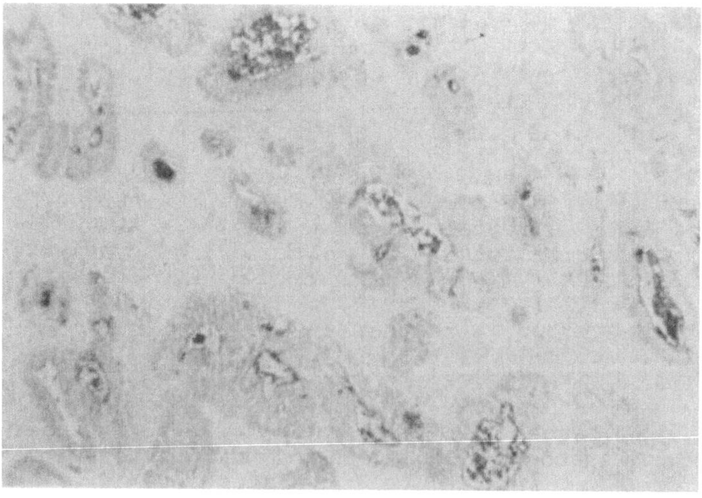

Fig. 3b. A colonic carcinoma with apical CEA expression pattern (IP x 150)

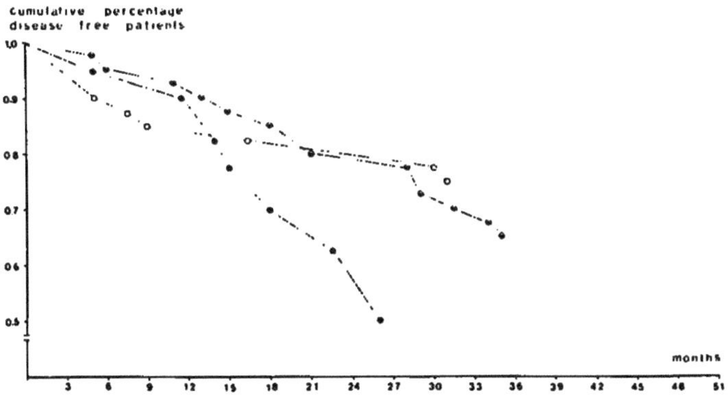

Fig. 4 Survival of patients with Ca 19-9 uniformly positive (●——●), focally positive (◒——◒) and negative tumours (○——○). P (Wilcoxon / Breslau) 0.33; P (Mantel / Cox) 0.25.

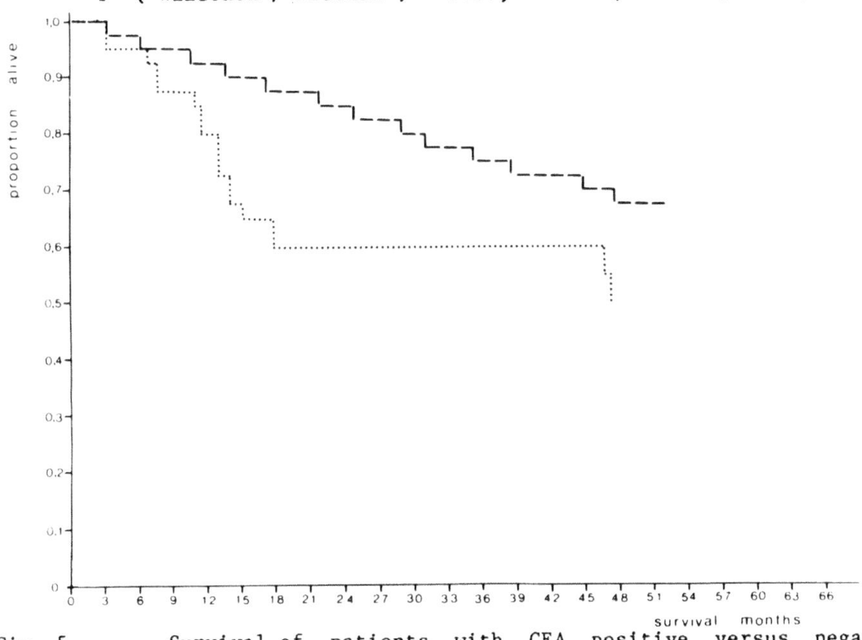

Fig. 5. Survival of patients with CEA positive versus negative tumours.

— — — — —positive

·············negative

TABLE II

MONOCLONAL ANTIBODIES RECOGNIZING ANTIGENS ASSOCIATED WITH LARGE BOWEL CARCINOMA

Designation	Immunizing agent	Immunocytochemical characterization on: cell lines	Immunocytochemical characterization on: tissue sections	Nature of antigen	Literature
1116					
19-9	SW colonic carcinoma	+	+	monosialoganglio-	10
52 a	cell line cells	+		side/mucin	
3 d		+	+	CEA 180.000	11
10		+			
38 a		+		LeB blood group	12
43		+			
3 a		+			
33 a		+		Neutral glycolipids	12
33 b					
WCDK	SW colonic	+		Not known	12
	carcinoma cell	+			
series	line cells	+			
YPC series	Not stated				
2/12.1					
				CEA mucin like	13
2/44.3		+(P)			
1083-17	SW colonic carcinoma	+(S)		Not known	14
1116-56	cell line cells	+(S)			
250-series	fresh colonic carcinoma	+	+	Not known	15
250.30 6	cells + Ht-29 cells				
C-series					
C 50	Colo-205 colonic	+ (S)		monosialoganglio-	16
C 51	carcinoma cell line	+ (S)		side complex	
C 53	cells	+ (S)			

S indicates, that the MoAb is reported to be large bowel carcinoma specific

\+ indicates, that the MoAb was screened in the system indicated at the top of the column.

P indicates, that the MoAb is reported to be reactive on paraffin sections.

potential interest for immunization seems to be an important prerequisite to obtain more useful MoAbs. In this respect, products of oncogenes may be suitable candidates as well as MoAbs generated against developmental stage specific antigens obtained by immunization with fetal intestinal epithelium, normal adult colonic crypt base cells and clones of undifferentiated large bowel carcinomas (2). Such antigens conceivably may help in the establishment of cell origin related classifications and in diagnosis of colorectal cancers.Application of panels of MoAbs for the simultaneous detection of multiple antigens might provide additional information in a multivariate analysis on large series of patients and increase the efficiency of MoAbs in the establishment of a differential diagnosis and assessment of prognosis.

6. CONCLUSIONS

1. Due to specificity problems, either in relation to the exclusiveness of antigen occurrence or related to the specificity of antigen detection, the application of MoAbs in diagnosis of large bowel cancer is as yet limited.
2. Application of MoAbs will be of great value to study the biology of large bowel cancer, especially the phenomenon of heterogeneity. Study of intertumor heterogeneity may enable the identification of subgroups of colorectal cancers of different histogenesis, each with a distinct biological behaviour and prognosis. Intratumor heterogeneity in contrast, may complicate the assessment of prognosis.
3. Despite this intratumor heterogeneity the initial results of the application of MoAbs in the assessment prognosis of patients with colorectal cancer appears to be encouraging.
4. A selective approach in the generation of MoAbs, especially directed towards the production of MoAbs recognizing developmental stage specific antigens, will probably result in MoAbs more useful for diagnostic and prognostic purposes than those generated so far.
5. Application of a panel of MoAbs in a multivariate analysis on large patient series is the proper setting to test their prognostic contribution.

REFERENCES

1. Koprowski H, Steplewski Z, Mitchell K, Herlyn M, Herlyn D, Fuhrer P. Colorectal carcinoma antigens detected by hybridoma antibodies. Som. Cell Genet. 1979; 5: 957-972.
2. Arends JW, Bosman FT, Hilgers J. Tissue antigens in large-bowel carcinoma. Biochem. Biophys. Acta 1985; 780: 1-19.
3. Thor A, Horan Hand P, Wunderlich D, Caruso A, Muraro R, Schlom J. Monoclonal antibodies define differential ras gene expression in malignant and benign colonic diseases. Nature 1984; 311: 562-565.
4. Primus FJ, Kuhns WJ, Goldenberg DM. Immunological heterogeneity of carcinoembryonic antigen: immunohistochemical detection of carcinoembryonic antigen determinants in colonic tumors with monoclonal antibodies. Cancer Res. 1983; 43: 693-701.
5. Wagner C, Joy Yang YH, Crawford FG, Shively JE. Monoclonal antibodies for carcinoembryonic antigen and related as a model system: a systematic approach for the determination of epitope specificaties of monoclonal antibodies. J. Immunol. 1983; 130: 2308-2315.
6. Haskell CM, Buchegger F, Schreyer M, Carrel S, Mach JP Monoclonal antibodies to carcinoembryonic antigen: ionic strength as a factor in the selection of antibodies for immunoscintigraphy. Cancer Res. 1983; 43: 3857-3864.
7. Verstijnen CPHJ, Arends JW, Moerkerk PTM, Warnaar S, Hilgers J, Bosman FT (in press) CEA-specificity of CEA-reactive monoclonal antibodies. Immunochemical and immunocytochemical studies. Anti Cancer Res.
8. Taylor-Papadimitriou J. Peterson JA, Arklie J, Burchell J, Ceriani RL, Bodmer WF. Monoclonal antibodies to epithelium-specific components of the human milk fat globule membrane; production and reaction with cells in culture. Int. J. Cancer 1981; 28: 17-21.
9. Hilkens J. Buys F, Hilgers J, Hageman Ph, Sonneberg A, Koldowski U, Karanda K, v. Hoeven RP, Feltkamp C, v.d. Rijn JM. Monoclonal antibodies against human milkfat globule membranes detecting differentiation antigens of the mammary gland. Prot. Biol. Fluids 1982; 29: 813-826.
10. Magnani JL, Nilsson B, Brockhaus M, Sopf D, Steplewski Z, Koprowski H, Ginsburg V. A monoclonal antibody-defined antigen associated with gastrointestinal cancer in ganglioside containing sialyted lacto-N-Fuco pentaose II. J. Biol. Chem. 1982; 257: 14365-14369.
11. Mitchell KF. A carcinoembryonic antigen (CEA) specific monoclonal hybridoma antibody that reacts only with high-molecular-weight CEA. Cancer Immunol. Immunother. 1980; 10: 1-5
12. Steplewski Z, Koprowski H. Monoclonal antibody development in the study of colorectal carcinoma-associated antigen. Methods Cancer Res. 1982;

10: 313.
13. Finan PJ, Grant RM, Mattos de D, Takei F, Berry PJ, Lennox ES, Bleehen NM. Immunohistochemical techniques in the early screening of monoclonal antibodies to human colonic epithelium. Br. J. Cancer 1982; 46: 917.
14. Herlyn M, Steplewski Z, Herlyn D, Koprowski H. Colorectal carcinoma-specific antigen: Detection by means of monoclonal antibodies. Proc. Natl. Acad. Sci. 1979; 76: 1438-1442.
15. Thompson CH, Jones SL, Pihil E, McKenzie IFC. Monoclonal anitobdies to human colon and colorectal carcinoma. Br. J. Cancer 1983; 47: 595-605.
16. Lindholm L, Holmgren J, Svennerholm L, Fredman P, Nilsson O, Persson B, Myrvold H, Lagergard. Monoclonal antibodies against gastrointestinal tumor-associated antigen isolated as monosialogangliosides. Int. Archs. Allergy Appl. Immun. 1983; 71: 178-181.
17. Gold P, Freeman SO. Demonstration of tumor-specific antigens in human colonic carcinoma by immunological tolerance and absorption techniques. J. Exp. Med. 1965; 121: 439-462.
18. Koprowski H, Herlyn M, Steplewski Z, Sears HF. Specific antigen in serum of patients with colon carcinoma. Science 1981; 212: 53-55.
19. Atkinson BF, Ernst CS, Herlyn M, Steplewski Z, Sears H, Koprowski H. Gastrointestinal cancer-associated antigen in immunoperoxidase assay. Cancer Res. 1982; 42: 4820-4823.
20. Arends JW, Verstijnen C, Bosman FT, Hilgers J, Steplewski Z. The distribution of 116 NS 19-9 monoclonal antibody defined monosialoganglioside in normal and cancerous human tissues. Hybridoma 1983; 2: 81-91.
21. Rogers GT. Heterogeneity of carcinoembryonic antigens: Implications on its role as a tumor marker subtance. Biochim. Biophys. Acta 1976; 458: 355-373.
22. Raux H, Labbe F, Fondanneche MC, Koprowski H, Burtin P. A study of gastrointestinal cancer-associated antigen (GICA) in human fetal organs. Int. J. Cancer 1983; 32: 315-319.
23. Arends JW, Wiggers T, Thijs Ct, Verstijnen C, Swaen GJV, Bosman FT. The value of secretory component (SC) immunoreactivity in diagnosis and prognosis of colorectal carcinomas. Am. J. Clin. Pathol. 1984; 82: 267-274.
24. Ten Kate J, Van den Ingh HFGM, Khan PM, Bosman FT (in press). Adenosine deaminase complexing protein (ADCP9 immunoreactivity in colorectal adenocarcinoma. Int. J. Cancer.
25. Arends JW, Wiggers T, Verstijnen C, Bosman FT. (in press) The occurence and clinicopathological significance of serotonin immunoreactive cells in large bowel carcinoma. J. Pathol.
26. Goldenberg DM, Kim EE, Deland FH, Bennett S, Primus FJ. Radioimmunodection of cance with radioactive antibodies to carcinoembryonic antigen. Cancer Res. 1980; 40:

2984-2992.

27. Mach FP, Buchegger F, Forni M, Ritschard J, Berche C, Lumbroso JD, Schreyer M, Girardet C, Accolla RS, Carrell S. Use of radiolabeled monoclonal anti-CEA antibodies for the detection of human cercinomas by external photoscanning and tomoscintography. Immunol. 1981; today: 239-249.
28. Berche C, Mach JP, Lumbroso JD, Langlais C, Aubry L, Buchegger P, Parmentier C, Tubiana M. Tomoscintigraphy for detecting gastrointestinal and medullary thyroid cancers: first clinical results using radiolabeled monoclonal antibodies against carcinoembryonic antigen. Br. Med. J. 1982; 285: 1447-1451.
29. Arends JW, Wiggers T, Verstijnen C, Hilgers J, Bosman FT. Gastrointestinal cancer-associated antigen (GICA) immunoreactivity in colorectal carcinoma in relation to patient survival. Int. J. Cancer 1984; 34: 193-196.
30. Arends JW, Wiggers T, Verstijnen C, Bosman FT, Swaen GJV, Hilgers J, Lennox E, Steplewski Z. (in press) Tumor cell heterogeneity in primary and metastatic colorectal carcinoma. Proceeding of the 31st Colloquium Protides of the Biological Fluids Ed. H. Peeters (Pergamon Press, Oxford) p.p. 587-595.
31. Wiggers T, Arends JW, Verstijnen C, Moerkerk PM, Bosman FT. Prognostic significance of CEA immunoreactivity patterns in large bowel carcinoma tissue. Br. J. Cancer.(in press)

12. MONOCLONAL ANTIBODIES REACTING WITH TUMORS OF THE UROLOGICAL TRACT OR PROSTATE.

S.O. WARNAAR, E. OOSTERWIJK

1. INTRODUCTION

The diagnoses of renal cell carcinoma (RCC) can be difficult. The primary tumor may be symptomless and a distant metastasis can present the first clinical manifestations. Also the variable aspects of cell morphology, such as clear cells, spindle cells and solid undifferentiated cells can lead to diagnostic problems in metastatic RCC, although in large sections the presence of all cell types mentioned above usually permits unequivocal identification.

The sites to which RCC metastasizes are mainly the lung (50%) and bone marrow (33%). In addition the regional lymph nodes, the liver and the adrenals are frequently involved, although RCC can be found at almost any location in the body. Growth into the renal vein is not always considered as metastatic as a continuous mass is usually formed with a primary site in the kidney. Considering the clinical and morphological aspects RCC can be mistaken for osteosarcoma, soft tissue sarcoma, various adenocarcinomas, clear cell sarcoma, undifferentiated melanoma and lymphoma. Therefore antibodies specific for RCC associated antigens can be of considerable help in establishing a differential diagnosis.

2.1 RENAL CELL CARCINOMA SPECIFIC ANTIBODIES

Renal cell carcinoma originates from the epithelium of proximal tubules (1,2,3). This is a highly specialized epithelium and it may therefore be anticipated to contain specific antigens. These antigens might to some extent be retained in the neoplastic situation and be used as markers for RCC. This anticipation is already suggested by older literature data that indicated that RCC could be detected by conventional antibodies raised against the tumor, after exhaustive absorption with normal tissue antigens (45). In the recent past a number of research groups have developed monoclonal antibodies with considerable specificity for RCC (6-12). These antibodies can be grouped into two categories. One category of antibodies reacts with RCC but does not react with normal renal tissues. In fact most of the antibodies in this category do not react with any other normal tissue, whether fetal or adult. The second category of antibodies does react with RCC and also with normal renal epithelia and with some other tissues, mainly epithelia.

A number of the antibodies described in the literature has been extensively characterized on normal tissues, primary and metastatic RCC and other non related tumors. Some have also been characterized on cell lines. Here we will summarize some relevant data on those antibodies that recognize RCC with sufficient specificity to merit closer scrutiny of their potential as diagnostic reagents.

Ueda et al (6) described a number of antibodies with specificity for RCC cell lines. These antibodies fell into four groups, based on staining results on cell lines, absorption analysis and immunoblotting. Some of these antibodies were characterized subsequently by Cordon-Cardo et al (11,13) and Finstad et al (7) on normal human tissues and tumor sections. The following discussion will be based on the data presented in these four papers.

Group 1, consists of antibodies S4, S7 and S11, all of subclass Ig2a and derived from one immunized mouse, and antibodies S24 and M1 both of subclass Igγ1, derived from two additional mice. Antibody S4 is identical to Uro2 in ref 13. These antibodies recognize a glycoprotein of 160 kilodalton. The prototype antibody S4 reacts with glomeruli and proximal tubuli up to the thin part of Henle's loop and also reacts with fibroblasts of interstitial matrix and with endothelium of blood vessels. This antibody does not react with cell lines from astrocytoma, melanoma, breast carcinoma or with various cell lines of hematopoietic malignancies. However the antibody reacted with cell lines derived from germ cell tumors as well as neuroblastoma, ovarian carcinoma, various sarcomas and a few other tumors in addition to reacting with RCC cell lines. When tested on frozen sections of tumors S4 antibody appeared to be more specific for RCC than expected from the results obtained on tumor cell lines. Whereas 80 percent of RCC were positive with this antibody only 5/65 of a variety of other tumors tested were positive. These tumors were 4 sarcomas and one mesothelioma. Therefore S4 (and presumably the other antibodies of this group) may have some utility in diagnosing RCC. A drawback is the reaction with fibrocytes in the tumor matrix.

Group 2 consists of antibodies S23 and S27 (=Uro4) both of subclass Igγ1 and derived from the same mouse. The antigen recognized was identified as a glycoprotein of 120 kilodalton, later shown to be the adenosine-deaminase binding protein ADA-BP (7). S23 and S27 recognize different epitopes of this protein.

In the kidney these antibodies react with the proximal tubulus and the thick descending part of Henle's loop. In normal kidney adjacent to RCC occasionally the glomerulus and Bowman's space were also positive. In normal tissues S27 was restricted to placentic trophoblast and prostatic epithelium whereas S23 was more widely distributed and also stained epithelial cells in breast, lung and colon. When tested on cell lines these antibodies were negative with melanoma, sarcoma, hematopoietic malignancies, neuroblastoma and breast carcinomas whereas other cell types showed variable staining results. When tested on frozen sections of tumors both antibodies stained about 90% of RCC including 4 RCC metastases. S23 stained 9/31 of the other carcinomas tested whereas S27 reacted weakly with 5/12 leukemias and lymphomas and only stained one carcinoma of the prostate out of 31 other carcinomas tested. For diagnostic purposes S27 seems therefore to offer greater specificity than S23.

Group 3 contains only antibody S22, subclass Igγ1. This antibody reacts with a glycoprotein of 115 kilodaltons. All normal tissue tested, whether fetal or adult were negative with S22 except normal kidney adjacent to RCC where in some cases a weak staining of Bowman's capsule was observed. When tested on frozen sections of RCC, 50% of the tumors tested were positive, the majority of which showed a heterogeneous staining reaction. Out of 65 other tumors of various origins only one bladder and one adrenal cortical carcinoma were positive with S22. This antibody appears therefore to offer a high specificity for diagnosing RCC, although the sensitivity is low.

Antibody S22 is the first antibody described that does not stain normal adult or fetal tissues and is highly specific for RCC. Other groups have described antibodies with similar characteristics. The nature of the antigen recognized is unknown, however it is tempting to speculate that it is related to an infectious agent, possibly a retrovirus (14).

Group 4 consists of antibody F23, subclass Ig2a that recognizes a glycoprotein of 140 kilodalton. In normal kidney the proximal tubulus and fibrocytes in the interstitium are stained. In other tissues fibrocytes and cartilage are stained. F23 reacts with 90% of RCC when tested on frozen sections. Of 31 other carcinomas 2 were positive and of 34 of a variety of other tumors tested 9 were positive.

In Minneapolis a group of workers (Vessela, Moon, Rei Kwan Chiou, Lange and others) have developed two antibodies (of Igγ1 subclass) A6H and D5D respectively that appear to be very promising as diagnostic reagents (8,9,10). Antibody A6H reacts with proximal tubular epithelium and does not react with the normal adult or fetal tissues tested. When tested on cell lines it was found to react with 14/14 RCC cell lines, with some colonic and testicular carcinoma cell lines and, more weakly, with a bladder and a breast carcinoma cell line. When tested on thin sections of various tumors 14/17 RCC and 6/12 colonic carcinomas were positive whereas 17 other tumors of various origins were negative.

The positive reaction of A6H on colon tumors makes this antibody less suitable for diagnostic purposes. However this antibody was found to be capable of locating small RCC tumors growing in nude mice by immune scintigraphy. This antibody may possibly be useful in detecting RCC metastases in patients.

Antibody D5D was found to be extremely specific for RCC. Normal adult or fetal tissues, including kidney, were negative with this antibody, as was also the case for all non RCC cell lines tested. When tested on tumors D5D stained 14/19 of RCC and did not stain any of 36 other carcinomas. The staining reaction on RCC appeared to be weak to moderate. Occasionally in normal kidney tissue adjacent to RCC Bowman's capsules were weakly stained. The determinant recognized was resistant to glutaraldehyde and on occasion could be demonstrated in formalin fixed and paraffin embedded RCC specimen. The antigen has not yet been characterized. The staining pattern of D5D seems similar to the S22 antibody described by the Sloan-Kettering group. It will be interesting to see whether or not the same antigen is recognized. Possibly D5D and S22 may complement each other on RCC, leading to a higher sensitivity of detection of RCC tumors.

In Mainz the group of Schärfe et al (12) have developed 4 monoclonal antibodies all (Igγ1) with overall staining patterns reminiscent of D5D and S22. No normal adult or fetal tissues were stained by any of these 4 antibodies whereas 92/97 RCC were positive. It appears that only 4 other carcinomas were tested, all negative with these 4 antibodies. A remarkable feature was the negative reaction with sarcomatous components of RCC.In this respect the 4 antibodies of Schärfe et al differed clearly from D5D and S22. Schärfe's antibodies may recognize two or more different determinants, based on intracellular localisation of stain. It was reported that the antigen(s) were excreted into patient's urine.

Wahlström et al (15) reported recently that a monoclonal antibody 12/1-2 against HTLV p19 reacted with 42/42 RCC, with 10/10 destructive hydatiform moles and with 10/10 choriocarcinomas. This antibody also reacted with normal syncytiotrophoblast, recognizing an antigen of 28KD, possibly related to endogenous human retrovirus. That a retroviral protein is recognized in RCC is supported by the fact that a conventional antibody against a synthetic peptide with a sequence based on a cloned human endogenous retroviral DNA sequence also reacted with 42/42 RCC and with syncytiotrophoblast cells and choriocarcinoma (14) . Syncytiotrophoblast cells have been reported to contain retroviral like particles. The antibody against the synthetic peptide reacts with a 75 kD component in these tissues. Normal kidney was negative as well as 82 other carcinomas consisting of Wilms' tumor, colonic carcinomas and tumors of the female genital tract.
The negative staining results on normal kidney resemble the data on D5D, S22 and the four antibodies described by Schärfe et al. It would be interesting to see whether D5D and Schärfes antibodies are positive on syncytiotrophoblast and choriocarcinoma, as this might indicate an endogenous viral component, similar to the antibody described by Wahlstrom. Such data may result in the recognition of retrovirus involvement with RCC.

Recently our Leiden group described a set of antibodies with specificity for RCC (16). Two antibodies, RC3 (Igγ1) and RC69 (IgGanna ιaained proximal tubuli in normal kidney sections and did not stain any other adult or fetal tissue tested. These antibodies stained approximately 35% of primary RCC but did not react with metastatic RCC nor with any other tumor tested.

As metastatic RCC is not stained by these antibodies they cannot be used for differential diagnostic purposes. A third antibody RC38 (Igγ1) appears to be better suited for this purpose. This antibody reacts with the glomerular and proximal tubular epithelium in normal kidneys and also reacts with the surface epithelium in jejunum and colon, the mucous cells of the foveolar and glandular layer of the stomach mucosa, the acini of sweat glands and with cells lining sinuses in liver and lymph nodes. Other tissues tested, whether adult or fetal were negative. This antibody stained 46/47 primary RCC and 8/13 of RCC metastases. In 70% of RCC more than 50% of cells were positive with RC38. No reaction was seen with a variety of 179 other tumors, indicating that this antibody may be of help in diagnosing difficult cases of RCC. RC38 can be used to immunoscintigraph human RCC growing in nude mice (to be published).

We also isolated an antibody, RC250 (Igγ1) that reacts with RCC but does not react with normal adult or fetal tissues except bile canaliculi and surface epithelium of jejunum and that resembles in this respect the antibodies D5D, S22 and the four antibodies of Schärfe et al. Antibody RC250 stained 47/48 primary RCC and 7/9 RCC metastasis. In 90% of primary RCC and in 51% of metastatic RCC more than 50% of the tumor cells were positive. Out of 118 other tumors 14 were positive. These positive tumors were 3/13 colonic carcinomas, 4/19 sarcomas, 6/20 ovarian carcinomas. In general these positive tumors contained less positive cells than RCC. RC250 can also be used for immunescintigraphy.

The data on the anti-RCC monoclonal antibodies are summarized in table 1.

Table 1
DISTRIBUTION OF RCC ASSOCIATED ANTIGENS RECOGNIZED BY MONOCLONAL ANTIBODIES

			STAINING RESULTS			
antibody	antigen	kidney	RCC prim.	RCC metas.	ca*	other tumors**
S4,S7,S11 (1)	gp160	G,PT	13/16	3/4	0/32	5/31
F23 (1)	gp140	PT,HL	14/16	4/4	2/32	8/31
S23 (1)	gp120	PT,HL	14/16	4/4	9/32	2/32
A6H (2)	-	PT	13/15	1/2	6/30	-
RC3 (5)	-	PT,HL	36/51	1/10	0/88	0/16
RC69 (5)	-	PT,HL	30/44	0/7	0/54	0/8
RC38 (5)	-	G,PT	46/47	8/13	0/127	0/51
S22 (1)	gp115	no react.	9/16	2/4	2/52	0/31
D5D (2)	-	"	12/17	2/2	0/35	0/1
C8/D8,E6/B7 (3)		"	92/97	6/6		
RC250 (5)	-	"	46/42	7/9	14/108	4/33
12/1-2 (4)			42/42	?	20/102	-

G=glomerulus, PT=proximal tubulus, HL=Henle's loop
*=carcinomas of non renal origin
**=lymphomas, sarcomas and melanomas
(1) lit.ref.6,7,11,13 (2) lit.ref. 8-10 (3) lit.ref.12
(4) lit.ref.15 (5) lit.ref.16

2.2 CYTOSKELETAL ANTIBODIES IN RCC

For a more complete discussion of the cytoskeleton as tumor marker see chapter 4 of this book.
In establishing a diagnosis of RCC it has been found that antibodies to cytokeratin and vimentin can be useful as RCC is a tumor in which it is usually possible to find tumor cells positive with anti-keratin as well as with anti-vimentin, see chapter 5. Herman et al (17) found 11/13 of RCC positive with anti keratin and 12/13 positive with anti vimentin, Holthöfer et al (18) found cytokeratin in 28/30 tumors whereas only 16/30 RCC were vimentin positive. This discrepancy in vimentin staining is difficult to explain. Data from our own lab indicated that 51/52 RCC were cytokeratin positive and 48/52 vimentin positive. These data are comparable to the data of Herman et al. The somewhat higher staining with anti cytokeratin may be due to differences in antibody used. No difference was found between primary and metastatic RCC.
With antivimentin clone V9 and anticytokeratin clone 80 (Sanbio B.V., see appendix) we found that almost all tumor cells were diffusely positive with anti vimentin whereas the anti cytokeratin in general stained more than 50% of tumor cells irrespective of the morphology of the tumor cells.
Both Holthöfer et al and we did not find any tumor cells positive with antidesmin. Also out of 53 tumors tested none was positive with specific anticarcinoembryonic (CEA) antigen (see chapter M.Nap for full discussion anti CEA antibodies). This can be helpful differentiating RCC from anaplastic lung, breast and colon tumors.

2.3 CONCLUSIONS AND FUTURE DEVELOPMENTS

In establishing a differential diagnosis of RCC on a metastatic tumor immunohistochemistry with anti vimentin and anti cytokeratin is at present the most useful combination as these antibodies are available commercially. Of the RCC related antibodies described in the literature S27, RC38 and D5D seem to be the most useful for diagnostic purposes.
The relatively large number of antibodies that recognize determinants on RCC and that do not react with any normal tissue support a viral origin of this tumor as was first suggested by the positive reaction with RCC of antibodies directed against various retroviral proteins.
The availability of RCC specific antibodies will most likely lead to the development in the near future of tests for monitoring tumor burden.
Some antibodies already available may be useful for immunoscintigraphy.

3 TRANSITIONAL CELL CARCINOMA (TCC) OF THE BLADDER

In the USA TCC of the urinary tract is responsible for approximately 1% of cancer deaths. The tumor is highly

variable and may be solid, papillary sessile or be present as carcinoma in situ (19,20). The course of the illness may also vary considerably.
Several investigators have tried to develop monoclonal antibodies to bladder tumor antigens (11,21,22).However none of the antibodies described appear to be useful for the differential diagnosis of metastatic TCC of the urinary tract.

The most specific of the antibodies described is the Uro 9 (=OM5) antibody described by Cordon-Cardo (11) This antibody reacted with about half of all bladder carcinomas and did not stain any of other tumors tested. These tumors included renal, colonic, lung and breast carcinomas, melanomas, lymphomas, squamous carcinomas and astrocytomas. Uro 9 is reported to stain some but not all urothelial tissues, and to be negative on all other normal human tissues tested.
On urothelial tumors it was found to stain 17/20 non invasive papillary bladder carcinomas, 6/8 non papillary carcinomas in situ, but only 3/15 invasive transitional carcinomas. Out of 6 bladder cancer metastases none was positive with Uro 9. This severy limits the usefulness of Uro 9 for diagnostic purposes.

Another possibly useful antibody is 3G2-C6 (22), an antibody of subclass Igγ1(k) that recognizes a protein of 90.000 dalton present in cultured bladder tumor cells. This antibody reacts with grade 3 and some grade 2 TCC but not with normal urothelium. The antibody will also react with some other tumors of the urogenital tract such as embryonal carcinoma, seminoma and an occasional renal cell carcinoma. No extensive screening on normal human tissues and other cancers has been performed. As normal urothelium is negative the antibody may be used for cytological examination of urine specimen.

For estimating patients prognoses by immunohistochemical analysis two markers have been found to be useful. The loss of bloodgroup antigens of the ABH(0) system and the abnormal expression of the Thomsen-Friedenreich antigen were found to be correlated with an unfavorable course (23).At present no monoclonal antibodies to these antigens have been evaluated for expression on normal and abnormal bladder epithelium.

3 CONCLUSION

No monoclonal antibody is recommendable as yet for differential diagnosis of bladder TCC.

4 PROSTATE CARCINOMA

Carcinoma of the prostate gland (PC) has the second highest cancer morbidity in males.Two antigens are highly specific markers for the diagnosis and monitoring of PC. These antigens have been extensively characterized and conventional and monoclonal antibodies reacting with these antigens have been prepared. The oldest and best known of

these is the prostate acid phosphatase, PAP, that was originally described by Gutman and Gutman (24). Jobsis et al (25) in an immunohistochemical study showed that 29/30 primary PC and 20/20 metastases were positive for PAP whereas 0/56 other carcinomas were stained with conventional anti PAP.
Recently Lillehoy et al(26) have described monoclonal antibodies against PAP. Three antibodies were of rat and three other of mouse origin, of varying subclasses. No immunohistochemical data were provided.

The second well characterized protein is the prostate specific antigen (PSA or PA) (27) a protein of 34 kilodalton. Nadji et al (28) showed that 73/73 primary PC and 49/49 metastases were positive with conventional anti PSA antibodies whereas 0/78 other tumors were positive. Purnell et al (20) also found that PC are positive with anti PSA antibodies. Recently Papsidero et al (30) described a monoclonal antibody, F5, Igγ1(k) that reacts with PSA. The epitope recognized was resistant to formalin fixation and paraffin embedding. F5 does not react with normal tissue except the ductal epithelium of the prostate gland.
When tested on 56 different tumors, mainly carcinomas, none was found to be positive.
In addition to F5 three other monoclonal antibodies to PSA have been described that were tested only for use in ELISA type tests for PSA in serum (31).

Two other monoclonal antibodies specific for PC have been characterized immunohistochemically. One antibody KR-P8 (32) subclass Igγ1 reacts with normal prostatic ductal epithelium but not with other normal epithelia. This antibody reacted with 15/15 PC and was negative on 2 colonic carcinomas. Although more tumors need to be tested before the usefulness of this antibody for differential diagnosis of PC can be evaluated the fact that the normal tissues tested were all negative suggests that this antibody is specific for prostate. The antigen recognized appears to be different from PAP or PSA and also different from an antigen recognized by antibody α Pro-3 (33)) an anti prostate antibody whose specificity was assayed by means of ELISA tests on tissue extracts.
Antibody KR-P8 will react with sections from formalin fixed and paraffin embedded PC and therefore may be a useful additional PC marker. Finally the antibody D83-21 can be mentioned. This antibody will stain proximal tubular epithelium but is negative with all other normal tissues tested, including the ductal epithelium of the prostate. When tested on PC sections 11/19 primary PC and 1/6 PC metastases were positive. Benign tumors and well differentiated regions of PC were negative or weakly positive with this antibody. Of 4 bladder carcinomas tested 1 was positive. Fifteen other carcinomas including 2 RCC were negative. The antibody also reacts with a cytomegalovirus antigen. The epitope recognized was shown to be present on two glycoprotein molecules of 60 and 28 kdalton respectively present in HCMV infected cells and in a

PC cell line. Possibly HCMV has a role in the induction of certain PC.

CONCLUSION

Monoclonal F5 directed against prostate specific antigen is a suitable reagent for immunohistochemical detection of prostate carcinoma.
Possibly KR-P8 and the monoclonal antibodies to prostate acid phosphatase are also suitable for this purpose.

REFERENCES

1. Oberling C, Riviere M, Haguenau F: Ultrastructure of the clear cells in renal carcinomas and its importance for the demonstration of their renal origin.
Nature 186: 402. 1960.
2. Bennington JL: Cancer of the kidney - Etiology, epidemiology and pathology.
Cancer 32: 1017, 1973.
3. Xipell JM: The incidence of benign renal nodules (a clinico pathologic study).
J.Urol.106:503. 1971.
4. Belitsky P et al: Radionuclide imaging of primary renal cell carcinomas by ^{131}J labeled antitumor antibody.
J.Nucl.Med. 19: 427. 1978.
5. Ghose T et al: Localisation of ^{131}J labeled antibodies in human renal cell carcinomas and in a mouse hepatoma and correlation with tumor detection by photoscanning.
Cancer Res. 40: 3018. 1980.
6. Ueda R et al: Cell surface antigens of human renal cancer defined by mouse monoclonal antibodies: Identification of tissue-specific kidney proteins.
PNAS 78: 5122-5126. 1981.
7. Finstad CL et al: Specificity analysis of mouse monoclonal antibodies defining cell surface antigens of human renal cancer.
PNAS 82: 2955-2959. 1985.
8. Moon TD et al: A highly restricted antigen for renal cell carcinoma defined by a monoclonal antibody.
Hybridoma 4: 163. 1985.
9. Vessella RL et al: Monoclonal antibodies to human renal cell carcinoma:recognition of shared and restricted antigens.
Cancer Res. 45: 6131. 1985.
10. Chiou RK et al: Localisation of human renal cell carcinoma xenografts with a tumor preferential monoclonal antibody.
Cancer Res. 45: 6140. 1985.
11. Cordon-Cardo C et al: Monoclonal antibodies in the diagnosis of solid tumors: studies on renal carcinomas, transitional cell carcinomas and melanoma.
In: Immunocytochemistry in tumor diagnosis. Jose Russo ed. Martinus Nijhoff 17: 281. 1984.
12. Schärfe T et al: Tumor-specific monoclonal antibodies for renal cell carcinoma.
Eur. Urol. 11: 117. 1985.
13. Cordon-Cardo C et al. Immunoanatomic dissection of the human urinary tract by monoclonal antibodies.
J. Histochem.Cytochem. 32: 1035. 1984.
14. Wahlstrom T et al: Mw 75000 protein, a tumor marker in renal adenocarcinomen reacting with antibodies to a synthetic peptide based on a cloned human endogenous retroviral nucleotide sequence.
Int. J. Cancer 36: 379. 1985.

15. Suni J et al: Monoclonal antibody to human T cell leukemia virus p19 defines polypeptide antigen in human choriocarcinoma cells and syncytiotrophoblasts of first trimester placentas.
Int.J. Cancer 33: 293. 1984.
16. Oosterwijk E et al: Immunohistochemical analysis of monoclonal antibodies to renal antigens:application in the diagnosis of renal cancers.
Am.J. Path. (in press).
17. Herman CJ: Is renal cell (Grawitz) tumor a carcinosarcoma? Evidence from analysis of intermediate type filaments.
Virchow's Archiv. (Cell Pathol) 44: 73. 1983.
18. Holthöfer H et al: Cellular origin and differentiation of renal carcinomas: a fluorescence microscopic study with kidney-specific antibodies anti intermediate filaments antibodies and lectins.
Lab.Invest. 49: 317. 1983.
19. Heterogeneity of superficial bladder cancer. G.R. Prout Jr. W.W. Bonney and G.R. Prout Jr.(eds.)In: AUA Monographs, Bladder Cancer 1: 149, 1982 Baltimore, Williams and Wilkers.
20. Slack NH, Prout GR Jr: Heterogeneity of invasive bladder carcinoma and different responses to treatment. In: AUA monograpgh (see)p.213.
21. Fradet Y et al: Cell surface antigens of human bladder cancer defined by mouse monoclonal antibodies.
PNAS 81: 224. 1984.
22. Young DA et al: Production and characterization of mouse monoclonal antibodies to human bladder tumor-associated antigens.
Cancer Res. 45: 4439. 1985.
23. Summers JL et al: Prognosis in carcinoma of the urinary bladder based upon tissue blood group ABH and Thomsen-Friedenreich antigen status and karyotype of the initial tumor.
Cancer Res. 43: 934. 1983.
24. Gutman AB, Gutman EB: An "acid" phosphatase occurring in the serum of patients with metastasizing carcinoma of the prostate gland.
J. Clin.Invest.17: 473. 1938.
25. A.C. Jobsis et al.Demonstration of the prostatic origin of metastases: an immunohistochemical method for formalin-fixed embedded tissue.
Cancer 41: 1788. 1978.
26. Lillehoj HS et al: Monoclonal anti-human prostatic acid phosphatase antibodies.
Mol.Immunol. 19: 1199. 1982.
27. Wang MC et al: Purification of a prostate specific antigen.
Invest.Urol. 17: 159. 1979.
28. Nadji M et al: Prostate-specific antigen an immunologic marker for prostatic neoplasms.
Cancer 48: 1229. 1981.
29. Purrel DM et al: Immunohistochemical evaluation of human prostatic carcinomas for carcinoembryonic

antigen, non specific crossreacting antigen, βHCG and prostate specific antigen.
Cancer Res. 44: 285. 1984.

30. Papsidero LD et al: Monoclonal antibody (F5)to human prostate antigen.
Hybridoma 2: 139. 1983.

31. Frankel AE et al: Monoclonal antibodies to a human prostate antigen.
Cancer Res. 42: 3714. 1982.

32. Raynor RH et al: Characterization of a monoclonal antibody KR-P8 that detects a new prostate specific marker.
J NCI 73: 617. 1984.

33. Ware JL et al: Production of monoclonal antibody α Pro 3 recognizing a human prostatic carcinoma antigen.
Cancer Res. 42: 1215. 1982.

34. Starling JJ et al: Monoclonal antibodies to human prostate and bladder tumor associated antigens.
Cancer Res. 42: 3084. 1982.

35. Campbell AE et al.Antiprostate carcinoma monoclonal antibody (D83-21)crossreacts with a membrane antigen expressed on cytomegalo virus-transformed human fibroblasts.
The Prostate 6: 205. 1985.

13.OVARIAN CANCER

G.J. FLEUREN

1. INTRODUCTION

Ovarian cancer is the most lethal of all gynecological cancers and is responsible for approximately 50% of all deaths resulting from malignancies of the gynecological tract (1). This is due to the fact that tumors localized in the ovary produce symptoms only late in the course of the disease. As a consequence more than 2/3 of ovarian carcinomas have metastasized by the time they are detected (2). In recent years combination chemotherapeutic regimens have improved the prognosis of patients with ovarian carcinomas. With modern treatment consisting of debulking surgery followed by cisplatin containing chemotherapeutic drugs, a 40% pathologically confirmed complete response rate can be obtained in patients with advanced ovarian cancer (3). Monitoring response of intraperitoneal disease to chemotherapy necessitates "second-look" procedures like laparoscopy and/or laparotomy. This surgical intervention for patients who are treated for malignancy for a long time is not without risk and cumbersome. Furthermore the morbidity of cisplatin-containing chemotherapy is considerable. Therefore it is desirable to discontinue this therapy at an appropriate time in patients with no evidence of persistant ovarian cancer or with no response to therapy. Therefore, it would be of great importance if reliable and practical methods for diagnosis and evaluation of treatment of ovarian carcinoma could be developed. In this way, the necessity of a second-look procedure could thus be reduced. A great deal of effort has been invested in finding markers for detection of occult disease, for staging or for more convenient monitoring of response to treatment (4).
Furthermore, immunochemical techniques have been applied to detect tumor associated antigens suitable as markers in surgical pathology.
Monoclonal antibodies specific for ovarian cancer can be used in surgical pathology to establish the nature of an ovarian tumor. It is important to distinguish primary ovarian tumors from metastases to the ovary, because the therapeutic approach of disseminated ovarian carcinoma differs from that used in the treatment of other malignancies (5,6). Approximately 5-10% of tumors in the ovary are of metastatic origin (7,8), mainly metastases of intestinal or breast carcinomas. The clinical presentation of primary and secondary ovarian cancers is often identical (7,8,9,10), and the histological distinction between primary ovarian cancer and ovarian metastases may be difficult or impossible (10,11). The use of monoclonal antibodies may be an improvement in this differential diagnosis of primary or metastatic malignancy of the ovary. Monoclonal antibodies can also be used for the diagnostic recognition of cancer

cells in serous peritoneal effusions by immuno-cytopathologic methods.
The purpose of this chapter is to review the specificity and sensitivity of monoclonal antibodies to ovarian tumor antigens of common epithelial tumors, germ cell tumors and sex cord-stromal tumors.

2. EPITHELIAL OVARIAN CANCER

2.1. Introduction

The histogenesis of ovarian tumors can be understood on the basis of the elements that constitute the ovary: the surface epithelium, the germ cells, and the supporting stroma. The germinal epithelium of the ovary develops from the Mullerian duct, as does the lining of the Fallopian tube, endometrium and cervix. Epithelial ovarian tumors are thought to arise from this germinal epithelium, that consists of modified peritoneal mesothelial cells that cover the surface of the ovary and line inclusion cysts present immediately beneath the ovarian surface (11). The epithelial ovarian neoplasms constitute the vast majority (80%) of all ovarian cancers and are classified into 6 histological subgroups according to cell type. Serous, endometrioid and mucinous tumors resemble the epithelial cells that line the inner aspects of fallopian tube, uterus and endocervix, respectively. Serous and endometrioid cystadenocarcinomas are observed most frequently, clear cell adenocarcinomas - containing abundant glycogen - and mucinous cystadenocarcinomas are the least common of the epithelial tumors. As far as prognosis is concerned, histological grade appears to be more important than type (11). Epithelial ovarian cancers metastasize along several different routes. Tumor cells can easily form serosal implants in the peritoneal cavity and can spread through lymphatic channels to the para-aortic, iliac or inguinal lymphnodes. Hematogenous metastases are rare, although they are seen with increasing frequency in patients who have prolonged survival after an initial response to chemotherapy (12).

2.2. Antigens and antibodies

With respect to ovarian carcinomas, one of the earliest tumormarkers was carcino-embryonic antigen (CEA). This marker appeared especially useful for the follow-up of patients with mucinous cystadenocarcinomas (13,14,15,16,17). Subsequently, polyclonal antibodies to ovarian cyst adenocarcinoma antigen (OCAA) developed by Bhattacharya and Barlow (18,19) and ovarian cancer antigen (OCA)(20,21) have been used in radio-immunoassay. Both markers were elevated in 50%-80% of patients with epithelial ovarian malignancy depending of the stage of the disease. The clinical use ,however, was limited to patients with mucinous and serous cystadenocarcinomas. None of the known polyclonal hetero-antisera was specific enough for use in surgical pathology.
The hybridoma technique (22) opened the possibility of production of more specific antibodies against ovarian

carcinoma antigens. Hitherto, several tumor associated antigens of non-mucinous ovarian carcinoma have been reported (Table 1). The best known monoclonal antibody is

TABLE 1. Monoclonal ab against epithelial ovarian tumors

			Specificity		
Monocl.Ab	Authors	Tumors	Low	Moder.	High
F36/22	Croghan et al	epithelial	+		
MOv1	Tagliabue	mucinous		+	+
MOv2	Tagliabue	mucinous	+		
ID3	Bhattacharya et al	mucinous	+		
OC125	Bast et al	nonmuc		+	
OVTL3	Poels et al	muc+nonmuc		+	
4C7	Tsuji et al	muc+nonmuc		+	
3C2	Tsuji et al	nonmuc			+
MH55	Mattes et al	nonmuc			+
OV632	Fleuren et al	nonmuc			+

OC125, developed by Bast et al. (23), which reacts with over 80% of serous, endometrioid and clear cell ovarian cancers and with some nongynecological malignancies (23,24,25). Monoclonal antibody OC125 was raised against serous cystadenocarcinomas (23). The antigenic determinant, CA125, detected by monoclonal antibody OC125 is associated with coelomic and amnion epithelium during embryonic development (25) and was found in fetal ovarian surface epithelium and in adult tissues derived from coelomic epithelium including the pleura, peritoneum (fig.1), pericardium and the epithelial cells lining the Fallopian tube, endometrium (fig. 2) and endocervix (24,25).

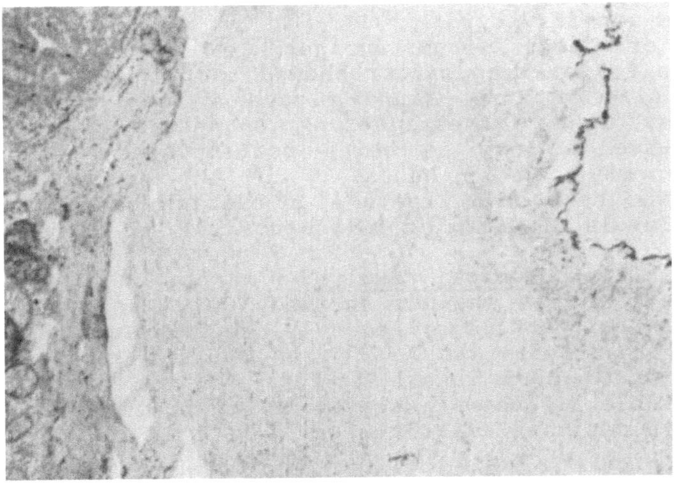

fig.1 Mesothelial lining cells of the peri-appendicular region show CA 125 positivity (Frozen section, X200).

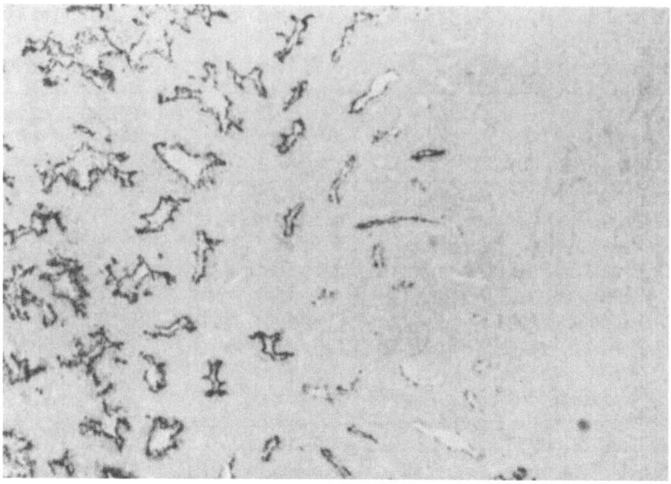

Fig.2 Normal secretory endometrium stained with OC125. Basal glands close to the myometrium (right) are stained less intensely or are negative (Frozen section, X65).

A radioimmunoassay was developed for estimation of CA125 antigen in blood samples using monoclonal antibody OC125 (26). It was demonstrated that in 42 out of 45 cases of ovarian carcinoma the antigen levels of blood samples reflected progression or regression of the malignancy. Also tumormarker NB/70 K was used for the follow-up of patients with carcinomas of the ovaries. The NB/70K and CA125 radioimmunoassays appeared to measure two different populations of antigenic substances (27) and showed a rather comparable sensitivity.
A study of CA125 serum antigen levels in second-look procedures for ovarian cancer showed that levels correlated with the size of tumor found at second-look or subsequent operations. These investigations suggested that, unless cytoreductive surgery is being contemplated, second-look procedures may not be necessary in the select group of patients who have been treated for ovarian cancer but have elevated levels of CA125 on follow-up (28).

2.3. Immuno-histochemical results
The question arises whether antibody OC125 is adequate for use in surgical pathology. Recently, we performed a study in which the reactivity of OC125 with ovarian tumors (n=49), and nongynecological tumors (n=104) was investigated. The results (table II) show that over 80% of nonmucinous ovarian tumors were positive (fig.3,4,5).

TABLE 2. Immunohistology on frozen sections of gynecological tumors

Epithelial ovarian-tumors	OV632	OC125
- Serous carcinoma	13/14*	14/14
serous borderline	1/2	2/2
serous benign	4/8	8/8
- mucinous carcinoma	3/5	4/5
mucinous borderline	2/5	4/5
mucinous benign	3/6	2/6
- endometrioid carcinoma	2/3	2/3
- clear cell carcinoma	1/3	3/3
- Brenner tumor	0/2	0/2
- undiff. carcinoma	1/1	1/1

* number positive/number stained

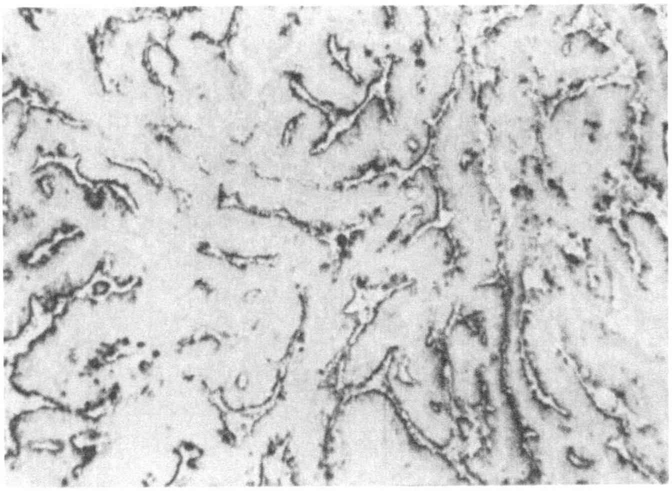

fig.3 Primary endometrioid adenocarcinoma of ovary, stained with OC125. The neoplastic cells show strongly membranous staining (Frozen section, x 200).

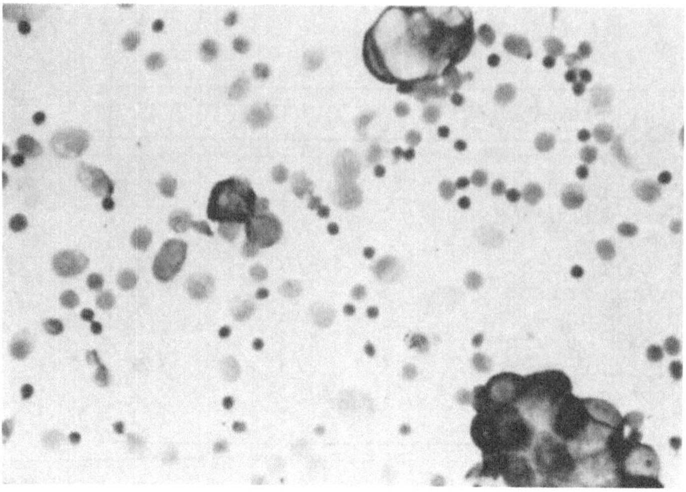

fig.4 Ascitic cells of a patient with a serous cystadenocarcinoma of the ovary show CA125 positivity (Imprint specimen, x 800).

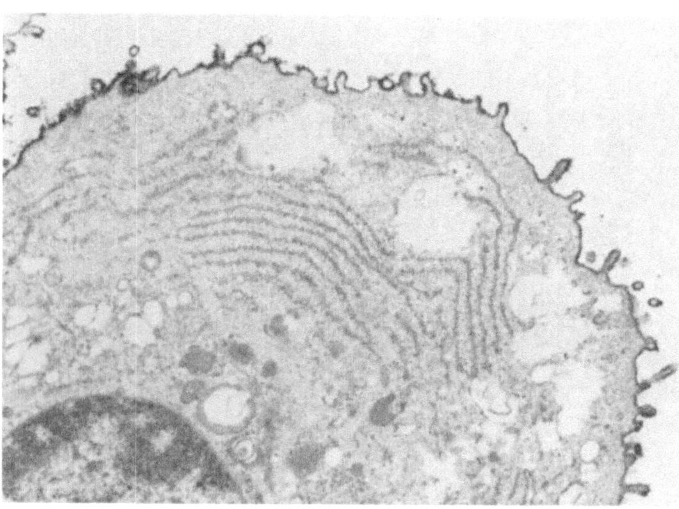

fig.5 Same patient as fig. 4. Immuno-electronmicroscopy shows intense membranous staining for CA125, x 10,350.

On the other hand nearly 25% of the nongynecological tumors (table 3) reacted with OC125: approximately 40% of adenocarcinomas of the breast and some colon and lung carcinomas were positive (25,29). Because of the presence of CA125 in adenocarcinomas of nongynecological origin, especially in breast carcinomas (fig.6) and incidentally in colon carcinomas, and because neoplasms derived from these

organs are a frequent secondary neoplasm of the ovary, OC125 seems to be of limited value in surgical pathology. However, OC 125 is valuable in immunohistology for comparison of tumor antigen content with serum values.
A comparison was made between staining of CA125 in frozen sections and in routinely formalin fixed paraffin-embedded tissue sections.The staining results of paraffin-embedded tissue sections obtained from nine different laboratories showed that 25/30 serous tumors were positive, whereas 24/24 serous carcinomas were positive using frozen sections. Moreover, the number of positive tumor cells was less in paraffin-embedded tissue as compared to frozen sections.
Recently, we developed a monoclonal antibody (OV632) against nonmucinous ovarian carcinomas, with a limited range of reactivity against nonovarian carcinoma tissues. Antibody OV632 stained approximately 80% of nonmucinous carcinomas including serous (fig.7), endometrioid, clear cell and undifferentiated carcinomas (table 2). Three out of 5 mucinous carcinomas were positive.

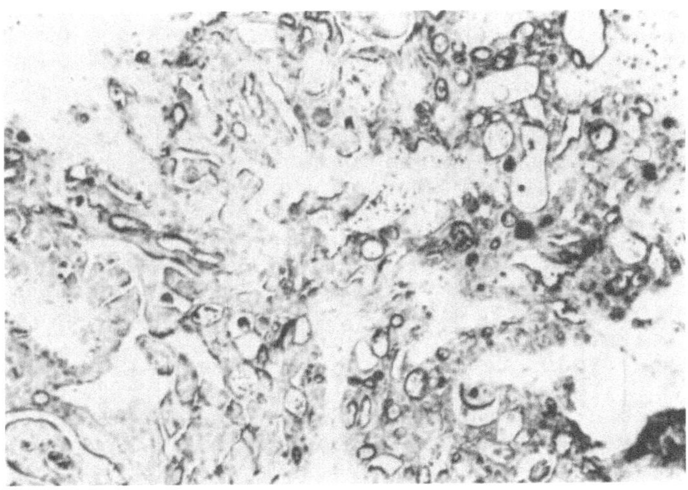

fig.6 Primary carcinoma of the breast stained with OC125 (Frozen section, x 200).

Also 5/9 adenocarcinomas of the endometrium showed a positive reaction with this antibody. The two cases of endocervical adenocarcinomas studied were negative. Several normal epithelia showed positive staining. The ciliated epithelium lining the fallopian tube and few cells lining the surface of the endometrium and endocervix were positive. In the ovary, OV632 stained cells lining follicular cysts. Outside the female genital tract positive staining was found in the appendix, prostate and in ganglion cells.

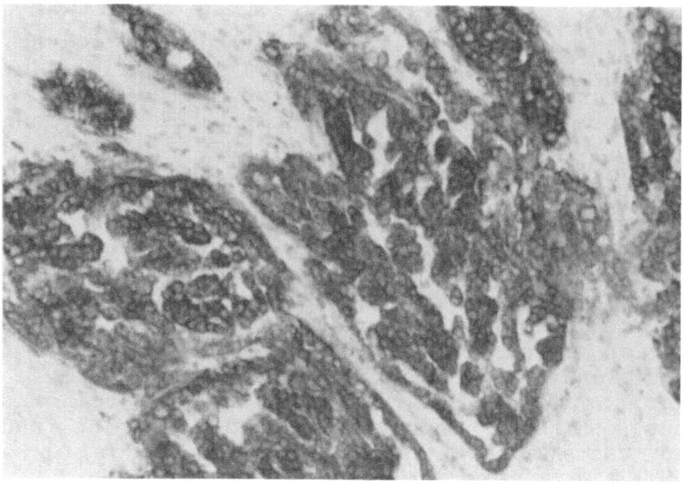

Fig.7 Serous cystadenocarcinoma of the ovary stained with OV 632. A strong cytoplasmic staining is present (Frozen section, X 400).

All other normal tissues tested were negative. In two-wave length indirect immunofluorescence studies it was found that different staining patterns were displayed by OV632 and OC125. Immunoperoxidase studies showed that antibody OV632 recognizes a cytoplasmic determinant, whereas CA125 appears to be present on the cell membranes (fig. 5). The pattern of staining reported here for antibody OV632 and the data in the literature show that this antibody is distinct from antibodies reactive to ovarian cancer antigens as reported by other workers (23,24,25,30-36).
Apparently, OV632 reacts with a normal differentiation antigen that is amongst others associated with epithelium derived from the Mullerian duct. The observation that epithelial ovarian cancers and endometrial carcinomas of the uterus are positive with OV632 may reflect the Mullerian origin of these tissues. In this respect, it is remarkable that fetal coelomic epithelium and the ovarian surface did not stain at all. Therefore the staining of coelomic epithelium and its derivates with this antibody seems maturation dependent. Only 7 out of 117 extra-genital malignancies, mostly adenocarcinomas from 14 different nongynecological organs, including breast, colon, lung and kidney were positive (Table 3).

TABLE 3. Immunohistology of nongynecological tumors

Tumors tested	Staining results on frozen sections		
	OV632	OC125*	OC125**
Carcinoma			
- Kidney	1/18	1/3	0/1
- Pancreas	0/1		0/1
- Thyroid	2/4	1/4	0/3
- Bladder	1/4	0/4	-
- Breast	0/38	20/38	3/15
- Lung	0/17	1/17	3/5
- Stomach	1/8	1/8	0/2
- Colon	0/18	1/21	0/6
- Carcinoid	1/1	0/1	
- Mesothelioma	0/1	0/1	
- Melanoma	1/4	0/4	1/4
- Seminoma testis	0/2	0/2	0/8
- Lymphoma	0/1	0/1	
Total	7/117	25/104	7/45

* present study

** Bast et al.(ref.23,24,25)

It is of importance to note, that colon carcinomas as well as breast carcinomas, together representing over 70% of the metastatic tumors in the ovary, did not react with OV632 at all.

Therefore, antibody OV632 can be a useful aid in routine surgical pathology in the discrimination between ovarian and nonovarian carcinomas both in the ovary itself as well as elsewhere in or outside the abdominal cavity.

Antibody OV632 did not react with paraffin sections. It was found that even a short fixation of frozen sections with 2% formalin completely abolished the staining .

Some other monoclonal antibodies directed against nonmucinous ovarian tumors have to be mentioned.Mattes et al. (32) reported five distinct antigens which were characterized using mouse monoclonal antibodies to several cell surface antigens of human ovarian and endometrial carcinoma. One epitope, MH55 antigen, appeared to be weakly expressed on ovarian and uterine cancer cell lines but not on other cells and tissues tested. Recently, Poels et al. (35) and Tsuji et al. (36) reported on monoclonal antibodies specific for both nonmucinous and mucinous epithelial carcinomas of the ovary. These antibodies need further histological studies on a large panel of carcinoma specimens to appraise their usefulness in surgical pathology.

Several monoclonal antibodies that recognize antigenic determinants present in mucinous cystadenocarcinomas of the

ovary have been described. Bhattacharya et al. (30) reported on an antibody (1D5) that did not react with any other gynecological or non-gynecological tumor or with any normal adult tissue.
Furthermore, less specific monoclonal antibodies against both mucinous and nonmucinous ovarian carcinomas have been described. Monoclonal antibody F36/22 (34), raised against breast carcinoma, recognizes high- molecular-weight glycoprotein components associated with breast carcinoma and with all adenocarcinomas of the ovary tested. F36/22 also reacted a small proportion of colon, lung and prostate adenocarcinomas. The monoclonal antibodies MOv1 and MOv2 (31) recognize two different molecules present on both malignant and benign ovarian mucinous tumors and colonic glands. In addition the antigen recognized by MOv2 was also detected in carcinomas of lung, colon, stomach and breast. MOv1 and MOv2 were raised against a membrane preparation of a mucinous ovarian cystadenocarcinoma. Gangopadhyay (33) reported the distribution of an antigen recognized by antibody 1D3. One hundred percent of ovarian mucinous cyst adenocarcinomas expressed high levels of the antigen, but relatively high proportions of colonic carcinoma, gastric carcinomas and pancreatic carcinomas were also positive.
Finally, the use of antibodies against CEA as a useful tool in the diagnosis of metastatic tumors to the ovary has to be mentioned. Because CEA is known to be present in almost all colonic adenocarcinomas, we studied the presence of CEA in 97 primary ovarian tumors and in 12 known metastatic ovarian adenocarcinomas of intestinal origin, using an absorbed monospecific commercial rabbit anti-CEA antiserum (37). In primary ovarian tumors CEA was present in foci of squamous differentiation of endometrioid carcinomas, and also focally in areas of intestinal differentiation of mucinous tumors. Serous tumors, clear cell carcinomas, undifferentiated carcinomas and 19 out of 22 mucinous tumors without intestinal differentiation were negative. In the metastatic ovarian adenocarcinomas of intestinal origin in all cases CEA was present in a characteristic diffuse staining pattern was present. This difference consisting of negative or focal versus diffuse staining for CEA is therefore useful in the differentiation between primary ovarian cancers and metastastic ovarian adenocarcinomas of intestinal origin.

2.4 Immuno-cytochemical results

Immuno-cytological methods can be used to detect epithelial tumor cells in effusions (fig.4,5), and are especially helpful if tumor cells are rare or admixed with inflammatory cells and reactive mesothelium. In a recent study monoclonal antibody B/2.3 was found on carcinoma cells in nearly 100% of the specimens containing adenocarcinoma cells identifiable by cytologic criteria (38). Mesothelial and lymphoid cells were negative. Similar results were obtained on methanol fixed cytospin cell preparations from serous effusions. The diagnostic application of B72.3 is useful in cytologic specimens as for example obtained at second look operations in differentiating adenocarcinoma cells from

reactive mesothelium and lymphoid elements. Furthermore, antibodies to human milk fat globule membranes have been used to differentiate carcinoma cells, which are positive, and reactive mesothelial cells (negative) (39, see chapters 9 and 16).
When antibody OC125 is used for these purposes, its reactivity with mesothelial cells is a drawback and has to be kept in mind (fig.1).

3. THE RELATIONSHIP BETWEEN OVARIAN TUMOR TISSUE ANTIGENS AND SERUM ANTIGEN LEVELS

Immunohistology is valuable to determine whether a certain tumormarker is produced by a malignant process. With such a screening method, an appropriate marker can be selected for serial plasma determinations as a means to monitor therapeutic response. Immunohistochemical staining of tissue specimens were shown to be useful to identify those patients whose tumors contain high antigen concentrations and who therefore should benefit most from sera plasma determinations following therapy (14). For example, in trophoblastic tumors, which characteristically contain a high percentage of HCG-producing cells, monitoring of ß-HCG is generally used. Plasma antigen concentrations are related also to tumor extent and to antigen metabolism. It has been demonstrated that absolute plasma CEA concentration is related to antigen concentration in the tumor, to the extent of disease and to antigen metabolism (40-43). A progressive increase in plasma CEA was found to accurately predict tumor recurrence in over 80% of patients whose tumors stained immunohistochemically for CEA (44). Immunoperoxidase staining was shown to be indicative of a tissue CEA concentration of at least 3 micro-gram per gram (44).
Recently, we performed a study to gain insight in the relationship between the presence of tumor antigens in ovarian tumor tissue and in the circulation. Patients with epithelial ovarian tumors are appropriate for such a study for three reasons. Firstly, most ovarian carcinomas are cystic and for instance high levels of CEA were demonstrated within ovarian cyst fluid, exceeding those in serum by 10-1000 fold (15). Secondly, patients with metastatic disease may develop ascites and therefore the unique possibility exists to quantitate and compare the levels of ovarian cancer antigens in ascites with the amounts in tissue, cyst fluid, and serum. Thirdly, CA125 is a useful ovarian tumor-associated antigen for such an investigation because it is known that elevated serum levels are found in 90% of patients with ovarian cancer (25,26). Immunohistology demonstrated, as mentioned above, that CA125 was present in the tumor tissue of 90% of malignant ovarian cancers and in 100% of benign serous cystadenomas. Forty percent of mucinous tumors were negative, whereas positive mucinous carcinomas only focally showed positive cells.
Quantitative analysis of CA125 contents of 70 cyst fluids of a wide variety of ovarian tumors revealed extremely high levels of this antigen. CA125 was present in a concentration

of approximately 300,000 U/ml in benign serous cyst adenomas, in a range of 20,000 to 2,140,000 U/ml in malignant non-mucinous epithelial ovarian tumors and in a range of 1,000 to 17,000 U/ml in both malignant and benign mucinous tumors. CA125 was detected in cyst fluids of 43 out of 45 tumors studied, which means that nearly all epithelial tumors produce the antigen. The fraction of positive cyst fluids is higher than may be expected from immunohistochemical studies and extends to all histological types of epithelial neoplasms, including mucinous tumors which originally were reported to be negative (23). These observations indicate that immunohistology is not sensitive enough to detect CA125 in tissue sections of 10-20% of non-mucinous epithelial tumors and approximately 60% of mucinous tumors. The amount of antigen in these cases is probably too low to be detected with immunohistological methods. The different levels of CA125 in cyst fluid content indicate that the proportion of antigen-releasing cells varies from tumor to tumor. This is consistent with the observed antigenic heterogeneity of ovarian neoplasms (24,25). It is conceivable that in those tumors that express and release high quantities of antigen per unit volume, even small changes in overall tumor size are accurately reflected in a corresponding change in serum antigen level. In this group the marker will be most accurate for the monitoring of therapy or for detecting a relapse (45).

4. GERM CELL TUMORS

4.1. Introduction

Germ cell tumors are neoplasms considered to be derived from the primitive germ cells. These tumors may develop both in the gonads or at extra-gonadal sites along the line of migration of the primitive germ cells. The remarkable homology between the various tumor types in the male and female is in agreement with the theory on the histogenesis of Teilum (46). Germ cell tumors of the ovary account for approximately 20% of ovarian tumors. The vast majority, about 97%, of all germ cell tumors is benign, mainly mature cystic teratoma. The remaining 3% are malignant and account for approximately 2% of all ovarian cancers in the western countries. Classification of germ cell tumors is based on the agreements reached by a panel of pathologists under the auspicies of the World Health Organizationy. This classification has the advantage that it is used worldwide and can lead to identical use of nomenclature between pathologists and clinicians, and is as follows (11): A. Dysgerminoma B. Endodermal sinus tumor C. Embryonal carcinoma D. Polyembryoma E. Choriocarcinoma F. Teratoma.

4.2. Immunohistology

Detection of tumor markers in germ cell tumors sometimes adds information for pathologic diagnosis. Moreover, studying tumor markers in tissue sections may establish a relation between the presence of markers in tissue and serum. Tumor markers which are associated with germ cell

tumors are either related to extra-embryonic cells (alpha fetoprotein (AFP), human chorionic gonadotropin (HCG), pregnancy-specific beta-1 glycoprotein, alpha 1 anti-trypsin) or to embryonic tissue (CEA and hormones). For example, thyreoglobulin is produced by a struma ovarii and can be used to identify this lesion. The most practical tumor markers in germ cell tumors are AFP and HCG. Approximately 60% of malignant germ cell tumors give rise to an elevation of either AFP or ß-HCG in the serum, giving the possibility to monitor the response to treatment. AFP can be identified in endodermal sinus tumor, foci of yolk sac differentiation within embryonal carcinomas and poly-embryonas. Antibodies have been used to demonstrate HCG in the syncytiotrophoblastic cells of choriocarcinomas, embryonal carcinomas, poly-embryomas and occasional dysgerminomas. Isolated mononucleated cells in occasional dysgerminomas and embryonal carcinoma, which are not recognizable as trophoblastic in haematoxylin and eosin stain, may also stain positively for HCG (47). Immunoperoxidase studies of choriocarcinomas have demonstrated that syncytiotrophoblast also contains placental lactogen.
In the following paragraph, the different germ cell tumors and their tumormarkers will be discussed.

4.3. Endodermal sinus tumor
The endodermal sinus tumor is an uncommon neoplasm, which is regarded as extra-embryonic, because of its relation to the yolk sac. The large vesicles, the goblet cells containing glands and the endodermal sinuses indicate an endodermal direction of differentation. In nearly all endodermal sinus tumors AFP and alpha 1-antitrypsin can be found, partly related to rather characteristic PAS-positive, diastase resistant hyalin droplets (48). The synthesis of AFP by these germ cell tumors gives further support to the view that endodermal sinus tumor is a germ cell neoplasm resulting from differentiation of primitive germ cell elements in the direction of yolk sac or amnion structures. The vast majority of patients with an endodermal sinus tumor have elevated AFP levels in the serum. CEA can be detected in endodermal sinus tumors cells, but has no value as a tumor marker in surgical pathology or clinical follow-up.

4.4. Embryonal carcinoma
Embryonal carcinoma is considered to consist of primitive cells which still may differentiate either toward somatic structures (teratomatous tumors) or toward extra-embryonal structures (endodermal sinus tumor, choriocarcinoma). HCG can be identified both in multinucleated giant cells and mononuclear cells whereas AFP is present within mononuclear embryonal cells in hyalin droplets as in endodermal sinus tumorcells. The presence of both AFP and HCG in embryonal carcinoma is in concordance with the observation that embryonal carcinoma cells can differentiate toward yolk sac or trophoblastic structures (48).

4.5. Dysgerminomas

Dysgerminomas are considered to represent abnormal growth of primordial germ cells and contain placental alkaline phosphatase. HCG may be present in syncytiotrophoblastic cells and in mononucleated dysgerminoma cells, which are otherwise indistinguishable from cells that stain negatively for HCG.

4.6. Teratoma

The category of the teratomas contains those tumors in which elements of the embryonic layers (endoderm, mesoderm and ectoderm) are found. The great majority of cases (98%) consists of the mature cystic neoplasms, known as dermoid cysts. In the dermoid cyst malignant transformation may occur, in which case a cancer of adult type develops in contrast to the malignancy due to immature (embryonal type) tissue as present in the immature teratoma. Neurohormonal peptides, HCG, AFP and CEA are present in benign cystic and solid teratomas.

It is noteworthy that at one hand AFP has been incidentally localized within cells of common epithelial ovarian tumors, whereas on the other hand we identified markers for epithelial ovarian cancer like CEA and CA125 within germ cell tumors like endodermal sinus tumor and teratoma.

5. GERM CELL-STROMA TUMORS

This category only represents 4% of ovarian tumors. Estradiol, progesterone and testosterone have been demonstrated in the four major cell types of sex cord-stromal tumors, i.e. granulosa cells, theca cells,

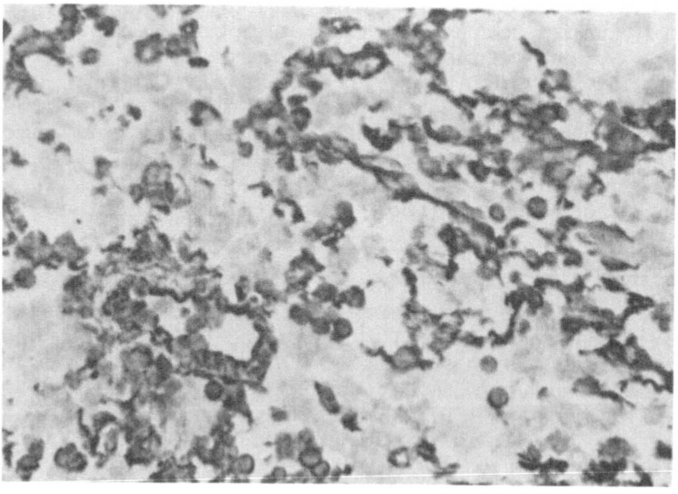

Fig. 8 Granulosa cell tumor showing abundant positive immunostaining for vimentin (Frozen section, x 400).

Sertoli cells and Leydig cells. In most cases of granulosa cells the diagnosis can be easily made on the coffee-bean aspect of tumor cells and the positivity of a fat stain. Sometimes, it is difficult to distinguish an undifferentiated common epithelial tumor from a solid granulosa-cell tumor. In these cases the use of antibodies to intermediate filaments is useful. Carcinomas are diffusely positive for keratin and may be positive for HMFG-2, whereas in 50% of cases CA125 is present. Granulosa-cell tumors only occasional contain keratin and mainly consist of vimentin positive cells (fig.8).

6. CONCLUSIONS

At present antibodies to a single tumor associated antigen have only limited value in surgical gynecopathology, not least because expression is frequently heterogeneous in a given neoplasm, regardless of the histological appearance. Therefore, batteries of antibodies seem more informative in individual cases. Furthermore, immunohistology is of value in studies that are needed to establish the temporal relation between changes in viable tumor burden and changes in serum antigen levels and to identify new markers for monitoring the disease.
In future studies, a greater specificity might be obtained by developing antibodies to different determinants on the same molecule of isolated cyst fluid antigens.

The author thanks Mr.L.J.C.M. van den Broek, Mrs.G.H.H.M. van Leeuwen-Herberts and Mr.F.A. Prins for excellent technical assistance and Dr.I.A. Koelma and Dr.C.J. Rodenburg for helpful advice. The secretarial assistance of Mrs.M.A.P. Kantebeen-Zoetemelk is greatly appreciated.

REFERENCES

1. Silverberg E, Lubera JA: A review of American Cancer Society estimates of cancer cases and deaths. CA:A Cancer J. Clin. 1983; 33: 2-8.
2. Griffiths CT. In Holland JF and Frei E III (eds.): Cancer Medicine 1982; pp. 1958, Lea and Febiger, Philadelphia.
3. Rodenburg CJ, Cleton FJ: Chemotherapy in advanced ovarian cancer. J. Cancer Res. Clin. Oncol. 1984; 107: 99-105.
4. Bast RC Jr, Knapp RC. Immunologic approaches to the management of ovarian carcinoma. Sem.Oncol. 1984; 11, 264-274.
5. Davis HL. Chemotherapy of large bowel cancer. Cancer 1982; 50: 2638-2646.
6. Vogl SE, Berenzweig M, Kaplan BH, Mouktar M, Bulkin W. The CHAD and HAD regimens in advanced ovarian cancer: combination chemotherapy including cyclosposphamide, hexamethylmelamine, adriamycin and cis-dichloro-diammineplatinum (II). Canc.Tr.Rep. 1979; 63: 311-317.
7. Kempson RL, Hendrickson MR. The female reproductive system. In Coulson WF (ed): Surgical Pathology, vol.1,

1978; pp.725-727, Lippincott, Philadelphia.
8. Fox H, Langley FA. In: Tumours of the ovary. Year Book Medical Publishers, 1976; pp.293-305, Chicago.
9. Johansson H. Clinical aspects of metastatic ovarian cancer of extragenital origin. Acta Obstet Gynecol Scand 1960; 39: 681-697.
10. Ulbright TM, Roth LM, Stehman FB. Secondary ovarian neoplasia. A clinico pathologic study of 35 cases. Cancer 1984; 53: 1164-1174.
11. Scully RE. Tumors of the ovary and maldeveloped gonads. In Atlas of Tumor Pathology, series 2, fascicle 16 (1980). Armed Forces Institute of Pathology, Washington DC.
12. Mayer RJ, Berkowitz RS, Griffiths CT. Central nervous system involvement by ovarian carcinoma. A complication of prolonged survival with metastatic disease. Cancer 1978; 41: 776-783.
13. Van Nagell JR, Meeker WR, Parker JC, Harralson JD. Carcinoembryonic antigen in patients with gynecologic malignancy. Cancer 1975; 35: 1372-1376.
14. Van Nagell JR, Donaldson ES, Hanson MB, Gay EC, Pavlik EJ. Biochemical markers in the plasma and tumors of patients with gynecologic malignancies. Cancer 1981; 48: 495-503.
15. Van Nagell JR, Donaldson ES, Gay EC, Sharkey RM, Rayburn P, Goldenberg DM. Carcinoembryonic antigen in ovarian epithelial cystadenocarcinomas. The prognostic value of tumor and serial plasma determinations. Cancer 1978; 41: 2335-2340.
16. Marchand A, Fenoglio CM, Pascal R, Richart RM, Bennett S: Carcinoembryonic antigen in human ovarian neoplasms. Cancer Res. 1975; 35: 3807-10.
17. Rutanen EM, Lindgren J, Sipponen P, Stenman UH, Saksela E, Seppala M: Carcinoembryonic antigen in malignant and nonmalignant gynecologic tumors: Circulating levels and tissue localization. Cancer 1978; 42: 581-90.
18. Bhattacharya M, Barlow JJ. Immunologic studies of human serous cystadenocarcinoma of ovary. Cancer 1972; 31: 588-595.
19. Bhattacharya M, Barlow JJ. Tumor markers for ovarian cancer. Int.Adv.Surg.Oncol. 1979; 2: 155-176.
20. Knauf S, Urbach GI. Ovarian tumor-specific antigens. Am.J.Obstet.Gynecol. 1974; 119: 966-970.
21. Knauf S, Urbach GI. The development of a double-antibody radioimmunoassay for detecting ovarian tumor-associated antigen fraction OCA in plasma. Am.J.Obstet.Gynecol. 1978; 131: 780-787.
22. Kohler G, Milstein C. Continuous cultures of fused cells secreting antibody of predefined specificity. Nature 1975; 256: 495-497.
23. Bast RC, Feeney M, Lazarus H, Nadler LM, Colvin RB, Knapp RC, Reactivity of a monoclonal antibody with human ovarian carcinoma. J. Clin. Invest. 1981; 68: 1331-1337.
24. Kabawat SE, Bast RC, Welch WR, Knapp RC, Colvin RB. Immunopathologic characterization of a monoclonal antibody that recognizes common surface antigens of

human ovarian tumors of serous, endometrioid, and clear cell types. Am. J. Clin. Pathol. 1983; 79: 98-104.
25. Kabawat SE, Bast RC, Bhan AK, Welch WR, Knapp RC, Colvin RB. Tissue distribution of a coelomic-epithelium-related antigen recognized by the monoclonal antibody OC125. Int.J.Gynecol.Pathol. 1983; 2: 275-285.
26. Bast RC, Klug TL, St John E, Jenison E, Niloff JM, Lazarus H, Berkowitz RS, Leavitt T, Griffiths CT, Parker L, Zurawski VR, Knapp RC. A radioimmunoassay using a monoclonal antibody to monitor the course of epithelial ovarian cancer. N Engl J Med 1983; 309: 883-887.
27. Knauf S, Anderson DJ, Knapp RC, Bast RC Jr. A study of the NB/70K and CA125 monoclonal antibody radioimmunoassays for measuring serum antigen levels in ovarian cancer patients. Am J.Obstet.Gynecol. 1985; 152: 911-913.
28. Niloff JM, Bast RC, Schaetzl EM, Knapp RC. Predictive value of CA125 antigen levels in second-look procedures for ovarian cancer. Am. J. Obstet. Gynecol. 1985; 151: 981-5.
29. Fleuren GJ, Koelma IA, Rodenburg CJ, v.d. Broek LJCM, van Leeuwen-Herberts GHHM, Nap M. Immunohistological characterization of two monoclonal antibodies directed against non-mucinous ovarian carcinomas (632 and OC125). XII Annual Meeting of the Int. Society for Oncodevelopmental Biology and Medicine, Paris, France, september 10-13,1985.
30. Bhattacharya M, Chatterjee SK, Barlow JJ, Fuji H. Monoclonal antibodies recognizing tumor-associated antigen of human ovarian mucinous cystadenocarcinomas. Cancer Res. 1982; 42: 1650-1654.
31. Tagliabue E, Menard S, Torre GD, Barbanti P, Mariani-Constantini R, Porro G, Colnaghi MI. Generation of monoclonal antibodies reacting with human epithelial ovarian cancer. Cancer Res. 1985; 45: 379-385.
32. Mattes MJ, Cordon-Cardo C, Lewis JL, Old LJ, Lloyd KO. Cell surface antigens of human ovarian and endometrial carcinoma defined by mouse monoclonal antibodies. Proc. Natl. Acad. Sci. USA 1984; 81: 568-572.
33. Gangopadhyay A, Bhattacharya M, Chatterjee SK, Barlow JJ, Tsukada Y. Immunoperoxidase localization of a high-molecular-weight mucin recognized by monoclonal antibody 1D3. Cancer Res. 1985; 45: 1744-1752.
34. Croghan GA, Wingate MB, Gamarra M,. Johnson E, Chu TM, Allen H, Valenzuela L, Tsukada Y, Papsidero LD. Reactivity of monoclonal antibody F36/22 with human ovarian adenocarcinomas. Cancer Res. 1984; 44: 1954-1962.
35. Poels L, Peters O, Van Megen Y, Vooijs GP, Verheyen R, Willemsen A, Van Niekerk C, Jap P, Mungyer G, Kenemans P. Monoclonal antibody against human ovarian tumor associated surface antigens. J.Natl.Cancer Inst. In press.
36. Tsuji Y, Suzuki T, Nishiura H, Takemura T, Isojima S. Identification of two different surface epitopes of human ovarian epithelial carcinomas by monoclonal

antibodies. Cancer Res. 1985; 45: 2358-2362.
37. Nap M, ten Hoor KA, Fleuren GJ. Crossreactivity with normal antigens in commercial anti-CEA sera, used for immunohistology. The need for tissue controls and absorptions. Am. J. Clin. Pathol. 1983; 79: 25-31.
38. Johnston WW, Szpak CA, Lottich SC, Thor A, Schlom J: Use of a monoclonal antibody (B72.3) as an immunocytochemical adjunct to diagnosis of adenocarcinoma in human effusions. Cancer Res. 1985;45:1894-1900.
39. Epenetos AA, Conti IG, Taylor-Papapdimitriou J: Use of two epithelium-specific monoclonal antibodies for diagnosis of malignancy in pleural effusions. Lancet II 1982;1004-1006.
40. Van Nagell JR, Donaldson ES, Wood EG, Goldenberg DM. The clinical significance of carcinoembryonic antigen in the plasma and tumors of patients with gynecologic malignancies. Cancer 1978; 42: 1527-1532.
41. Lurie BB, Lowenstein MS, Zamcheck N. Elevated carcinoembryonic antigen levels and biliary tract obstruction. JAMA 1975; 233: 326-330.
42. Primus FJ, Hansen HJ, Goldenberg DM: Altered metabolism of carcinoembryonic antigen in hamsters bearing GW-39 tumors. Nature 1974; 249: 837-838.
43. Shuster J, Silverman M, Gold P: Metabolism of human carcinoembryonic antigen in xenogeneic animals. Cancer Res. 1973; 33: 65-68.
44. van Nagell JR, Donaldson ES, Gay EC, Rayburn P, Powell DF, Goldenberg DM. Carcinoembryonic antigen in carcinoma of the uterine cervix. 1. The prognostic value of serial plasma determinations. Cancer 1978; 42: 2428-2434.
45. Canney PA, Wilkinson PM, James RD, Moore M. CA 19-9 as a marker for ovarian cancer: Alone and in comparison with CA 125. Br.J.Cancer 1985; 52: 131-133.
46. Teilum G. Tumours of germinal origin. In: Gentil F, Junqueira AC (eds). Ovarian Cancer, U.I.C.C. Monograph Series vol. II, pp.58-73, 1968. Springer Verlag, Berlin, Heidelberg,New York.
47. Kurman RJ, Norris HJ. Embryonal carcinoma of the ovary. A clinicopathologic entity distinct from endodermal sinus tumor resembling embryonal carcinoma of the adult testis. Cancer 1976; 38: 2420-2433.
48. Blaustein A (Ed.) Pathology of the female genital tract. Springer Verlag, New York, Berlin, Heidelberg, Tokyo, 1982.

14. ENDOCRINE TUMORS.

A.C. NIEUWENHUIJZEN KRUSEMAN

1. INTRODUCTION

The introduction of immunocytochemical techniques in diagnostic histopathology has been of major importance for the recognition and characterization of endocrine tumors. Although previously applied morphological light - and electron microscopical methods permitted the identification of endocrine (neurosecretory) granules in tumors derived from endocrine and non-endocrine tissues, the results of these studies have often given rise to controversy about the relationship between structure and function of neoplastic endocrine cells. With the application of immunocytochemistry the confusion concerning the functional classification of endocrine tumors has been eliminated almost completely.

The first immunocytochemical studies conducted on endocrine tumors were directed to the identification of hormones in the tumor cell cytoplasm. These studies involved mainly the investigation of peptide hormone producing tumors, since it appeared technically difficult to detect steroid hormones in tissue sections. Immunostaining of peptide hormones has proved to be rather easy since these hormones, whether or not coupled to a carrier, are fairly immunogenic and the generation of antibodies therefore poses no major problems. In addition, peptide hormones are usually stored in large quantities in cytoplasmic neurosecretory granules and can withstand fixation and subsequent·paraffin embedding, which promotes the identification of these hormones in routinely processed tissue specimens. With some exceptions, all immunocytochemical studies concerning the identification of hormones in tumor cells were performed with polyclonal antisera. Only in recent years studies with monoclonal antisera were undertaken. These studies, however, involved mainly the identification of nonhormonal membrane or cytoplasmic constituents of endocrine cells. In this chapter the significance of these studies for diagnostic histopathology will be elucidated. In addition, some aspects of immunocytochemical studies with polyclonal antisera will be discussed, as far as these are relevant for further development of monoclonal antibody studies.

2. CLASSIFICATION OF ENDOCRINE TUMORS

Endocrine tumors can be subdivided into:

2.1. Tumors derived from the neuroendocrine Amine Precursor Uptake and Decarboxylation (APUD) cell system. These tumors are summarized in table 1 and are usally called apudomas or after their main secretory product (e.g. gastrinoma, vipoma, insulinoma).

TABLE 1. Neuroendocrine neoplasms (apudomas)

gangliocytoma
paraganglioma
chemodectoma
neuroblastoma
anterior pituitary adenoma
medullary thyroid carcinoma
anaplastic small cell lung carcinoma
carcinoid
pancreatic islet cell tumor
pheochromocytoma
Merkel cell carcinoma
melanoma
thymoma

2.2. Tumors derived from endocrine tissues without neuroendocrine characteristics, such as papillary and follicular thyroid carcinomas, tumors from steroid producing tissues and germ cell tumors.
In addition, in a substantial number of non-endocrine tumors hormone-like compounds have been identified with immunocytochemistry. In particular material with human chorionic gonadotropin-like immunoreactivity has been demonstrated in a majority of tumors studied (1). Concanavalin A-Sepharose affinity chromatography revealed however that this hCG-like immunoreactivity is probably different from placental hCG in its carbohydrate moiety (2,3).

Apudomas can occur as sporadic cases or in combination with other apudomas as part of the multiple endocrine neoplasia syndromes type I and type II. In the latter situation the tumors are usually familial due to an autosomal dominant inheritance. Immunostaining of apudomas may reveal a variety of neuropeptides in a given tumor and also in individual neoplastic cells (4,5).

3. PROBLEMS INVOLVED IN IMMUNOCYTOCHEMICAL STAINING OF ENDOCRINE TUMORS

If immunocytochemistry is used for the identification of hormones in tumorcells, the results should be interpreted with some reservation. Immunocytochemistry only demonstrates the presence or absence of hormones within the cytoplasm, which does not necessarily imply that absent immunostaining excludes the synthesis and secretion of the hormone being examined. When the tumor cells are not reactive with the antiserum a high secretion rate with minimal storage may be responsible. Absent immunostaining may also be due to the synthesis of substances biologically but not immunologically identical to the hormone under investigation or due to storage in the granules in a way that masks the antigenic determinants for the antibodies. Another problem in interpreting immunocytochemical staining of endocrine tumors concerns the specificity of antisera applied. In endocrine immunocytochemistry a two-fold specificity of the relevant antisera is required: the antiserum should only react with the hormone against which the antiserum is raised, and the binding should be restricted to unique antigenic determinants that are not present in other portions of the prohormone from which the relevant hormone or other related hormones are derived. Even when polyclonal antisera are used, these specificity problemes can usually be overcome to some degree when synthetic hormonal fragments and a proper model system are used for specificity testing (6). If synthetic hormonal fragments are not available, the results of specifity testing of either polyclonal or monoclonal antibodies remain inconclusive as to the nature of the hormone identified in the tissue section.

4. IMMUNOSTAINING OF NEUROENDOCRINE TUMORS (Apudomas)

Like non-neoplastic neuroendocrine or APUD-cells, the majority of apudomas produces peptide hormones that can be demonstrated with immunocytochemical methods. It appears that many of these tumors are plurihormonal, producing a variety of peptide hormones eu- and ectopically. These various hormones can be revealed in one cell or in different cell types (4,5). In recent years several non-endocrine compounds have been identified in apudomas with either polyclonal or monoclonal antibodies. These include the enzyme neuron - specific enolase, chromogranins and intermediate filaments.

Neuron-specific enolase (NSE) was originally extracted from bovine brain and was later characterized as a glycolytic enzyme that catalyzes the interconversion of 2-phosphoglyceric acid and phosphoenolpyruvic acid (7). This enzyme was initially identified in neurones but was later found to be present in most APUD-cells and tumors of the APUD-series. NSE was therefore considered as one of the best markers for identification of the neuroendocrine APUD system and of derivative neoplasms (8,9). Some investigators, however, convincingly showed that NSE-immunoreactivity in neoplasia is not restricted to nervous system neoplasms or apudomas. They found NSE in several types of central nervous system tumors as well as in lymphoma and in carcinoma of for instance the ovary and breast (10,11).

Chromogranins comprise a group of acidic polypeptides of various sizes which form a major part of the soluble proteins in the secretory granules of the adrenal medulla (12). Several studies indicated that chromogranin helps to stabilize the soluble portion of the secretory granule through interaction with ATP and catecholamines (13). The ubiquitous distribution of chromogranin in APUD-cells suggests that it may have a general role in storage or release of hormones and other substances from neurosecretory granules (14). Wilson et al. (1984) recently developed a monoclonal antibody (LK2 H10) against a chromogranin-like substance and demonstrated that this antibody reacts specifically with a wide range of tissues and tumors of the diffuse neuroendocrine APUD system as well as parathyroid tumors (15,16). The immunoreactivity with parathyroid cells is probably due to the structural and immunological similarities between chromogranin A and parathyroid secretory protein I (17). No reactivity was found with non-endocrine tissues and tumors. For unknown reasons reactivity was neither found in hypothalamic neurones, posterior pituitary tissue and prolactinomas (16). Together with the observation that many patients with peptide-producing neoplasms have elevated concentrations of plasma chromogranin A (18), it is likely that chromogranins will become useful markers for the characterization of neuroendocrine neoplasms.

The majority of studies on the identification of intermediate filaments in neuroendocrine tumors have been performed with monoclonal antibodies (19). In one of the first studies neurofilaments (NF) were found in certain tumors originating from the sympathic nervous system, e.g. ganglioneuroblastoma, pheochromocytoma and at least some neuroblastomas (19). These results suggested that NF-staining might be a useful tool for the recognition of neuroendocrine neoplasms. Lehto and coworkers (20) demonstrated NF in bronchopulmonary apudomas, a result which could however not be confirmed by other investigators. Instead, these investigators demonstrated cytokeratins in these tumors and in other apudomas as pituitary adenomas and cutaneous Merkel cell tumors (21,22,23,24). Apart from the fact that these observations may have important implications for the ideas on the histogenesis of neuroendocrine neoplasms, the identification of intermediate filaments is not very helpful for the recognition of these tumors.

In addition to the well defined epitopes mentioned above, Sappino and coworkers (25) produced a monoclonal antibody, named LICR-LON-E36 to the acidic fraction of soluble protein extracts of human brain. With immunocytochemistry affinity of this antibody for peripheral nerves, adrenal medulla, pancreatic islets and enterochromaffin cells was demonstrated, but not for other members of neuroendocrine APUD-cells, such as those in the skin, bronchial mucosa and thyroid. In addition the antibody recognized an intracytoplasmic epitope in pheochromocytomas, carcinoid tumors, some small cell anaplastic lung carcinomas and a few breast carcinomas, but not in the medullary thyroid carcinomas studied. The potential use of this antibody as an immunological probe for neural and neuroendocrine differentiation will therefore probably be restricted to certain types of neuroendocrine neoplasms.

5. IMMUNOSTAINING OF NON-NEUROENDOCRINE TUMORS

As mentioned before non-neuroendocrine tumors derived from endocrine tissues comprise papillary and follicular thyroid carcinomas, tumors from steroid producing tissues and germ cell tumors. Anaplastic thyroid carcinomas can be of follicular origin, but several studies have shown that some of these contain immunoreactive calcitonin, which means that this tumor type may be also derived from neuroendocrine parafollicular cells (26,27).

Almost all differentiated follicular and papillary thyroid carcinomas contain thyroglobulin immunoreactivity (28). This antigen is exclusively found in thyroid carcinomas of follicular origin and is therefore superior to any other marker used for the recognition of these types of thyroid carcinoma. In contrast, in the distinction of undifferentiated thyroid carcinoma from malignant lymphoma the application of a panel of selected antibodies to lymphoid and epithelial cells may be very useful. In this situation staining for thyroglobulin and calcitonin is often negative. Reactivity for either cytokeratins or epithelial membrane antigens is usually maintained (29).

Tumors of steroid producing tissues comprise tumors from the adrenal cortex from Leydig cells of the testis and the endocrine cells of the ovary. Up till now it has been very difficult to demonstrate steroid hormones in these tissues with immunocytochemical techniques. This is mainly due to the fact that steroid hormones are easily dissolved during the embedding procedure. Various steroid hormones have however been demonstrated in certain gonadal tumors, and it is expected that this area will progress in the coming years (30,31,32).

Germ cell tumors may contain a number of tumormarkers as for instance human chorionic gonadotropin, human placental lactogen, placental-like alkaline phosphatase (Regan isoenzyme) and alpha-fetoprotein. These antigens are however not restricted to germ cell tumors and can be found in a variety of other carcinomas as well, which means that they are of little help in differential diagnosis. Very few investigations on localization of intermediate filaments in cases of germ cell tumors have been performed (33,34). More studies are needed before one can conclude whether characterization of intermediate filaments is helpful or not in the histopathological diagnosis of these tumors.

6. CONCLUSIONS

Up till now very few immunocytochemical studies on endocrine tumors have been performed using monoclonal antibodies directed to hormones. Since in many instances synthetic preparations of hormonal fragments are available, specificity testing and purification by the absorption of antihormone antisera is easy to perform and therefore often does not necessitate the application of monoclonal antibodies. However, in those situations in which properly purified hormonal preparations are not available, use of monoclonal rather than polyclonal antibodies may enable the differentiation between certain endocrine cell types. For instance, the glycoprotein pituitary hormones LH, FSH and TSH have a species specific α-chain in common. These hormones are not available in synthetic form and preparations of β-chains of these hormones obtained by extraction of pituitary tissue are usually contaminated with traces of the common α-chain, which may give rise to unwanted cross-reactivities in immunocytochemical staining of gonadotropic and thyrotropic cells (35).

Some of the recent advances in immunocytochemistry on endocrine tumors are probably the development of monoclonal antibodies to chromogranin to characterize neuroendocrine neoplasms, and the use of monoclonal antibodies to cytokeratins and epithelial membrane antigens to characterize undifferentiated thyroid carcinomas. Since, however, many markers are not specific for certain tumor types, application of panels of antisera are at present the best way to characterize endocrine tumors with immunocytochemistry (table 2). It is expected that in the near future development of monoclonal antibodies to defined and undefined epitopes of endocrine cells will further improve the accuracy of histopathological classification of endocrine neoplasms.

TABLE 2. Antigens characteristic for endocrine neoplasms

tumortype	antigen
neuroendocrine tumors (apudomas)	peptide APUD hormones neuron-specific enolase chromogranin epitope E36
parathyroid tumor	chromogranin
thyroid tumor	
- follicular and papillary ca.	thyroglobulin
- medullary ca.	calcitonin, CEA
- undifferentiated ca.	thyroglobulin, calcitonin cytokeratins epithelial membrane antigen
ovarium granulosa and theca cell tumor	estradiol
testicular sertoli and Leydig cell tumor	testosterone
germ cell tumors	alpha-fetoprotein human chorionic gonadotropin placental lactogen

REFERENCES

1. Hattori M, Fucase M, Yoshimi H: Ectopic production of human chorionic gonadotropin in malignant tumors. Cancer 42: 2328-2333, 1978.
2. Yoshimoto Y, Wolfsen AR, Odell WD: Glycosylation, a variable in the production of hCG by cancers. Am J Med 67: 414-420, 1979.
3. Rodenburg CJ, Nieuwenhuijzen Kruseman AC, de Maaker HA, Fleuren GJ, van Oosterom AD: Immunocytochemical localization and chromatografic characterization of human chorionic gonadotrophin in a bladder carcinoma. Arch Pathol Lab Med 109: 1046-1048, 1985.
4. Asa SL, Kovacs K, Killinger DW, Marcon N, Platts M: Pancreatic islet cell carcinoma producing gastrins, ACTH, ß-endorphine, somatostatin and calcitonin. Am J Gastroentrology 74: 30-35, 1980.
5. Heitz PU, Karper M, Polak JM, Kloppel S: Pancreatic endocrine tumors: immunocytochemical analysis of 125 tumors. Human Pathology 13: 263-271, 1982.
6. Nieuwenhuijzen Kruseman AC: Application of ELISA for assessment of antiserum immunoreactivity in endocrine immunocytochemical studies. J Clin Pathology 36: 406-410, 1983.
7. Bock E, Dissing J: Demonstration of enolase activity connected to the brain specific protein 14-3-2. Scand J Immunology 4 (suppl 2): 31-36, 1975.
8. Schmechel D, Marangos PJ, Brightman M: Neuron-specific enolase is a molecular marker for peripheral and central neuroendocrine cells. Nature 276: 834-836, 1978.
9. Tapia FJ, Polak JM, Barbosa AJA, Bloem SR, Marangos PJ, Dermody C, Pearse AGE. Neuron-specific enolase is produced by neuroendocrine tumors. Lancet i: 808-811, 1981.
10. Wick MR; Scheithauer BW, Kovacs K: Neuron-specific enolase in neuroendocrine tumors of the thymus, bronchus and skin. Am J Clin Pathology 29: 703-707, 1983.
11. Vinores SA, Bonnin JM, Rubenstein LJ, Marangos PJ: immunohistochemical demonstration of neuron-specific enolase in neoplasms of the CNS and other tissues. Arch Pathol Lab Med 108: 536-540, 1984.
12. Winkler H: The composition of adrenal chromaffin granules: an assessment of controversial results. Neuroscience 1: 65-80, 1976.
13. Sharp RR, Richards EP: Molecular mobilities of soluble components in the acqueous phase of chromaffin granules. Biochem Biophys Acta 497: 260-271, 1977.
14. O'Connor DT, Burton D, Deftos LJ: Immunoreactive human chromogranin A in diverse polypeptide hormone producing human tumors and normal endocrine tissues. J Clin Endocrinol Met 57: 1084-1086, 1983.
15. Lloyd RV, Wilson BS: Specific endocrine tissue markers defined by a monoclonal antibody. Science 222: 628-630, 1983.
16. Wilson BS; Lloyd RV: Detection of chromogranin in neuroendocrine cells with a monoclonal antibody. Am J Pathology 115: 458-465, 1984.
17. Kruggel W, O'Connor DT, Lewish RV: The amino terminal sequences of bovine and human chromogranin A and secretory protein I are identical. Biochem Biophys Res Commun 127: 380-383, 1985.

18. O'Connor DT, Deftos LJ: Secretion of chromogranin A by peptide-producing endocrine neoplasms. New Eng J Med 314: 1145-1151, 1986.
19. Osborn M, Weber K: Tumor diagnosis by intermediate filament-typing: a novel tool for surgical pathology. Lab Investigation 48: 372-3794, 1983.
20. Lehto VP, Stenman S, Miettinen M, Dahl D, Virtanen I: Expression of a neural typ of intermediate filament as a distinguishing feature between oatcell carcinoma and other lung cancers. Am J Pathology 110: 113-119, 1983.
21. Höfler H, Denk H, Walter GF: Immunohistochemical demonstration of cytokeratins in endocrine cells of the human pituitary gland and in pituitary adenomas. Virchows Arch (Pathol Anat) 404: 359-368, 1984.
22. Blobel GA, Gould VE, Moll R, Lee I, Huszar M, Geiger B, Franke WW: Coexpression of neuroendocrine markers and epithelial cytoskeletal proteins in bronchopulmonary neuroendocrine neoplasms. Lab Investigation 52: 39-51, 1985.
23. Van Muijen GNP, Ruiter DJ, van Leeuwen C, Prins FA, Rietsema C, Warnaar SV: Cytokeratin and neurofilament in lung carcinomas. Amer J Pathol 116: 363-369, 1984.
24. Höfler H, Kerl H, Lackinger E, Helleis G, Denk H: the intermediate filament cytoskeleton of cutaneous neuroendocrine carcinoma (Merkel cell tumor). Virchows Arch (Pathol Anat) 406: 339-350, 1985.
25. Sappino AP, McIlhinny RAJ, Ellison M, Monaghan P, Neville AM: A monoclonal antibody detecting neural and neuroendocrine differentiation. J Histochem Cytochemistry 32: 1041-1047, 1984.
26. Nieuwenhuijzen Kruseman AC, Bosman FT, van Bergen Henegouw JC, Cramer-Knijnenburg G, Brutel de la Rivière G: Medullary differentiation of anaplastic thyroid carcinoma. Am J Clin Pathology 77: 541-547, 1982.
27. Ljungberg O, Bondeson L, Bondeson AG: Differentiated thyroid carcinoma, intermediate type. Hum Pathology 15: 218-228, 1984.
28. Logmans SC, Jöbsis AC: Thyroid associated antigens in routinely embedded carcinomas. Cancer 54: 274-279, 1984.
29. Myskov MW, Krajewski AS, Dewar E, Millar ES, Mclaren K, Fabre JW. The role of immunoperoxidase techniques on paraffin embedded tissue in determining the histogenesis of undifferentiated thyroid neoplasms. Clin Endocrinology 24: 335-341, 1986.
30. Taylor CR, Kurman RJ, Warner NE: The potential value of immunohistologic techniques in the classification of ovarium and testicular tumors. Hum Pathology 9: 417-427, 1978.
31. Gaffney EF, Majmudar B, Hertzler GL, Zane R, Furlong B, Breding E: Ovarium granulosa cell tumors - immunohistochemical localization of estradiol and ultrastructure, with functional correlation. Obstet. Gynecology 61: 311-319, 1983.
32. Kovacs, K. Immunocytology of endocrine tumors. In: Immunocytochemistry in tumor diagnosis. Ed. Jose Russo. Martinus Nijhoff Publishing, Boston/Dordrecht/Lancaster, 183-201, 1985.
33. Miettinen M, Lehto VT, Virtanen: Expression of intermediate filaments in normal ovarium and ovarium epithelial, sex cord-stromal, and germinal tumors. Int J Gynecol Pathology 2: 64-71, 1983.

34. Battifora H, Sheibani K, Tubbs RR, Kopinsk MI, Sun TT: Anti-keratin antibodies in tumor diagnosis. Distinction between seminoma and embryonal carcinoma. Cancer 54: 843-848, 1984.
35. Nieuwenhuijzen Kruseman AC, Bots GThAM: The role of microscopic examination of pituitary tumors in clinical decision making. In: Trends in diagnosis and treatment of pituitary adenomas. Eds. SWJ Lamberts, FJH Tilders, EA van der Veen, J Assies. Free University Pres Amsterdam, 389-400, 1984.

15. APPLICATION OF MONOCLONAL ANTIBODIES IN CYTOPATHOLOGY.

G.P. VOOIJS, A.C.L.M. HUYSMANS, M.H.J. SALET-V.D.POL, A.J.M. ASPERT-VAN ERP, F.C.S. RAMAEKERS

1. INTRODUCTION

The diagnosis of pathologic changes by cytologic examination of exfoliated or aspirated cellular material is becoming an increasingly important part of diagnostic pathology.

The most frequent application has become the identification of cells with a premalignant or malignant change. However, in view of progressive improvements in therapy and therefore in prognosis of the patients it has become increasingly important to establish an accurate diagnosis of the histogenetic origin and the degree of differentiation of the neoplasm under investigation. The importance of a correct decision as to the cell type from which the tumor originates cannot be overestimated since the preferred treatment protocol as well as the prognosis is often critically dependent on this diagnosis.

Usually conventional cytology offers more information than the mere presence or absence of tumor cells. It may provide evidence for the nature of the malignant process e.g. carcinoma, sarcoma or malignant lymphoma and a number of sub-classes therefrom.

However, frequently the cytopathologist is confronted with severe problems concerning recognition and characterisation of cancer cells. Often a diagnosis of malignancy can not be made on cytomorphological criteria alone. Techniques which can provide objective evidence for malignancy in such cases, have therefore long been awaited.

Through the years a number of techniques have been introduced to augment the information obtained by conventional cytologic examination. These have included chromosomal analysis, histochemistry, tissue culture and more recently the application of flow cytometric and image cytometric analysis. Immunocytochemical staining procedures demonstrating various cellular antigens offer another means of increasing the accuracy of cytodiagnosis in problem cases, especially when monoclonal antibodies are used.

Another important value of cytochemical techniques lies in their use as a means of objectively verifying the accuracy of the cytopathologists' diagnosis. This contribution to quality control may prove to be one of the most important results of the introduction of immunocytochemistry in cytopathology(3).

In the following paragraphs a review will be given on the application of monoclonal antibodies in the cytopathological diagnosis of tumors.

2. METHODOLOGY

2.1. Specificity and sensitivity of antibodies

When the morphological diagnosis in high quality conventional preparations is uncertain(40), additional diagnostic techniques can prove their value.
In most investigations sofar polyclonal antibodies have been used. The reproducibility of the results obtained with such antibodies is not as high as that obtained with monoclonal antibodies(1).

No antibody fully specific to cancer cells has been identified to date. Even when using an antibody with a high specificity it is unwise to place complete reliance on a single immunocytochemical test.

The first step to achieve a definite diagnosis should consist of the application of a small panel of monoclonal antibodies for a primary subclassification. These panels should be composed in such a way that positive and negative results reinforce each other (see chapter 17).

The additional information obtained is much more than simply additive, since the different results confirm and control each other. The use of multiple well characterized monoclonal antibodies will in the future increasingly be used to determine the type of a primary tumor. Future efforts in cytochemistry may ultimately contribute to a major change in the current concepts of cell classification and assessment of cell function(3).

Sometimes immunochemical reactivity is present in cytopathologic specimens but is sporadic or completely absent in tissue sections of the same tumor. This suggests that the examination of cellular specimens by the availability of intact cells has a high sensitivity and may therefore offer significant advantages over similar studies in tissue sections and frozen section specimens(21).

2.2. Processing of cell specimens

The methodology for immunocytochemical staining on different types of cytological specimens needs further development and standardization(40).

Discrepancies in findings may be due to differences in the fixation technique and the staining procedure used. Furthermore, the antibody preparations may vary considerably. These differences emphasize the need to use well defined conditions in immunohistochemical staining procedures (see chapter 2), since the spectrum of reactivity of a certain antibody may be determined by these conditions(38). For instance, smears prepared from effusions with a high protein content, which often is the case in malignant effusions, may have a dirty, heavy background staining if the cells are not washed in normal saline. This background staining makes microscopical analysis unreliable.

False negative staining results may be obtained when an epitope is no longer recognized by the antibody. This occurs when the epitope is masked or its three-dimensional organization is destroyed by fixation- and embedding procedures. False negative results may be avoided by combining a number of different monoclonal antibodies that react with various epitopes of the same antigen or by establishing the proper fixation conditions for every individual moAb.

Determinants recognized by monoclonal antibodies may be inactivated in cytologic material, which has been fixed in 95% ethylalcohol or in air dried smears that have been kept at room temperature. It is therefore suggested when preparing smears from cytologic specimens, that may be used for immunocytochemical staining, to store some air dried smears at -70°C. This enables the application of all available procedures. When the cytologic material is sparse and most likely not sufficient for the preparation of a series of smears, which often happens with fine needle aspiration specimens or bronchial brushing specimens, it is advised to collect the entire specimen in phosphate buffered saline. This enables the cytotechnician to prepare smears by a cytocentrifuge or a pressure fixation technique and can thus control the number of cells per volume or per slide(28,29,30). Conventional staining procedures can be applied after fixation of the preparation.

3. EFFUSIONS

Cytopathologic diagnosis of cells in serous effusions, although widely practiced and even when handled by an expert cytopathologist, may have significant limitations and pitfalls.

It has been generally recognised for many years that the serous effusion is an exceedingly complex biologic system in which multiple cellular and dissolved molecular components engage in endless permutations of interactions(38). Both benign and malignant cells may undergo structural and functional changes secondary to environmental factors, that may complicate cytopathologic diagnosis(38).

Monoclonal antibodies raised against tumor associated antigens may be of great value when applied to specimens of questionably malignant effusions. By "marking" cancer cells these may be conclusively distinguished from any non-neoplastic cells, particularly reactive mesothelial cells. Specific monoclonal antibodies may also reveal the tissue or organ of origin of the neoplasm(6). However, antibodies that are not tumor specific but recognise certain subtypes of tissues may also help in establishing the differential diagnosis.

Therefore, a suitably chosen panel of monoclonal antibodies can be of great value in identifying neoplastic cells in serous effusions(17).

Cytologic examination of effusions is primarily concerned with the question whether the effusion is caused by a benign (reactive or inflammatory) process or is the result of a malignancy. This malignancy may originate in the mesothelial surface or may be a metastasis to a body cavity.

Malignant lymphocytes generally are difficult to differentiate from other malignant cells or reactive lymphocytes by routine cytologic examination. The application of antibodies to lymphocytic surface antigens may reveal the lymphocytic phenotype of the cells. In addition, the monoclonality of staining for immunoglobulins indicates the lymphoproliferative character of the effusions(6).

One of the major pitfalls in the cytopathologic examination of effusions is the differential diagnosis between reactive atypical mesothelial cells and single malignant cells.

In establishing the malignant character of the effusion it is often possible to recognise the squamous or adenomatous origin of carcinoma cells. It is often difficult, however, to positively identify the tissue of origin of the neoplastic cells(38).

The frequency of non-malignant effusions in different series is reported to range from 40-90% in several series[16,32], differences most likely being caused by selective sampling of the patients. In a recent survey of 5888 consecutive pleural effusions examined over a 14 year period, 9.8% of the pleural fluid specimens were found to contain malignant cells. In pleural effusions diagnosed as malignant, adenocarcinoma is the most frequent cancer identified (48%) followed by large cell undifferentiated carcinoma (14%) and lymphoma/leukemia (15%)[19]. For all malignant pleural effusions taken together tumors of the lung (36%), breast (15%) and female genital tract (8%) comprised 59% of all primary tumor sites considered.

Of even greater importance are those effusions from patients in whom there is no previous history of underlying cancer. In the above series[19] the patient group without known prior or extant cancer constituted approximately 10% of all malignant effusions studied. Of these, adenocarcinoma of the breast, ovary and lung constituted the majority of malignant effusions.

Gosh et al(16) reported that 16% of their patients presenting with pleural effusions had unknown primaries at the time of diagnosis.

In our own series of 254 patients with a cytologically malignant effusion, at the time of the cytological diagnosis of the effusion, in 30% of patients the primary localisation was not evident. For pleural effusions the four most frequent sites of the primary malignant process were breasts (26%), lungs (25%), lymph nodes and bone marrow (23%), and ovaries (7%). These comprised 81% of patients with malignant pleural effusions. For peritoneal effusions the most frequent sites were ovaries (34%), stomach (12%), breasts (10%) and pancreas (7%). These comprised 63% of patients with malignant peritoneal effusions (unpublished results).

These data clearly illustrate the need for tissue and organ specific markers in the cytodiagnosis of effusions, particularly in those cases where the primary localisation of the malignant process is not known.

Several reports in the literature describe the application of monoclonal antibodies in the cytologic diagnosis of effusions (Table I).

Gosh et al(16,17) applied the Ca-1, HMFG-2 and anti CEA MoAbs and increased the detection of carcinoma cells in serous effusions by 30%. According to these authors mesothelial cells stained rarely with Ca-1 and more frequently with HMFG-2.

However Pallesen and coworkers(31) found weak to moderate positive Ca-1 staining in mesothelial cells. Leucocytes and macrophages remained unstained. They concluded that the use of the Ca-1 antibody did not provide significant additional information over conventional cytology of serous effusions.

Table I **Reaction pattern of monoclonal antibodies in benign and malignant effusions**

Author (ref)	Mo.Ab	Epithelial cancer cells	Normal adult tissue cells	Mesothelial cells	Leukocytes Macrophages	Endothelial cells
Gosh et al. (16,17)	Ca-1 HMFG-2	30% increase in detection of malignant cells		weakly to moderately positive	negative	
Pallesen et al. (42)	Ca-1	positive		negative		
To et al. (39,40)	anti CEA	positive		negative		
Epenetos et al. (13)	HMFG-2 AUA-1	positive positive		negative negative		negative negative
Johnston et al. (19)	B72.3	positive breastcarcinoma 50% coloncarcinoma 100%	negative	negative	negative	negative
Szpak et al. (38)	B72.3	adenocarcinoma positive		negative	negative	
Yam et al. (43)	534F-8	oat cell carcinoma positive		negative		
Peters et al. (32)	GIGA SSEA anti CEA			negative negative negative		
Mariani Constantini et al. (25)	MBRI	breastcarcinoma positive		negative		

Woods et al(42) applied the Ca-1 MoAb to smears from 50 effusions and reported that this antibody could distinguish malignant from non-malignant cells in 21 out of 25 malignant effusions.

Additional support for distinction between benign and malignant effusions might be derived from the use of EMA (epithelial membrane antigen)[18,39,40]. EMA is only weakly and inconsistently visualised on mesothelial cells, while being strongly expressed by most malignant epithelial cells.

Mesothelial cells and inflammatory cells were also negative for the anti-CEA serum used by these authors and therefore this MoAb was thought to be an extremely useful tool for the differential diagnosis between atypical mesothelial cells and adenocarcinoma cells in effusions.

2D1, an anti leucocyte antibody was used to differentiate between white blood cells and undifferentiated small (cancer) cells.

Epenetos et al(13) used two MoABs (HMFG-2 and AUA1), raised against epithelial cell determinants. Both MoAbs were reported by these authors to react with cancer cells, but not with mesothelial or endothelial cells.

Johnston et al(19) have used a series of MoAbs raised against membrane enriched or crude extracts of metastatic breast carcinomas. Of these B72.3 has shown a selective reactivity for carcinomas over normal human adult tissues(27). B72.3 was reported to react with 50% of all breast carcinomas and nearly 100% of all colon carcinomas examined.

The ability of B72.3 to distinguish between adenocarcinomas and other malignant neoplasms is of particular interest when it is recalled that on occasion, particularly in the early phase of dissemination to body cavities, adenocarcinomas may occur predominantly as small cells with a propensity of single occurrence. This causes potential confusion with a wide variety of non adenocarcinomas, carcinoids, lymphomas, small cell undifferentiated carcinomas, leukemias, neuroblastomas, Ewing sarcomas and embryonal rhabdomyosarcomas. Adenocarcinomas that may have this small cell type of presentation include lobular carcinoma of the breast, adenocarcinoma of stomach and pancreas, adenocarcinoma of the endometrium, adenocarcinoma of the prostate and follicular carcinoma of the thyroid. Szpak et al(38) and Johnston et al(19) reported no reactivity of the B72.3 antibody with any cell type in benign effusions and apparent negativity with mesothelial cells in malignant effusions. They stated that "the monoclonal antibody B72.3 may function as a highly selective marker in recognizing a cancer cell versus a mesothelial cell and an adenocarcinoma cell versus other malignant tumor cells". B72.3, moreover, showed no reactivity to leukemic or lymphomatous effusions (see chapter 16).

Yam and coworkers(43) applied an oat cell specific monoclonal antibody 534F-8, raised and characterised by Cuttitta and coworkers[11] to a pleural effusion in a patient with a mediastinal mass of unknown origin. Cytologic examination of the effusion was inconclusive and the question remained whether the tumor cells originated from a lymphoma or from a small cell anaplastic carcinoma. Immunocytochemical staining showed the tumor cells to react with the MoAb 534F-8, indicating their oat cell nature. Subsequent clinopathological analysis confirmed the diagnosis.

Peters et al(32) evaluated MoAbs against a gastrointestinal carcinoma antigen (GICA), a stage specific embryonic antigen (SSEA) and against a portion of the carcinoembryonic antigen (CEA) molecule for their ability to differentiate between mesothelial cells and tumor cells.
They concluded that a strong reaction with any one or a combination of these MoAbs provides strong evidence against a diagnosis of benign mesothelial cells.
Mariani Constantini et al(25) applied antibody MBRI, raised against the membrane fraction of the breast cancer cell line MCF 7, to serous effusions. Preliminary data indicated that this MoAb is able to discriminate between mesothelial cells and breast carcinoma cells in effusions.

Another type of tissue-specific markers are the intermediate filament proteins, which are part of the cytoskeleton.
Nucleated cells contain an intracellular matrix of fibrous elements recognised as microfilaments, microtubules and intermediate-sized filaments (IF). These IF often constitute a considerable part of the cytoskeleton and are composed of different types of proteins that are specific for the various cell types (see chapter 5).

Antibodies to the different protein components of the IF can be of use in cytopathological diagnosis when a definitive diagnosis can not be made on the basis of conventional cytopathologic features(33).

In cytological preparations from body cavity fluids, antibodies to IF proteins are of a restricted value since, so far, no IF markers specific for mesothelial cells have been prepared. Furthermore, Ramaekers et al(37) have reported that keratin and vimentin may be coexpressed in (malignant) cells in effusions. Apparently part of the epithelial tumor cells in body fluids adapt to their new growth conditions by the development of a vimentin cytoskeleton. The presence of such an additional cytoskeleton may have influence on the mitotic and motile activity of the cells and thus influence the growth rate, agressive behaviour and spread of metastasizing cells. It is noteworthy in this respect that cells from squamous cell carcinomas did not coexpress vimentin when in body fluids, which may be explained by the highly differentiated state of these cells or because of a less rapid expression of vimentin in cells from squamous cell carcinomas.

However antibodies to different types of IF proteins, especially those directed against cytokeratins and vimentin can be useful in the differential diagnosis of epithelial and non-epithelial tumor cells. All non-epithelial cells present in effusions are negative with the cytokeratin antiserum but positive with the antiserum against vimentin. Macrophages and lymphocytes, as well as tumor cells of mesenchymal origin, could be shown to exclusively express vimentin type intermediate sized filaments. These neoplastic cells included lymphomas, leukemias, fibrosarcomas, melanomas and neurofibrosarcomas(34,35).

Once the cells under study, by positive identification of

one of five groups of intermediate filaments proteins, are subclassified as to the direction of differentiation, the use of further markers, capable of subdividing particular tumor types, may be appropriate. Obvious choices include surface markers specific for different lymphoma subtypes and antibodies that recognise subsets of cytokeratins or a single cytokeratin polypeptide(22). The latter are able to distinguish between different types of epithelial tumor metastases. For example the monoclonal cytokeratin antibody RGE 53 can distinguish between cells derived from adenocarcinomas and cells derived from squamous cell carcinomas (Table II)(36). Unfortunately this antibody does not distinguish between benign or malignant mesothelial cells or adenocarcinoma cells.

Table II Patterns of cytokeratin and vimentin expression in benign and malignant cells in body cavity effusions

Cytological diagnosis	keratin (common determinant)	keratin 18*	vimentin
squamous cell carcinomas	+++	-	-
adenocarcinomas	++	++	++/-
mesothelioma	+++	+++	++
lymphomas	-	-	+/++
leukemias	-	-	++
melanomas	-	-	++
fibrosarcomas	-	-	++
benign mesothelial cells	++	++	+
macrophages & lymphocytes	-	-	++

* recognized by monoclonal antibody RGE 53

In the interpretation of preparations, stained with these IF antibodies it may be of help that cell nuclei can be counter-stained with haematoxylin. This staining procedure may however, influence the fluorescence pattern in sofar that erythrocytes show non-specific fluorescence. Furthermore, for optimal results preparations should be viewed within a few hours.

We have occasionally observed that clusters of epithelial like tumor cells in effusions were negative for cytokeratin, while single tumor cells showed a positive reaction for this antibody. This result may be partially explained by the compact nature of these clustered tumor cells.

4. FINE NEEDLE ASPIRATIONS

In the last decade the reemergence of fine needle aspiration cytology has created a greater accessibility of potential malignancy bearing tissues(21).

The advantages of fine needle aspiration cytology are obvious. The method is fast and needs no anaesthesia, it bears little risk of causing bleeding or infection and is usually accompanied by only slight discomfort to the patient(2).

A cellular specimen obtained by fine needle aspiration is an adequate sample for determining the antigenic phenotype of a tumor(20). The significance of monoclonal antibodies in this area of cytopathology lies in their potential usefulness in the major diagnostic dilemma posed by poorly differentiated and undifferentiated cancers. There remains a significant number of patients whose metastatic neoplasms appear as undifferentiated cancers by conventional light microscopy and whose clinical history or examination fails to reveal or suggest a primary site(21).

A promising approach to the differential diagnosis of undifferentiated neoplasms has been the search for antibodies to tumor associated antigens (TAA) that would provide information on the degree of differentiation and derivation from a certain tissue type. Among such TAA's several melanoma associated antigens have demonstrated high specificity(21).

MoAb B72.3 was used in the analysis of benign and malignant lung tumors by Johnston and coworkers(20). Adenocarcinomas, adenosquamous - and squamous cell carcinomas were all positive with B72.3, wherease various benign tumors, carcinoid tumors and six small cell anaplastic carcinomas were all negative for B72.3. Staining patterns with this antibody in fine needle aspirates were found to be highly predictive for the antibody reactivity patterns in the comparable surgically resected specimens(20).

Antibodies to intermediate filaments proteins have been shown to distinguish the major tumor groups (see chapter 5). Altmansberger and coworkers(2) and Ramaekers et al(2,34,35,36, 37) investigated smears from fine needle aspirations using well characterized antibodies, each specific for only one of the five types of IF proteins.

Tumor cells of different carcinomas, thymomas and the epithelial part of pulmonary blastomas were postive with antibodies recognizing cytokeratins. Tumor cells in non muscle sarcomas, including Ewing sarcoma and malignant lymphomas could be specifically identified with antibodies to vimentin. Tumor-cells from muscle sarcomas were desmin positive. Tumor cells in phaeochromocytoma and bronchus carcinoid were positive with antibodies specific for neurofilaments(2). IF-typing, was therefore considered a useful method for the determination of the histogenetic origin of cancer cells in aspirates.

In our hands IF typing in aspirates from pleomorphic adenomas of the parotid gland, which normally co-express cytokeratin and vimentin, has been most helpful in confirming or establishing the cytologic diagnosis of such neoplasms. In frozen sections of these tumors several cell types have been detected, which differ in their IF pattern. Amongst these are cells co-expressing cytokeratin and vimentin, which are negative for RGE 53. Another cell type is positive for the polyclonal cytokeratin antiserum, as well as for RGE 53, but does not contain vimentin. These two combinations are typical for solid pleomorphic adenomas. When examining thin needle aspirates from such neoplasms, these two cell types can be detected on the basis of their IF pattern in the cytological preparation.

Droese et al(12) have shown that also in cases of

ultrasound-guided percutaneous fine needle aspiration biopsies of intraperitoneal and retroperitoneal malignancies, routine cytologic examination can be supplemented by IF typing.

Auerbach and associates[4] applied antidesmin antibodies to a fine needle aspiration performed under CT guidance.

Also in brain tumor cytodiagnosis IF antibodies have been applied. Collins(10) and Collins et al(9) reported on the application of fine needle aspiration cytology in the diagnosis of brain tumors. Combined methods of computertomography and stereotaxis have been refined considerably in the last decade. This has created the possibility of obtaining a cytologic specimen from most suspect lesions in the brain. In central and vital areas a specimen may only be obtainable by thin needle aspiration cytology.

Furthermore, the application of the smear technique to neurosurgical biopsies is a rather useful procedure to obtain a rapid diagnosis of intracranial neoplasms[1]. In all tumortypes studied sofar the presence or absence of GFAP was in accord with previous reports following similar studies on sections of paraffin embedded material[10]. The demonstration of GFAP positive cells will establish the astrocytic nature of primitive or highly anaplastic tumors, even when fibril formation is scanty or absent. A major advantage of this method is the exclusion of non-glial tumors, such as malignant lymphomas and metastases of anaplastic carcinomas, which morphologically may resemble astrocytomas in routine preparations.

Bigner et al(7) using three MoAbs that were specific for GFAP, were able to demonstrate complete separation between non-glial tumors and glioblastomas in cerebrospinal fluid specimens or brain aspirates and tumor imprints. Another useful application is the use of GFAP antibodies in the differential diagnosis between fibrous meningiomas and astrocytomas.

Coakham and coworkers(8) have applied a panel of monoclonal antibodies consisting of markers for neuroectodermal tissue (UJ13A), epithelial tissue, i.e. cytokeratin (LE 61), leucocytes (2D1) and neoplastic neuroblasts (UJ 181.4) to cerebrospinal fluid from 17 patients with suspected neoplastic meningitis. The results were compared with those obtained from routine cytological preparations. They concluded that immunocytochemical testing of cerebrospinal fluid greatly increased the accuracy of identification and typing of malignant cells.

Good results were also obtained by Garson and coworkers[14]. Applying a panel of four monoclonal antibodies (LE 61, UJ 13A, UJ 181.4 and 2D1) they were able to considerably improve the accuracy of conventional light microscopical diagnosis. In 21 out of 22 cases, malignant cells were correctly diagnosed in cerebrospinal fluid specimens. In all cases these cells could be correctly identified as derived from carcinomas, neuroectodermal tumors (exept melanoma), melanomas or malignant lymphomas, respectively.

One of the areas in cytology where IF antibody application seems most promising is in lymph node aspirates.
The immunocytochemical data obtained with lymph node aspirates are similar as those with effusion specimens (see Table II). In all cases lymphocytes are negative for cytokeratin antibodies,

but (weakly) positive for vimentin. When examining frozen sections of total lymph nodes, we have found no cytokeratin-positive cells in normal lymph follicles.

As a result, the detection of cytokeratin-positive cells in aspirates from lymph nodes is a very strong indication for the presence of metastatic carcinoma cells. Normally no cytokeratin-positive cells can be observed in cases of chronic lymphadenitis or malignant lymphomas. Instead the cells are vimentin positive.

When using the monoclonal cytokeratin antibody RGE 53 no reaction with cells from metastatic squamous cell carcinomas or with lymphocytes is seen. A rather strong reaction, however, is seen in cells from metastases of adenocarcinomas. These reaction patterns are consistent with our results in frozen sections of several types of epithelial tumors.

Application of the immunocytochemical techniques described above thus seems promising in those cases where lymph node aspirates have to be evaluated. Epithelial tumor cells present in these preparations mostly contain exclusively cytokeratin IF and do not co-express vimentin (as in the case of ascites and pleural fluids). Moreover, since the monoclonal antibody directed against cytokeratin from glandular epithelial tissues (RGE 53) can distinguish between cells derived from adenocarcinomas and squamous cell carcinomas it is obvious that application of this antibody in cytopathology can help to make a more precise differential diagnosis and can thus give valuable information with respect to the nature of a primary tumor.

5. EXFOLIATIVE CYTOLOGY

5.1. Cervical Cytology

Koprowska and coworkers(23), in search for immunologic markers of epithelial cells derived from cervical carcinoma, applied a panel of monoclonal antibodies to cervical cytologic smears. They observed that antigenic determinants shared with other tumors, became more pronounced as cervical intraepithelial neoplastic lesions progressed to invasive carcinoma. Four monoclonal antibodies, found to identify tumor antigens but with different specificity were studied in greater detail for their potential diagnostic value in the differential diagnosis between progressive and stationary intraepithelial lesions that are morphologically similar(24).

5.2. Pulmonary Cytology

Memoli and coworkers(26) have described the application of a murine monoclonal antibody directed against an antigen associated with small cell anaplastic lung carcinoma (SCCL 175) to cytologic specimens of 21 cases of pulmonary small cell anaplastic carcinomas (SCC) and 78 cases of primary adeno-squamous-, bronchioloalveolar - and undifferentiated carcinomas of the lung. Nineteen of the 21 SCC cases showed some cytoplasmic or cell surface reactivity with the antibody, whereas none of the non-SCC cases showed reactivity with this MoAb. These results demonstrate the potential utility of this monoclonal antibody in the differential diagnosis between small

cell and non-small cell pulmonary cancers.
Banner and associates(5) applied a monoclonal antibody raised against a human lung adenocarcinoma cell line (NCA 44-3A6) to destained cytologic smears of bronchial brushings originally stained by the Papanicolaou method. They concluded that NCA 44-3A6 could be valuable in the precise classification of pulmonary carcinomas. Ten of 12 adenocarcinomas immunostained strongly, while two were focally positive. Squamous carcinomas were consistently negative. Noteworthy was the immunostaining frequently observed in the large cell undifferentiated carcinomas, which emphasizes the heterogeneous character of this tumor class. Occasional immunostaining in neuroendocrine carcinomas suggests focal exocrine differentiation in this type of tumor as previously documented by electron microscopy.

6. CONCLUSIONS

There are many problems in cytopathology for which immunocytochemical identification of tissue specific surface markers or cytoplasmic antigens may prove useful(40). Sofar the value of this approach has occasionally been tested in the cytodiagnosis of serous effusions. The available immunocytochemical techniques will be adapted to complement the traditional morphological assessment in many other types of cytological material.
It can be expected that the application of these techniques in fine needle aspiration cytology will become a most important procedure in solving differential diagnostic problems in cancer diagnosis(17).

ACKNOWLEDGEMENTS

The authors thank Mrs. Janny van Rennes for excellent secretarial support.

Figure 1

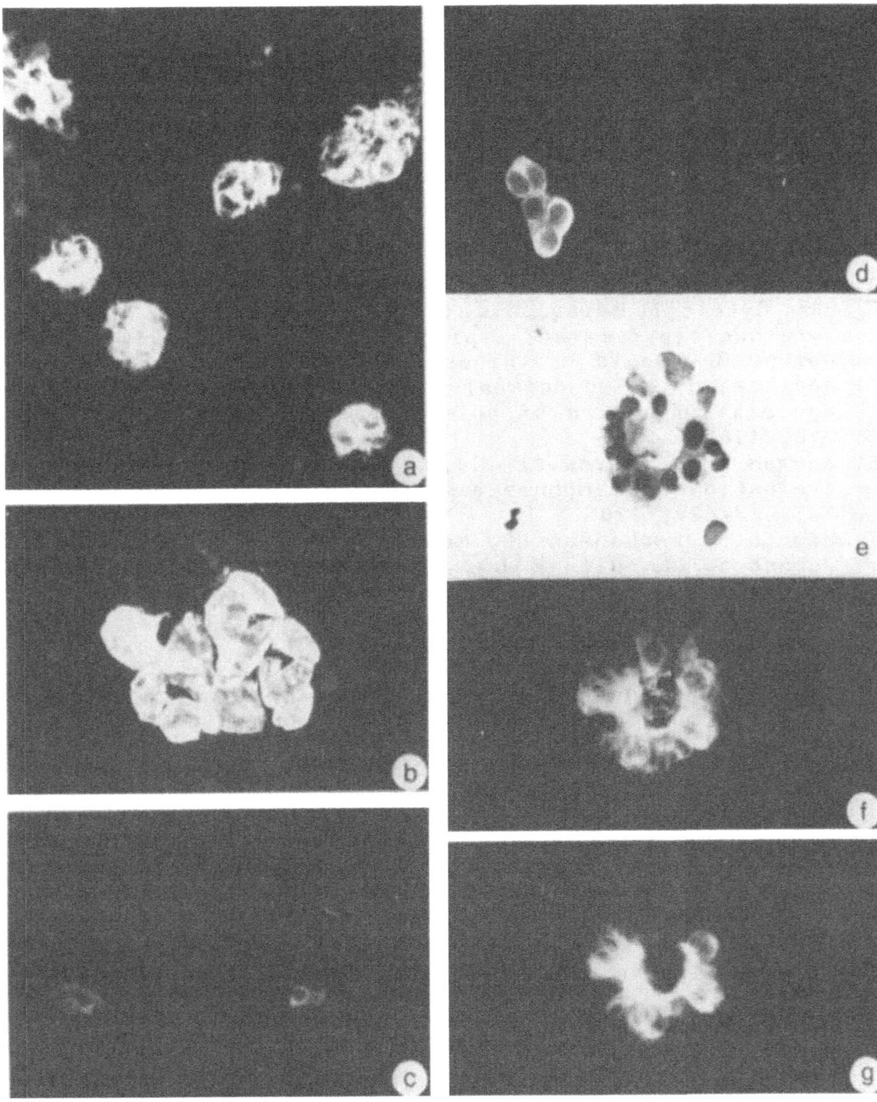

a) detection of metastatic tumor cells from a ductal breast carcinoma in a lymph node frozen section with a rabbit antiserum to skin keratins. **b-d)** fine needle aspiration biopsies of lymph nodes containing a squamous cell carcinoma metastasis (b, cytokeratin; c, vimentin) or an adenocarcinoma metastasis from the GI-tract (d, cytokeratin 18 positivity as detected by RGE 53; note negative cluster of lymphocytes).
e-g) ovarian carcinoma cells (e; hematoxylin) present in an effusion from ascites, positive for both cytokeratin (f; detected with the monoclonal antibody RGE 53) and vimentin (g; as detected with the rabbit antiserum to bovine lens vimentin; double label indirect immunofluorescence).

REFERENCES

1. Adams HJ, Graham DI, Doyle D: Brain biopsy: the smear technique for neurosurgical biopsies. Chapman & Hall, London, 1980, pp 1-22.
2. Altmannsberger M, Osborn M, Droese M, Weber K, Schauer A: Diagnotic value of intermediate filament antibodies in clinical cytology. Klin Wochenschr **62:** 114-123, 1984.
3. Ashall F, Bramwell ME, Harris A: A new marker for human cancer cells. 1: The Ca antigen and the Ca 1 antibody. Lancet ii: 1-6, 1982.
4. Auerbach HE, Atkinson BF, Ernest CS, Brooks KK, Filstein MR: Cytologic diagnosis of a retroperitoneal mass using intermediate filament typing. Acta Cytol **28:** 634, 1984.
5. Banner BF, Gould VE, Radosevich JA, MA Y, Lee I, Rosen ST: Application of monoclonal antibody 44-A3A6 in the diagnosis and classification of pulmonary carcinomas. Acta Cytol **29:** 946, 1985.
6. Bauman MD, Borowitz MJ, Johnston WW: Immunocytologic evaluation of lymphoid aspirates and effusions. Acta Cytol **28:** 628-629, 1985.
7. Bigner SH, McLendon RE, Mensi DW, Wikstrand CJ, Pegram CN, Johnston WW, Bigner DD: Expression of glial fibrillary acidic protein in cytologic specimens from the central nervous system as demonstrated by monoclonal antibodies. Acta Cytol **29:** 919, 1985.
8. Coakham HB, Brownell B, Harper EI, Garson JA, Allan PM, Lane EB, Kemshead JT: Use of monoclonal antibody panel to identify malignant cells in cerebrospinal fluid. Lancet i: 1095-1097, 1984.
9. Collins VP, Moser R: Monoclonal antibodies to glial fibrillary acidic protein. I. Characterization. Acta Pathol Microbiol Immunol Scand (A) **91:** 269-279, 1983.
10. Collins VP: Monoclonal antibodies to glial fibrillary acidic protein in the cytologic diagnosis of brain tumors. Acta Cytol **28:** 401-406, 1984.
11. Cuttitta F, Rosen S, Gazdar AF, Minna JD: Monoclonal antibodies that demonstrate specificity for several types of human lung cancer. Proc Natl Acad Sci USA **78:** 4591-4595, 1981.
12. Droese M, Altmannsberger M, Kehl A, Lankisch PG, Weiss R, Weber K, Osborm M: Ultrasound-guided percutaneous fine needle aspiration biopsy of abdominal and retroperitoneal masses. Accuracy of cytology in the diagnosis of malignancy, cytologic tumor typing and use of antibodies to intermediate filaments in selected cases. Acta Cytol **28:** 368-384, 1984.
13. Epenetos AA, Canti G, Taylor-Papadimitriou J, Curling M, Bodmer WF: Use of two epithelium-specific monoclonal antibodies for diagnosis of malignancy in serous effusions. Lancet **2:** 1004-1006, 1982.
14. Garson JA, Coakham HB, Kemshead JT, Brownell B, Harper E, Allan P, Bourne S: The role of monoclonal antibodies in brain tumour diagnosis and cerebrospinal fluid (CSF) cytology. J Neuro Oncol **3:** 165-171, 1985.
15. Gatter KC, Abdulaziz Z, Beverly P, Corvalon JRF, Ford C,

Lane EB: Use of monoclonal antibodies for the histopathological diagnosis of human malignancy. J Clin Pathol **35:** 1253-1267, 1982.
16. Gosh AK, Mason DY, Spriggs AI: Immunocytochemical staining with monoclonal antibodies in cytologically "negative" serous effusions from patients with malignant disease. J Clin Pathol **36:** 1150-1153, 1983.
17. Gosh AK, Spriggs AI, Taylor-Papadimitriou J, Mason DY: Immunocytochemical staining of cells in pleural and peritoneal effusions with a panel of monoclonal antibodies. J Clin Pathol **36:** 1154-1164, 1983.
18. Heyderman E, Steele K, Ormerod MG: A new antigen on the epithelial membrane: HE immunoperoxidase localization in normal and neoplastic tissue. J Clin Pathol **32:** 35-39, 1979.
19. Johnston WW, Szpak CA, Lottich SC, Thor A, Schlom J: Use of a monoclonal antibody (B72.3) as an immunocytochemical adjunct to diagnosis of adenocarcinoma in human effusions. Cancer Res **45:** 1894-1900, 1985.
20. Johnston WW, Spzak CA, Tello JW, Thor A, Schlom J: Immunocytochemical studies in fine needle aspirates from lung cancers by means of a monoclonal antibody (B27.3). Acta Cytol **29:** 930, 1985.
21. Johnston WW, Borowitz MJ, Stuhlmiller GM, Seigler MD: Expression of a melanoma-tumor associated antigen as demonstrated by a monoclonal antibody (D6.1) in cytopathologic preparations of human tumor cells from effusions and needle aspirates. Anal Quant Cytol & Histol **7:** 73-80, 1985.
22. Kahn HJ, Hanna W, Yeger H, Baumal R: Immunohistochemical localization of prekeratin filaments in benign and malignant cells in effusions. Am J Pathol **109:** 206-214, 1982.
23. Koprowska I, Zipfel S, Himes T, Herlyn M: Use of monoclonal antibodies and immunoperoxidase staining for demonstration of antigenic cross reactivity of exfoliated uterine cervical neoplastic cells with other human tumors. Acta Cytol **28:** 653, 1984.
24. Koprowska I, Zipsel S, Himes T, Herlyn M: The search for monoclonal antibodies to identify uterine epithelial neoplastic cells. Acta Cytol **29:** 920, 1985.
25. Marianni-Constantini R, Menard S, Clemente C, Tagliabue E, Colnaghi MI, Rilke F: Immunocytochemical identification of breast carcinoma cells in effusions using a monoclonal antibody. J Clin Pathol **35:** 1037, 1982.
26. Memoli VA, Jordan AG, Predmore L, Sullivan MM, Ball E: Use of a novel monoclonal antibody (MoAB SCCL 175) in the diagnosis of small cell carcinoma. Acta Cytol **29:** 919, 1985.
27. Nutti M, Teramoto YA, Mariani-Constantini R, Horan Hand P, Colcher D, Schlom J: A monoclonal antibody (B72.3) defines patterns of distribution of a novel tumor-associated antigen in human mammary carcinoma cell populations. Int J Cancer **293:** 539-545, 1982.
28. Oud PS, Zahniser DJ, Haag DL, Van Boekel MCG, Hermkens HJ, Herman CJ, Vooijs GP: A new disaggregation device for

cytology specimens. Cytometry **5:** 509-514, 1984.
29. Oud PS, Zahniser DJ, Garcia GL, Van Boekel MCG, Haag DJ, Hermkens HJ, Pahlplatz MMM, Vooijs GP, Herman CJ: Pressure fixation method of transferring cells from polycarbonate filters to glass slides. Anal Quant Cytol **6:** 131-138, 1984.
30. Oud PS, Haag DJ, Zahniser DJ, Ramaekers FCS, Huysmans ACLM, Veldhuizen JAM, Verheijen RHM, Verrijp K, Broers JLV, Herman CJ, Vooijs GP: Cytopress: automated slide preparation of cytologic material from suspension. Cytometry **7:** 8-17, 1986.
31. Pallesen G, Jepsen FL, Hastrup J, Ipsen A, Hvidberg N: Experience with the Oxford tumour marker (Ca 1) in serous fluids. Lancet i: 1326, 1983.
32. Peters J, Atkinson BF, Ernst CS, Chianese D, Aquino M, Perry MD, Herlyn M, Koprowski H: Gastrointestinal tumor antigen as a marker for malignancy in effusions. Acta Cytol **28:** 635, 1984.
33. Puts JJG, Vooijs GP, Huysmans A, Van Aspert A, Ramaekers FCS: Cytoskeletal proteins as tissue specific markers in cytopathology. Exp Cell Biol **54:** 73-79, 1986.
34. Ramaekers FCS, Puts JJG, Moesker O, Jap PHK, Vooijs GP: Use of antibodies to intermediate filaments in the characterization of human tumors. Cold Spring Harbor Symp Quant Biol **46:** 331-339, 1981.
35. Ramaekers FCS, Puts JJG, Moesker O, Kant A, Huysmans A, Haag D, Jap PHK, Herman C, Vooijs GP: Antibodies to intermediate filament proteins in the immunohistochemical identification of human tumours. An overview. Histochem J **15:** 691-713, 1983.
36. Ramaekers FCS, Huysmans A, Moesker O, Kant A, Jap PHK, Herman C, Vooijs GP: Monoclonal antibodies to keratin filaments, specific for glandular epithelia and their tumors. Use in surgical pathology. Lab Invest **49:** 353-361, 1983.
37. Ramaekers F, Haag D, Jap P, Vooijs P: Immunochemical demonstration of keratin and vimentin in cytological aspirates. Acta Cytol **28:** 385-392, 1984.
38. Szpak CA, Johnston WW, Lottich SC, Kufe D, Thor A, Schlom J: Patterns of reactivity of four novel monoclonal antibodies (B27,3, FS, B1,1 and B6.2) with cells in human malignant and benign effusions. Acta Cytol **28:** 356-367, 1984.
39. To A, Dearnaley DP, Ormerod MG, Canti G, Coleman DV: Epithelial membrane antigen. Its use in the cytodiagnosis of malignancy in serous effusions. Am J Clin Pathol **78:** 214-219, 1982.
40. To A, Coleman DV, Dearnaley DP, Ormerod MG, Steele K, Neville AM: Use of antisera to epithelial membrane antigen for the cytodiagnosis of malignancy in serous effusions. J Clin Pathol **34:** 1326-1332, 1981.
41. Von Koskull H: Rapid identification of glial cells in human amniotic fluid with indirect immunofluorescence. Acta Cytol **28:** 383-400, 1984.
42. Woods JC, Spriggs AI, Harris H, McGee JD: A new marker for cancer cells III. Immunocytochemical detection of malignant cells in serous fluids with the CA_1 antibody. Lancer ii,

512-515, 1982.
43. Yam LT, Winkler CF: Immunocytochemical diagnosis of oat-cell carcinoma in pleural effusions. Acta Cytol **28**: 425-429, 1984.
44. Garson JA, Coakham HB, Kemshead JT, Brownell B, Harper E, Allan P, Bourne S: The role of monoclonal antibodies in brain tumour diagnosis and cerebrospinal fluid (CSF) cytology. J Neuro Oncol **3**: 165-171, 1985.

16. TUMOR ASSOCIATED ANTIGENS AND ONCOGENE PRODUCTS DEFINED BY MONOCLONAL ANTIBODIES.

A. THOR, N. OHUCHI, P. HORAN HAND, M.O. WEEKS, W.W. JOHNSTON, C.A. SZPAK AND J. SCHLOM

1. INTRODUCTION

The advent of hybridoma/monoclonal antibody technology in 1975 (1) and gene cloning procedures have drastically influenced both the understanding and practice of pathology. Using these methodologies and reagents, applications have been developed in the research laboratory, distributed to the clinical setting, and now often impact on the diagnosis and management of human disease. It is the authors' intent to focus this chapter on some recently developed monoclonal antibody applications in human pathology using immunohistochemical techniques. The text will be roughly divided into three parts: background information and general principles, practical applications, and monoclonal antibodies as probes to investigate tumor biology and oncogene expression.

2. BACKGROUND INFORMATION

2.1. Development of Monoclonal Antibodies to Tumor Associated Antigens

Tumor associated antigens (TAAs) can be broadly divided into several categories, including: oncofetal antigens, hormones, growth factors and other cellular products. To detect these markers, biochemical as well as immunologic assays have been devised (2-8). Radioimmunoassays (RIA), enzyme linked immunoabsorbant assays (ELISA), dot blot techniques, gel separation methods, Western blot analysis, immunoprecipitations, immunohistochemical techniques, and fluorescence activated cell sort analysis (flow cytometry) have all been utilized. Immunohistochemical methods and flow cytometry have been particularly useful in the evaluation of human tissues submitted for either histologic or cytologic evaluation because they facilitate simultaneous routine morphologic analysis and antigenic phenotyping of specific cells using immunologic probes.

Monoclonal antibodies (MAbs) and immunohistochemical techniques may also be used to detect and define other cell associated markers including: receptors, developmental or differentiation stage specific antigens, structural elements (e.g., filaments), enzymes, proto-oncogene or oncogene products, and cell associated immunoglobulins. These cell associated antigens are often expressed by malignant as well as benign cell types, and can be used to investigate various aspects of cellular biology as well as to differentiate histologic cell types. MAbs directed against these epitopes as well as to tumor associated antigens have been utilized in an attempt to correctly diagnose and subclassify human carcinomas, sarcomas, neural tumors, and hematopoietic malignancies. New MAbs are now being developed using *in vivo* immunization as well as *in vitro* B-lymphocyte stimulation. These reagents, as well as many which are currently available, are rapidly being evaluated for potential applications. The most intense areas of investigation include the use of MAb to: (a) phenotype and differentiate malignant cell populations, (b) differentiate benign from malignant cell types, (c) recognize "preneoplastic" cellular alterations, (d) define the malignant phenotype in terms of structural and biologic variation from normal, (e) identify and characterize oncogenes, proto-oncogenes, and other cellular or genetic elements which may affect carcinogenesis, and (f) define the role that growth factors, tumor factors and other biologic response modifiers play in the development and maintenance of the transformed phenotype.

2.2. Immunohistochemical Analyses of Human Carcinomas

Malignant epithelial cell tumors (carcinomas) cause significant morbidity and mortality (approximately 400,000 deaths per year in the United States), and account for greater than 80% of human malignancy. Of these, the most common primary sites of carcinoma development are the lung, colon and breast. Therapeutic intervention is often not successful once metastases of these cancers have occurred, hence new diagnostic and therapeutic modalities are being sought.

To date, more than 100 MAbs against human carcinomas have been reported in the literature which are unique with respect to range of reactivity and reactive antigen. Of these, most have been directed against glycoprotein antigens found in breast, lung, colon, pancreatic, and ovarian carcinomas. These monoclonal antibodies have been produced using a variety of tumor homogenates, extracts, or cultured cell lines for immunogens. Several important concepts have emerged from these studies, including: (a) most of these MAbs demonstrate preferential binding to the immunogen against which they were produced, although they often bind to other benign and malignant cell types, (b) most carcinoma associated antigenic determinants (as defined by MAbs) are found on a wide variety of malignant epithelial cells, hence are "pancarcinoma" antigens, (c) a great deal of antigenic heterogeneity exists in the expression of a given TAA (both among cells of a given tumor mass, and between tumor masses from the same or different patients) which may affect the sensitivity of a given MAb assay, (d) established cell lines may not reflect the phenotype or even genotype of surgically resected carcinomas, (e) cross reactivity or specificity of a given MAb must be carefully evaluated using defined assay conditions and a wide variety of benign and malignant tissues before it can be utilized as an immunohistochemical adjunct for tumor diagnosis, and (f) assay conditions must be rigorously controlled and defined for each MAb, as variance may affect tissue reactivity and reproducibility of results. In a practical sense, availability of each MAb to the medical community at large, as well as the stability of a given antigen in various fixative and tissue preparations are also critical issues. Hence, the utility and potential applications of a single MAb in immunopathology may be affected by a variety of factors.

2.3. Evaluation of Potential Diagnostic Applications

To illustrate how MAbs can be utilized with surgical and cytologic specimens, several recent investigations using MAb B72.3 will be discussed. MAb B72.3 is reactive with a high molecular weight ($\geq 10^6$) mucin-like molecule termed tumor associated glycoprotein (TAG)-72. It was generated using a membrane-enriched extract of a breast carcinoma metastasis, and previous immunohistochemical studies have demonstrated the reactivity of this MAb with formalin-fixed, paraffin-embedded human tissues (9-12). The antigen recognized by B72.3 TAAG-72 has been detected at the cell surface (as well as within the cytoplasm) in various carcinomas but rarely in malignant human epithelial established cell lines (12).

The TAG-72 antigen was recently characterized by Johnson et al. (13) who obtained partially purified antigen from xenograft tumors of a human colon carcinoma cell line (LS-174T). A tumor homogenate was fractionated by Sepharose CL-4B chromatography, and then subjected to two sequential passages through B72.3 antibody affinity columns. This three step procedure produced a nearly pure preparation of TAG-72 antigen with minimal contamination as shown by polyacrylamide gel electrophoresis followed by staining with Coomassie Blue or periodic acid/Schiff reagent. The density, as determined by cesium chloride gradient ultracentrifugation, was found to be 1.45 g/ml. This density determination, together with the high molecular weight ($\geq 10^6$), resistance to chondroitinase digestion, presence of blood group related oligosaccharides, and sensitivity to shearing into lower molecular weight forms suggest that TAG-72 is a novel mucin-like glycoprotein distinct from carcinoembryonic antigen.

Expression of the TAG-72 antigen can be influenced by the spatial configuration of some carcinoma cell populations (13), is rapidly lost with passage into primary cell culture (14), and can be enhanced by incubation of tumor cells with recombinant α interferon (15). In addition, studies using ^{131}I-MAb B72.3 have demonstrated prolonged MAb binding to human carcinoma xenografts allowing in situ radioimmunodetection in the nude mouse model (16-18). Prior to the initiation of in vivo human trials, however, extensive studies were conducted to better define the distribution of the TAG-72 antigen in adult and fetal tissues.

2.4. TAG-72 Antigen Distribution

Using high concentrations of purified MAb B72.3 and overnight incubation conditions to enhance assay sensitivity, a variety of formalin-fixed, paraffin-embedded human tumors and normal tissues were analyzed for TAG-72 expression using avidin-biotin-peroxidase complex (ABC) immunohistochemical techniques. Adenocarcinomas demonstrated the most MAb B72.3 reactivity, whereas human neoplasia of non-epithelial origin failed to express detectable TAG-72 antigen as defined by MAb B72.3 (Table 1).

Thirty normal adult tissues, in contrast, failed to demonstrate significant MAb B72.3 immunoreactivity with the exception of uterine epithelium from the secretory phase of the menstrual cycle using formalin-fixed tissue sections (19). To eliminate the possibility of antigen denaturation during tissue fixation and processing (hence a false negativity of normal tissues), frozen section preparations of benign and malignant human tissues were also tested for MAb B72.3 reactivity. In all cases immunoreactivities with frozen non-processed tissues were equivalent to their respective formalin-fixed, paraffin-embedded counterparts. Of interest was the reconfirmation that specific benign disease states, particularly of the breast, colon (19), and ovary (20), may be associated with an increase in MAb B72.3 reactivity. This was particularly noted in 3 tumors of the ovary which were histologically interpreted as borderline in malignant potential (20). A preliminary survey of fetal tissues using MAb B72.3 also yielded interesting results, in that fetal colon, stomach and esophagus from a 300 gram fetus were immunoreactive. Hence, TAG-72 antigen was demonstrated to be both pan-adenocarcinoma and oncofetal in nature.

3. PRACTICAL APPLICATIONS

3.1. Tumor Screening and Detection

Phase I clinical trials to determine the applicability of radiolabeled MAb B72.3 in radioimmunoscintigraphy for the in situ detection of colonic carcinoma have recently been completed. Preliminary data suggest that ^{131}I-MAb B72.3 (injected intravenously in patients with metastatic adenocarcinoma of the colon) successfully binds to malignant cells, with

TABLE 1

IMMUNOREACTIVITY OF MALIGNANT HUMAN TISSUES WITH MAB B72.3[a]

Organs	Histologic Tumor Types	Number Reactive/ Number Tested
Brain	Glioblastoma Multiforme	0/1
Breast	Invasive Ductal Carcinoma	37/44
Bone	Osteogenic Sarcoma	0/1
Bone Marrow	Leukemia	0/1
Colon	Adenocarcinoma	51/54
Esophagus	Squamous Cell Carcinoma	2/2
Lung	Adenocarcinoma	28/29
	Large Cell Carcinoma	1/1
	Squamous Cell Carcinoma	3/3
	Small Cell Carcinoma	0/5
Lymph Node	Lymphoma	0/10
Ovary	Common Epithelial (Mucinous, serous, endometriod, clear cell and undifferentiated)	40/40
Pancreas	Adenocarcinoma	3/3
Skin	Melanoma	0/6
Stomach	Adenocarcinoma	3/4
Thymus	Thymoma	0/1

[a]Further detail given, ref 19, 20.

a tumor to normal tissue binding ratio of $\geq$3:1 in the majority of patients (n=27). In addition, gamma scans demonstrated increased uptake by tumor masses with successful radiolocalization of lesions in nearly one-half of the patients (21). In addition, an immunoradiometric assay has been developed to assay serum levels of the TAG-72 antigen (22). Using this assay, elevated levels of TAG-72 have been detected in patients with adenocarcinoma of the colon, as compared to patients with benign inflammatory bowel disease and normal volunteers. Hence, MAb B72.3 may be a useful marker for the detection of the TAG-72 antigen in serum of carcinoma patients which is distinct from CEA, CA19.9, and DF3 and CA125 antigen detection assays.

3.2. Detection of Occult Carcinoma in Cytology Preparations

The correct diagnostic recognition of cancer cells in serous effusions (pleural, pericardial, or peritoneal) by cytopathologic methods may be difficult, particularly if the malignant cells are rare, single without clusters, or admixed with inflammatory cells including macrophages or reactive mesothelium. If neoplastic cells are recognized, the cellular classification or organ of tumor origin may be difficult to determine. In a study at Duke University Medical Center, 5888 consecutive pleural effusions obtained over a 14 year period were reviewed (23). Of these, 576 specimens (9.8%) contained malignant cells; adenocarcinoma was the most frequent cancer identified (48%), followed by large cell undifferentiated carcinoma (14%) and lymphoma/leukemia (15%). The most common carcinomas which metastasized to the pleural space were tumors from the lung (36%), breast (15%), and female genital tract (8%). Of particular importance are the 10% of patients with a malignant effusion in which a previous diagnosis of cancer had not been made. In these patients, the correct diagnosis of tumor type as well as a differential diagnosis regarding the organ of tumor origin were critical to the patient management. In addition, other cases were also identified which were "suspicious," although a definitive diagnosis or malignancy could not be made because a distinction between reactive mesothelium and malignant epithelial cells could not be made using standard cytologic criteria.

Several MAbs were initially evaluated for the detection of malignant cells in cytology preparations including DF3 (24-26), B72.3, and anti-carcinoembryonic antigen MAb B1.1. A preliminary study demonstrated that only B72.3 selectively stained tumor cells and failed to react with benign effusions or mesothelial cells (27). MAb B72.3 was then utilized on a wide variety of formalin-fixed, paraffin-embedded cell block preparations of malignant and benign serous effusions to determine its reactivity with each cell type (28). The reactive antigen TAG-72 detected by MAb B72.3 was found on carcinoma cells in nearly 100% of the specimens obtained from patients with metastatic adenocarcinoma identifiable by cytologic criteria (Table 2). Benign mesothelial and lymphoid cells in the same cell block preparation did not react with MAb B72.3. Benign effusions from patients without cancer (n=24), or with prior or extant cancer in other body sites (n=17) were also non-reactive (Table 2). Malignant hematopoietic cells (from specimens containing lymphoma/leukemia) also failed to demonstrate MAb B72.3 reactivity (Table 2).

TABLE 2

REACTIVITY OF MAB B72.3 WITH FORMALIN-FIXED, PARAFFIN-EMBEDDED CELL PREPARATIONS FROM SEROUS EFFUSIONS[a]

Type of Effusion	Malignant Cell Reactivity/ Number Tested	Mesothelial Reactivity/ Number Tested
Benign		
Patients without Cancer	0/24	0/24
Patients with Prior or Extent Cancer in Other Body Sites	0/17	0/17
Malignant		
Breast Carcinoma	22/23	0/23
Ovarian Adenocarcinoma	28/28	0/28
Lung Adenocarcinoma	19/19	0/19
Adenosquamous carcinoma	1/1	0/1
Squamous cell carcinoma	2/4	0/4
Small cell carcinoma	0/3	0/3

[a]For further detail, please refer to ref. 20 and 28.

MAb B72.3 and immunocytochemical techniques have also been applied to cytospin preparations by Martin et al. (29). Similar results were obtained (i.e., reactivity with adenocarcinomas and lack of reactivity with mesothelial and lymphoid elements as well as benign effusions) using methanol fixed cytospin preparations of serous effusions. Cell block preparations and cytospins from the same effusion sample have consistently demonstrated similar B72.3 immunoreactivity (Thor, et al. unpublished data). Each method may have distinct advantages for the cytologist. Cytospin preparations can be made quickly, and the entire immunoperoxidase assay can be completed within 3 hours. Cell block preparations, provide a permanent cell block from which multiple sections can be made, and allow better visualization of cellular detail. They do, however, require at least twenty four hours for fixation, embedding and processing in addition to several hours for the immunoperoxidase assay.

The diagnostic applications of MAb B72.3 with cytologic specimens are made possible by this MAb's selective recognition of adenocarcinoma cells compared to non-reactive methothelium and lymphoid elements. A prospective study of "suspicious" cytology specimens thought to contain occult adenocarcinoma cells is now underway. Preliminary data presented above suggest that MAb B72.3 may be useful in immunocytochemical assays, either by itself or in a panel with other MAbs, for the reliable detection and differentiation of adenocarcinoma from mesothelial and lymphoid elements in malignant effusions.

3.3. Fine Needle Aspiration Biopsy

Specimens obtained by fine needle aspiration biopsy (FNAB) are similar to those obtained by exfoliative cytology, although cellular relationships and architectural patterns may be somewhat better preserved. The diagnostic distinction between malignant and benign cell types is again the primary diagnostic dilemma. However, FNAB specimens often requires the differentiation of malignant and benign phenotypes of the same histologic cell type (for example, hyperplasia vs. carcinoma of the breast epithelium), rather than differentiation of epithelial cells from mesothelium or macrophages. As one might expect, this adds another requirement to MAb probes which might be useful, as a selective reactivity for the malignant versus benign phenotype is required.

The immunoreactivity of MAb B72.3 with cells obtained by FNAB has recently been evaluated, and compared to that of surgically resected tissues obtained from the same body site, in an attempt to define the following parameters: (a) the reactivity of malignant and benign cells with MAb B72.3 in each specimen, and (b) the correlation of TAG-72 antigen expression between the specimens obtained by these two methods (30). The results obtained were roughly similar to those previously noted for surgically resected tissues and cytology preparations. MAb B72.3 was strongly reactive with formalin-fixed, paraffin-embedded cell preparations of FNAB containing adenocarcinoma of the breast, lung and colon (Table 3). In contrast, small cell carcinomas of the lung, melanomas, lymphomas and sarcomas were non-reactive. Aspiration biopsies of benign lesions (n=21) from breast, lung, and pancreas showed no immunoreactivity with the exception of apocrine metaplasia in one breast specimen. In addition, in 94% of patients (n=66) the reactivity of cells obtained by FNAB was predictive of the reactivity in surgically resected tissue sections.

Further studies by Lundy et al. (31) and Nuti et al. (32) have evaluated a large number of benign and malignant breast lesions using MAb B72.3 and aspiration smears. Their data reconfirms that obtained by Johnston et al. in our preliminary study (30). Benign lesions were generally non-reactive with MAb B72.3 (fibrocystic disease, fibroadenomas, papillomas etc.) with the rare exception of apocrine metaplasia. Malignant epithelial cells, in contrast, were reactive in greater than 75% of the cases. Further evaluation of various breast lesions including hyperplasia and atypical hyperplasia of the duct and lobular epithelium using FNAB techniques are in progress. These studies suggest that MAb B72.3 may be a useful immuno-

TABLE 3

REACTIVITY OF MAB B72.3 WITH FINE NEEDLE ASPIRATION BIOPSY CELL PREPARATIONS

Tissue Type	Cytologic Diagnosis	Specimens Reactive/ Specimens Tested
Breast	Benign	1/10[a]
	Adenocarcinoma	17/21
Lung	Benign	0/10
	Adenocarcinoma	27/27
	Squamous carcinoma	25/31
	Large cell carcinoma	7/13
	Small cell carcinoma	0/6
	Carcinoid	0/1
Colon	Adenocarcinoma	6/6
Pancreas	Benign	0/1
	Adenocarcinoma	5/8
Skin and Soft tissue	Melanoma	0/13
Lymph node	Lymphoma	0/2
Soft tissue	Sarcoma	0/2

[a]Apocrine metaplasia only, for further details see ref. 30.

histochemical adjunct for fine needle aspiration biopsies, either by itself or with a panel of MAbs. Using these techniques MAb B72.3 may be used to phenotype carcinoma cells, and serve as an adjunctive tool for the diagnosis and differentiation of malignant from benign cells.

3.4. Malignant Mesothelioma versus Adenocarcinoma

In light of the above data, which demonstrates the selective reactivity of MAb B72.3 for adenocarcinoma over mesothelium, Szpak et al. (33) evaluated potential applications in the diagnosis of malignant mesotheliomas. Classically, the distinction between malignant mesothelioma and adenocarcinoma is complex, and often encompasses clinical, radiological, surgical and pathologic data (including light and electron microscopies). This diagnostic "dilemma" is critical because of therapeutic, prognostic, and litigious implications (34,35). Immunohistochemical probes to differentiate the two tumor types have previously been reported using various antisera to carcinoembryonic antigen, keratins, and epithelial markers such as EMA (36-39).

MAb B72.3 was incubated with 19 malignant mesotheliomas (diagnosed according to strict pathologic criteria) as well as 22 cases of adenocarcinoma of the lung using ABC immunohistochemical techiques and formalin-fixed, paraffin-embedded tissues (33). No expression of the TAG-72 antigen was detectable in 10 of 19 mesotheliomas while $\leq 1\%$ of tumor cells were focally immunoreactive in the remaining eight cases (membranous staining only). Conversely, 19 of 22 adenocarcinomas of the lung demonstrated at least 10% of the malignant cells reactive with

MAb B72.3 (predominantly cytoplasmic reactivity). Thus, the presence of TAG-72 was significant in distinguishing adenocarcinoma from malignant mesothelioma ($p<.0001$). Hence, MAb B72.3 may be of potential utility when faced with the differential diagnosis of mesothelioma versus adenocarcinoma (particularly if tissue or facilities do not permit electron microscopy and mucin stains are negative).

Recent studies have demonstrated that MAb B72.3 may also be very useful in poorly differentiated tumors to distinguish between small cell carcinoma (negative for MAb B72.3) and non-small cell carcinoma of the lung (Johnston, personal communication), as well as lymphoma versus carcinoma.

4. MABS AS PROBES TO STUDY CELLULAR BIOLOGY

4.1. Antigens With Defined Function

Immunologic probes reactive with specific epitopes of biologic interest can now be produced using hybridoma technology. These MAbs can then be utilized with normal, benign, and malignant tissues to define the epitope expressed in various disease states. As an example studies involving the laminin receptor will be discussed. Liotta et al. (40-43) have suggested that the process of carcinoma attachment, invasion, and metastasis are complex, involving a variety of cellular as well as extracellular factors. One necessary step in this process is the movement of tumor cells through the extracellular matrix (which is composed of basement membranes and interstitial stroma). It has been hypothesized that the laminin receptor (which interacts with laminin, a glycoprotein component of basement membrane) may play a role in the multistep phenomenon of tumor invasion and metastases (43,44). To further investigate this theory, we generated MAbs using purified human laminin receptor as immunogen (44,45). Initial characterization of these MAbs (n=14) demonstrated their reactivity to purified laminin receptor (44). Selected human mammary and colon carcinomas (approximately 30%) were shown to bind more anti-laminin receptor MAb than their respective normal or dysplastic tissue counterparts using immunohistochemical methods and surgically resected human tissues(45). In addition, this choice of methodologies facilitated a correlation between histologic and immunohistochemical data. A consistent difference in the distribution of immunoreactivity between the benign and malignant cells was noted. The benign cells appeared to express laminin receptor immunoreactivity at the basal location adjacent to the formed basement membrane. In contrast, the carcinoma cells exhibited staining over the entire surface of the cell, including more pronounced cytoplasmic reactivity compared to the benign cells. This observation suggested that the surface distribution, state of internalization, and/or processing of the receptor may be altered in the actively invading cells (45). Hence, in addition to diagnostic utility, MAb probes may be useful to the pathologist for the definition, phenotyping, or identification of various cell populations based on biologically relevant markers.

4.2. Proto-Oncogenes, Oncogenes and MAb Probes

Oncogenes and proto-oncogenes are usually defined by their ability to mediate transformation via (a) DNA transfection assays using the established murine fibroblast 3T3 cells, (b) chromosome translocation, (c) gene amplification, or (d) promotor activation, i.e., the oncogene or proto-oncogene is located near a promotor sequence which regulates its level of transcription. Oncogenes usually have homology to the genomes of known RNA tumor viruses of animals. Proto-oncogenes are defined as endogenous elements of cellular DNA of a given species. Lists of the approximately 30 oncogenes and their proposed mechanisms of action have been detailed in numerous reviews (46,47) and thus will not be addressed here.

Recent investigations have demonstrated the expression or amplification of oncogenes (or proto-oncogenes), particularly of the ras gene family in a variety of carcinomas. Although originally recognized as the transforming genes of two rat derived viruses, the Harvey and Kirsten strains of the murine sarcoma virus, molecular cloning studies have identified Ha-, Ki-, and N (Neuroblastoma) ras as members of a gene family present in a wide range of species including humans (46). At least two mechanisms exist by which ras activation can mediate transformation, (a) a point mutation resulting in an alteration of the 21,000 dalton protein product p21, or (b) increased expression of ras p21. Point mutated ras genes, however, have only been found in a small percentage of a given type of carcinoma, usually less than 10% (46,47). In light of the provocative findings which demonstrated ras gene activation in selected colon carcinoma cell lines (48), a breast carcinosarcoma cell line (49), and bladder carcinomas (50), we sought to further investigate the expression of ras p21 in human carcinomas. Utilizing the known DNA sequence of the Ha-ras gene, MAbs were made using a synthetic peptide reflecting amino acids 10-17 of the human T24 bladder cancer cell line (Hu-ras^{T24}). These murine MAbs have been shown to react with both the normal cellular Ha, Ki, and N-ras p21, as well as with p21 molecules with a substitution (point mutation) at position 12 (51,52). In addition, they preferentially react with denatured, fixed cell extracts known to contain high levels of ras p21 in comparison to non-fixed extracts (51,52). This is most likely because the determinants detected by the RAP (RA:ras, P:peptide) MAbs (positions 10-17) have been predicted to be internally located in the tertiary structure of the p21 molecule (53), hence not as available for MAb binding in the non-denatured form. These MAbs, however, were ideally suited for the evaluation of ras p21 expression in formalin-fixed, paraffin-embedded tissues using immunoperoxidase techniques.

Immunohistochemical analyses of individual cells within fixed tissue sections revealed an increase in ras p21 expression in $\geq$60% of breast, and nearly 50% of colon adenocarcinomas as compared to normal or benign tissues from the same body sites (Table 4). Subsequent studies of "premalignant" breast lesions have demonstrated that an incremental increase in ras p21 is generally observed as the severity of histologic abnormality increases, ie., non-atypical hyperplasia, atypical hyperplasia, carcinoma in situ, and carcinoma respectively (Ohuchi et al., submitted for publication).

Other studies by Viola et al. (54) have utilized the same MAb to evaluate ras p21 expression in bladder and prostate lesions. Some dysplastic and all high grade bladder carcinomas studied (n=11) demonstrated increased p21 as compared to normal bladder epithelium (54). These data contrast with previous studies (55,56) showing ras activation (mutation) in <10% of bladder carcinomas. These findings, however, are similar to those observed for colon and breast carcinomas, suggesting an increased production of cellular ras p21 rather than point mutations in the p21 molecule. In addition, ras expression in prostate carcinomas has also been evaluated (57). Briefly, increased ras p21 was found to correlate with nuclear dysplasia and be inversely related to glandular differentiation.

Hence, MAbs directed at a specific peptide sequence from the T24 bladder carcinoma cell line and histochemical methods have clearly defined ras p21 expression on a cellular level, and have demonstrated ras gene amplification in a significantly higher percent of these tumors than had been detected utilizing NIH 3T3 transfection assays. Enhanced ras p21 levels

TABLE 4

ANTI-ras p21 MAB RAP-5 REACTIVITY WITH BREAST AND COLON SPECIMENS

Tissue	Diagnosis	>20% Tumor Cells Reactive/ Number of Tumors Tested
Breast	Benign	2/21[a]
	Invasive Ductal Carcinomas	19/30 (63%)
Colon	Normal	0/18
	Benign	0/39
	Adenocarcinoma	22/47 (47%)

[a]From 2 patients with multiple fibroadenomas
For further detail please refer to references 51,52.

have also been reported in human breast and colon carcinomas using RNA spot hybridization (58,59) and Western blotting analysis (60,61). The data generated using these various methodologies, however, may be considered qualitative or, at best, semiquantitative. The immunohistochemical assays, however, allow a direct comparison between routine pathologic parameters and cellular expression of an oncogene or proto-oncogene product. The expression of these products may also be used to better phenotype tumor cell populations with regard to oncogene expression, which ultimately may or may not correlate with other biologic parameters including metastatic potential.

An alternative approach which yields information complementary to that obtained using immunohistochemical analyses is provided by the development of a liquid binding competition radioimmunoassays (RIAs) for the p21 ras oncogene and proto-oncogene products (62). Using purified recombinant ras p21 from Escherichia coli expressing the full length T24 mutant human Ha-ras gene protein product as a standard, we have used these RIAs to define the absolute amounts of ras p21 in Escherichia coli expressing the point mutated or proto-ras p21 and mammalian cell lines of human and murine origin (62). The adaptability of these RIAs to various assay conditions and their ease of methodology facilitate their use for the study of several parameters associated with ras p21 expression. These RIAs when used in conjunction with (a) immunohistochemical analyses to define ras p21 expression at the single-cell level, and (b) specific c-DNA probes to define the specific ras oncogene or proto-oncogene being expressed now provide the means for further delineation of the association between ras p21 expression and cellular transformation.

5. CONCLUSIONS

The MAbs developed thus far against human carcinomas have led to a more systematic study of specific human carcinomas. For the first time, one now has tools other than morphology or the presence of hormone receptors to characterize different tumors, or distinquish between cell populations within a given tumor mass. The number of these tumor "fingerprints" is now in the process of being expanded. MAbs are now available which recognize a wide variety of epitopes including tumor associated antigens, oncofetal antigens, hormones, metabolic products, glycoproteins, glycolipids, receptors, growth factors, and oncogene products. While some of these antigens may be selective for tumors or specific cell types, others are widely reactive but can be used to investigate specific facets of cellular biology. Advances in many areas of basic science including immunology, molecular biology, genetic engineering, and others are rapidly changing the understanding and practice of human pathology. Hybridoma/monoclonal antibody technology and gene cloning techniques, in particular, are finding new uses in applied as well as basic pathology. MAb research involving human disease is proceeding in two directions simultaneously -- one toward the mechanisms of oncogenesis and basic cellular biology, and the other toward more immediate clinical applications.

REFERENCES

1. Kohler M, Milstein C: Continuous cultures of fused cells secreting antibody of predefined specificity. Nature 256: 495, 1975.
2. Sell S: Cancer Markers, Diagnostic and Developmental Significance. Clifton, NJ, Human Press, 1980.
3. Stefarti M: Enzymes, isoenzymes, and enzyme variants in the diagnosis of cancer. Cancer 55: 1391, 1985.
4. Van Lente F, Shamberger RJ: Defining a role for enzymes in cancer diagnosis. Diag Med 47, June 1983.
5. Wu JT: Applications of enzymes: tumor markers, new enzymes, and atypical isoenzymes. J Med Technol 7: 438, 1985.
6. Mirecki DM, Jordan VC: Steroid hormone receptors and breast cancer. Lab Med 16: 287, 1985.
7. Hakomori S: Tumor-associated carbohydrate antigens. Ann Rev Immunol 2: 103, 1984.
8. Ohosh BC (ed): Tumor Associated and Other Related Markers: McGraw Hill Publishers (in press).
9. Colcher D, Horan Hand P, Nuti M et al.: A spectrum of monoclonal antibodies reactive with mammary tumor cells. Proc Natl Acad Sci USA 78: 3199, 1981.
10. Nuti M, Teramoto YA, Mariani-Costantini R et al.: A monoclonal antibody (B72.3) defines patterns of distribution of a novel tumor-associated antigen in human mammary carcinoma cell populations. Int J Cancer 29: 539, 1982.
11. Stragmignoni D, Bowen R, Atkinson B et al.: Differential reactivity of monoclonal antibodies with human colon adenocarcinomas and adenomas. Int J Cancer 31: 543, 1983.
12. Horan Hand P, Colcher D, Salomon D, Ridge J, Noguchi P, Schlom J: Influence of spatial configuration of carcinoma cell populations on the expression of fa tumor-associated glycoprotein. Cancer Res, 45: 833-840, 1985.
13. Johnson VG, Schlom J, Paterson AJ et al.: Analysis of a human tumor-associated glycoprotein (TAG-72) identified by monoclonal antibody B72.3. Cancer Res, 46: 850, 1986.
14. Friedman E, Thor A, Horan Hand P, Schlom J: Surface expression of tumor-associated antigens in primary cultured human colonic epithelial cells from carcinomas, benign tumors and normal tissues. Cancer Res, 45: 5648, 1985.
15. Greiner J, Horan Hand P, Pestka S, Noguchi P, Fisher P, Colcher D, Schlom J: Selection and enhancement (by recombinant interferon) of carcinoma cell surface antigens using monoclonal antibodies. In: Cancer Cells 1: The Transformed Phenotype, pp. 285-292, Cold Spring Harbor

Lab., 1984.
16. Colcher D, Zalutsky M, Kaplan W et al.: Radiolocalization of human mammary tumors in athymic mice by a monoclonal antibody. Cancer Res, 43: 736-742, 1983.
17. Schlom J, Greiner J, Horan Hand P, Colcher D, Inghirami G, Weeks M, Pestka S, Fisher PB, Noguchi P, Kufe D: Monoclonal antibodies to breast cancer-associated antigens as potential reagents in the management of breast cancer. Cancer 54: 2777-2794, 1984.
18. Keenan AM, Colcher D, Larson SM, Schlom J: Radioimmunoscintigraphy of human colon cancer xenografts in mice with radioiodinated monoclonal antibody B72.3. J Nucl Med 25: 1197-1203.
19. Thor A, Ohuchi N, Szpak CA, Johnston WW, Schlom J: The distribution of oncofetal antigen TAG-72 defined by monoclonal antibody B72.3. Cancer Res (in press).
20. Thor A, Gorstein F, Ohuchi N, Szpak CA, Johnston WW, Schlom J: Monoclonal antibody B72.3 defines tumor associated antigen (TAG-72) in ovarian carcinoma. JNCI (in press).
21. Colcher D, Carrasquillo JA, Sugarbaker P, Bryant G, Esteban J, Simpson D, Thor A, Reynolds JR, Horowitz M, Larson SM, Schlom J: Biodistribution of monoclonal antibody B72.3 (I-131) in colon cancer patients. Proc of Society of Nuclear Medicine. P15, 1985.
22. Paterson AJ, Schlom J, Sears NF, Bennett J, Colcher D: A radioimmunoassay for the detection of a human tumor-associated glycoprotein (TAG-72) using monoclonal antibody B72.3 Cancer Res (in press).
23. Johnston WW: The malignant pleural effusion: a review of cytopathological diagnoses on 584 specimens from 472 consecutive patients. Cancer 56: 905, 1984.
24. Kufe D, Inghirami G, Abe M et al.: Differential reactivity of a novel monoclonal antibody (DF3) with human malignant versus benign breast tumors. Hybridoma, 3: 223, 1984.
25. Sekine H, Ohno T, Kufe DW: Purification and characterization of high molecular weight glycoprotein detectable in human milk and breast carcinoma. J Immunol, 135, 1985.
26. Lundy J, Thor A, Maenza R et al.: Monoclonal antibody DF3 correlates with tumor differentiation and hormone receptor status in breast cancer patients. Br Cancer Res and Treat, 5: 269, 1985.
27. Szpak CA, Johnston WW, Lottich SC, Kufe D, Thor A, Schlom J: Patterns of reactivity of four novel monoclonal antibodies (B72.3, DF3, B1.1 and B6.2) with cells in human malignant and benign effusions. Acta Cytol, 28: 356, 1984.
28. Johnston WW, Szpak CA, Lottich SC, Thor A, Schlom J: Use of a monoclonal antibody (B72.3) as an immunocytochemical adjunct to diagnosis of adenocarcinoma in human effusions. Cancer Res, 45: 1894-1900, 1985.
29. Martin SE, Moshiri S, Thor A, Vilasi V, Chu EW, Schlom J: Identification of adenocarcinoma in cytospin preparations of effusions using monoclonal antibody B72.3. Am J Clin Path (in press).
30. Johnston WW, Szpak CA, Thor A, Schlom J: The use of monoclonal antibody (B72.3) as a novel immunocytochemical adjunct for the diagnosis of carcinomas in fine needle aspiration biopsies. Human Path (in press).
31. Lundy J, Lozowski M, Mishriki Y: Monoclonal antibody B72.3 as a diagnostic adjunct in fine needle aspirates of breast masses. Ann Surg (in press).
32. Nuti M, Mottolese M, Viora M, Donnorso RP, Schlom J, Natali PG: Use of monoclonal antibodies to human breast tumor associated antigens in fine needle aspirate cytology. Int J Cancer (in press).

33. Szpak CA, Johnston WW, Roggli V et al.: The diagnostic distinction between malignant mesothelioma of the pleura and adenocarcinoma of the lung defined by a monoclonal antibody (B72.3). Am J Path (in press).
34. Antman KH, Blum RH, Greenberger JS et al.: Multimodality therapy for malignant mesothelioma based on a study of natural history. Am J Med, 68: 356, 1980.
35. Legha SS, Muggia, FM: Pleural mesothelioma: clinical features and therapeutic implications. Ann Intern Med, 87: 613, 1977.
36. Wang N, Huang SN, Gold P: Absence of carinoembryonic antigen-like material in mesothelioma. An immunohistochemical differentiation from other lung cancer. Cancer, 44: 937, 1979.
37. Corson JM, Pinkus GS: Mesothelioma: Profile of keratin proteins and carcinoembryonic antigen. An immunoperoxidase study of 20 cases and comparison with pulmonary adenocarcinomas. Am J Pathol, 108: 80, 1982.
38. Said JW, Nash G, Tepper G et al.: Keratin proteins and carcinoembryonic antigen in lung carcinoma: An immunoperoxidase study of 54 cases, with ultrastructural correlations. Hum Pathol, 14: 70-76, 1983.
39. Holden J, Churg A: Immunohistochemical staining for keratin and carcinoembryonic antigen in the diagnosis of malignant mesothelioma. Am J Surg Pathol, 8: 277, 1984.
40. Liotta LA: Tumor invasion and metastases: role of the basement membrane. Am J Path, 117: 340, 1984.
41. Liotta LA, Rao CN, Barsky SH: Tumor invasion and the extracellular matrix. Lab Invest, 49: 636, 1983.
42. Barsky SH, Rao CN, Hyams D, Liotta LA: Characterization of a laminin receptor from human breast carcinoma tissue. Breast Cancer Res Treat, 4: 181, 1984.
43. Barsky SH, Rao CN, Williams JE, Liotta LA: Laminin molecular domains which alter metastasis in a murine mode. J Clin Invest, 74: 0001, 1984.
44. Liotta LA, Horan Hand P, Rao CN, Bryant G, Barsky SH, Schlom J: Monoclonal antibodies to the human laminin receptor recognize structurally distinct sites. Expt Cell Res, 156: 117, 1985.
45. Horan Hand P, Thor A, Schlom J, Rao CN, Liotta LA: Expression of laminin receptor in normal and carcinomatous human tissues as defined by a monoclonal antibody. Cancer Res, 45: 2713, 1985.
46. Land H, Parada L, Weinberg RA: Cellular oncogenes and multistep carcinogenesis. Science, 222: 771, 1983.
47. Shih TY, Weeks MO: Oncogenes and cancer: the p21 ras genes. Cancer Invest, 2: 109, 1984.
48. Pulciani S, Santos E, Lauver AV, Long LK, Aaronson SA, Barbacid M: Oncogenes in solid human tumours. Nature (London), 300:, 539-542, 1982.
49. Kraus MH, Yuasa Y, Aaronson SA: A position 12-activated H-ras oncogene in all HS578T mammary carcinoma cells but not normal mammary cells of the same patient. Proc Natl Acad Sci USA, 81: 5384, 1984.
50. Fujita J, Srivastava SK, Kraus MH, Rhim JS, Tronick SR, Aaronson SA: Frequency of molecular alterations affecting ras protooncogenes in human urinary tract tumors. Proc Natl Acad Sci USA, 82: 3849, 1985.
51. Horan Hand P, Thor A, Wunderlich D et al.: Monoclonal antibodies of predefined specificity detect activated ras gene expression in human mammary and colon carcinomas. Proc Natl Acad Sci, 81: 5227, 1984.
52. Thor A, Horan Hand P, Wunderlich D et al.: Monoclonal antibodies define differential ras gene expression in malignant and benign colonic disease states. Nature, 311: 562, 1984.
53. McCormick F, Clark BFC, La Cour TF, Kjeldgaard M, Norskov-Lauritsen L, Nyborg J: A model for ther tertiary structure of p21, the product of

the ras oncogene. Science, 230: 78, 1985.
54. Viola MV, Tromowitz F, Oravez S, Deb S, Schlom J: ras oncogene p21 expression is increased in premalignant lesions and high grade bladder carcinoma. J Expt Med, 161: 1213, 1985.
55. Feinberg A, Vogelstein B, Droller M, Baylin S, Nelkin, B: Mutations affecting the 12th amino acid of c-Ha-ras oncogene product occur infrequently in bladder cancer. Science, 220: 1175.
56. Fujita J, Yoshida O, Yuasa Y, Rhim J, Hatanaka M, Aaronson S: Ha-ras oncogenes are activated by somatic alterations in human urinary tract tumours. Nature, 309: 464, 1984.
57. Viola MJ, Tromowitz F, Oravez S, Deb S, Sinkel G, Lundy J, Horan Hand P, Thor A, Schlom J: Expression of ras oncogene p21 in prostate cancer. NEJM 314: 133, 1986.
58. Spandidos DA, Kerr IB: Elevated expression of the human ras oncogene family in premalignant and malignant tumours of the colorectum. Br J Cancer 49: 681, 1984.
59. Spandidos DA, Agnantis NJ: Human malignant tumors of the breast, as compared to their respective normal tissue have elevated expression of the Harvey ras oncogene. Anticancer Res, 4: 269, 1984.
60. DeBortoli ME, Abou-Issa H, Haley BE, Cho-Chung YS: Amplified expression of p21 ras protein in hormone-dependent mammary carcinoma of humans and rodents. Biophys Res Commun, 127: 699, 1985.
61. Gallick GE, Kurzrock R, Kloetzer WS, Arlinghaus RB, Gutterman JU: Expression of p21 ^{ras} in fresh primary and metastatic human colorectal tumors. Proc Natl Acad Sci USA, 82: 1795, 1985.
62. Horan Hand P, Thor A, Caruso A, Wunderlich D, Muraro R, Weeks MO, Vilasi V, Schlom J: Comparisons of qualitative and quantitative immunoassays for ras p21. In: Monoclonal Antibodies and Cancer Therapy, p 23-36, Alan R. Liss, Inc., 1985.

III. *PRACTICAL APPLICATION AND CASE PRESENTATIONS*

17. PRACTICAL APPLICATION OF MONOCLONAL ANTIBODIES TO DIAGNOSTIC TUMORPATHOLOGY AND SOME FUTURE PERSPECTIVES.

C.J.L.M. MEIJER, H. MULLINK, S.C. HENZEN-LOGMANS

1. Introduction

Accurate classification of malignant tumors is important in predicting the clinical course and in selecting therapeutic strategies. Although conventional light-microscopic examination of representative tumor tissue specimens often results in a definite diagnosis, in quite a number of cases only a differential diagnosis can be made. Then "special" techniques such as plastic embedding, electronmicroscopy, and immunocyto/histochemistry can be helpful.

The wide availability of monoclonal antibodies against the intermediate sized filament proteins of the cytoskeleton, oncofetal antigens, mucins, cell surface antigens and other differentiation antigens has largely extended the use of immunohistochemistry in diagnostic tumor pathology.

The use of 'special' techniques in surgical pathology laboratories requires special handling of the tumor tissue. Ideally, fresh specimens of tumor tissue should be processed as depicted in table 1.

If small tissue specimens are received, or if specimens have to be collected from other hospitals, the minimal number of different treatments are formalin fixation and deep-freezing of unfixed tissue. In addition, imprint preparations should be made.

The main problem in the use of monoclonal antibodies in surgical tumor pathology is that their specificity is often incompletely defined because tissue distribution studies were not exhaustive. For instance, BA2, a monoclonal antibody directed against an antigen (p24) present on certain B cells and lympho-haemopoietic progenitor cells in bone marrow (1), also stains neuroblastoma cells. Another example is Leu3a, a monoclonal antibody originally described as being specific for T-helper/inducer lymphocytes, also reacts with the cytoplasm of Langerhans cells (2)

In addition, it is our experience that monoclonal antibodies specific for one tumor type do not exist or are very rare. Perhaps such monoclonal antibodies are those against prostate specific antigen. Therefore, before monoclonal antibodies can be used as an aid in surgical pathology the specificity of each monoclonal antibody has to be determined by immunohistochemistry on a broad range of normal tissues and different lesions. Moreover it is preferable as the antigen, defined by the antibody is also characterized biochemically. In practice too many monoclonal antibodies are used with specificities only determined on tissue sections of a few organs by immunohistochemistry.

1.2. Tissue prerequisites

The demonstration of antigens in cells of smears, imprints or tissue sections by immunohistochemistry needs proper treatment of the tissues and cell preparations. For detailed information one is referred to the review article of Brandtzaeg (3) and the

TABLE 1. SCHEME OF TISSUE PROCESSING FOR TUMOR SPECIMENS

tumor specimen

fixation:	buffered formalin	sublimate formol/B5	Burkhardt's and others	freezing	buffered glutar aldehyde	paraform-aldehyde	cell suspensions/ imprint preparations
embedding medium:	paraplast	paraplast	methacrylate (glycol,methyl)	cryo-preservative	Epon	Lowicryl	-
morphology:	'normal' histology	normal histology excellent nuclear detail	optimal histological and cytological details	poor	optimal ultra-structure	normal ultra-structure	good cellular detail
immunohisto/ cytochemistry:	hormones some cytoplasmic antigens, some mucins. In general: no membrane ag, poor intracyto-plasmic IgG	hormones intracellular antigens, mucins intracytoplas-mic immuno-globulins etc In general: no membrane Ig	some intra-cellular antigens have been reported Reproducibility: in general poor	nearly all membrane and intracytoplas-mic antigens	some intracellular antigens	most membrane and intracellular antigens	cytoplasmic and nuclear antigens, some membrane antigens

volume of Polak and Van Noorden (4). Some general remarks will be made here. In order to demonstrate cytoplasmic immunoglobulins, mucins and oncofetal antigens, a sublimate-formol mixture as fixative gives better results than buffered (pH 6.8-7.2) formalin. Surface membrane antigens, such as lymphocyte differentiation markers, can best be demonstrated in frozen sections which are air-dried and fixed in acetone.

When the tissue is embedded in paraffin one has to be sure that the temperature will not exceed 60C since this will destroy most immunoreactivity. This means that in paraffin embedded tissues only positive results are relevant and absence of reactivity can only be interpreted as negative when fixation and embedding procedures in that particular laboratory are well known. This is especially important for reference laboratories in interpreting immunohistochemical results obtained from tissue blocks or unstained sections, sent in from elsewhere.

1.3. Applications of monoclonal antibodies

In this review we will discuss the following topics concerning the use of monoclonal antibodies in diagnostic tumor pathology: 1) the role of monoclonal antibodies in the classification of neoplasms, 2) the use of monoclonal antibodies in the detection of low numbers of tumor cells, 3) prediction of the site of primary tumor by immunohistochemical investigation of the metastatic tumor tissue, 4) some future perspectives for the application of monoclonal antibodies in diagnostic tumor pathology.

2.1. Classification of neoplasms by monoclonal antibodies

When neoplasms are difficult to classify we always make a differential diagnosis by light microscopic investigation of routinely stained representative sections of tumor tissue. In order to obtain a more exact classification in a given situation, if possible we use small panels of monoclonal antibodies. These panels are composed in such a way that the positive and negative staining results reinforce each other to achieve a more definite diagnosis. The antibodies selected for these panels have all been extensively tested immunohistochemically on a broad range of normal and tumor tissues. In the following we will discuss the fields in which these panels can be helpful.

2.1.1. Analysis of large cell tumors

Anaplastic carcinoma, large cell lymphoma, amelanotic melanoma and undifferentiated sarcoma belong to this group of tumors. Differentiation of these tumors is important because it is clinically relevant (5, 6). For the differentiation of these tumors we use a panel of 5 antibodies (table 2). All of these antibodies react with paraplast embedded tissue routinely fixed in buffered formalin, B5 or a sublimate-formol mixture. However, for the demonstration of vimentin in paraplast-embedded formalin-fixed tissue pretreatment with pronase is necessary. The monoclonal anti MAM-6 antibody 115D8 is also included in this panel. The specificity for epithelium is somewhat higher if compared to cytokeratins, because certain sarcomas that react with anti-cytokeratin do not react with monoclonal antibody 115D8. Moreover the MAM-6 antigen is more resistent to improper fixation. However, its sensitivity is less than that of anti-cytokeratins. The polyclonal antibody against vimentin, mentioned here, also reacts with lymphoid cells in contrast to the monoclonal antibody 43ßE8 against vimentin described by Gown and Vogel (7).

The least specific antibody used here is NKI/C3 directed against a melanoma associated antigen (8, 9). We found this antigen also to be present in some mononuclear phagocytes, mesothelial cells and some normal and neoplastic epithelial cells, especially those with a secretory function, as can be seen amongst others in breast carcinomas, thyroid carcinomas and apudomas. However, when used in our panel it gives valuable information.

In this context it is important to know that in our hands the monoclonal antibodies against common leucocyte antigen are not reactive with all lymphoid cells. Some centroblastic and lymphoblastic lymphomas do not stain with these antibodies, even when amplifying staining procedures are used. Results obtained with this panel are described in table 3. When the neoplastic cells show a staining pattern suggestive of melanoma (vimentin +, NKI/C3 +, cytokeratin -, common leucocyte antigen - and 115D8 -) additional immunohistochemistry is necessary. A diagnosis of melanoma is further supported by the presence of S100 protein on paraffin embedded tissue and 653.40S (10) and M-2-2-4 (11) and NKI/BV (12) on frozen sections. See also Ruiter et al (13) (Chapter 8, this volume).

Table 2. Panel of antibodies used to differentiate large cell tumors*

Antibody	Determinant	Main cell specificity
anti-cytokeratin	cytokeratins (broad spectred) MW 45-68 KD	epithelial cells
anti-vimentin	vimentin MW 57 KD	mesenchymal cells
115D8	MAM-6 antigen MW 400 KD	epithelial cells
NKI/C-3	melanoma associated antigen MW 25-110 KD	melanocytic cells
anti-common leucocyte antigen (2B11, PD7/26)	common leucocyte antigen MW 200 KD	leucocytes

* The panel can be used on formalin fixed paraffin embedded tissue sections. For vimentin staining pretreatment with pronase is necessary.
MW = molecular weight, KD = kilo Dalton
See for source of the antibodies the appendix.

Table 3: SCHEME FOR DIFFERENTIATION OF ANAPLASTIC LARGE CELL TUMORS

LIGHT MICROSCOPY:
anaplastic large cell tumor:
DD lymphoma, carcinoma, sarcoma, melanoma

use panel

Anti-cytokeratins	+	+	-	-	-
Anti-vimentin	-	+	+	+	+
115D8	+/-	+/-	-	-	-
NKI/C-3	+/-	+/-	+	-	-
Anti-common-leukocyte antigen	-	-	-	+	-
	definitely carcinoma	probably carcinoma; exclude (histologically and clinically): .epithelioid sarcoma .synovial sarcoma .mesothelioma	probably melanoma; exclude histologically (most cases) or immunohistochemically (some cases) or ultrastructurally (some cases): .chemodectoma .clear cell sarcoma .neuroblastoma	definitely lymphoma	sarcoma or lymphoma (lymphoblastic, centroblastic) and a single melanoma additional immunohisto-chemistry and electronmicroscopy required for classification

2.1.2. Analysis of round cell tumors

Ewing sarcoma, neuroblastoma, lymphoblastic lymphoma, and embryonic rhabdomyosarcoma are the round cell tumors of childhood which can pose problems for the diagnostic pathologist. In addition, small-cell carcinoma may be included in this group of tumors, although it is rare in childhood. In table 4 a panel is given from which the antibodies against cytokeratins, vimentin and leucocyte common antigen can be used on paraffin embedded tissue. Remarkable in this context is the staining of neuroblastoma cells with BA2 and the presence of neurofilament in a few small cell carcinomas (7, 8).

Although with this panel the presence of desmin and vimentin in a round cell tumor is very suggestive for embryonic rhabdomyosarcoma, the demonstration of skeletal muscle myosin yields definite proof (19). However, since this type of myosin is not always present in the poorly differentiated cells of myogenic origin, the staining for desmin is more sensitive than for skeletal muscle myosin. Myoglobin is less suitable in these cases because it is present in more differentiated cells.

Table 4: Small round cell tumors

	cyto-keratin	vimentin	NF	desmin*	CLA	BA2
Ewing sarcoma	-	+	-	-	-	-
Neuroblastoma	-	-	+**	-	-	+
Lymphoma	-	+	-	-	+(-)	+/-
Small-cell carcinoma	+	-	(+)/-	-	-	-
Embryonic rhabdo-myosarcoma	-	+	-	+	-	-

NF = neurofilament
CLA = common leucocyte antigen
*Instead of anti-desmin anti-skeletal muscle myosin can be used (14).
(+)/- negative, sometimes +
+/(-) positive, sometimes -
**On frozen sections always +, on paraplast embedded tissue immunoreactivity is partly lost resulting in false negative staining (15, 16, 17).

2.1.3. Discrimination between adeno- or squamous cell carcinoma by different types of cytokeratins.

The presence of cytokeratins has become a decisive criterion for the characterization of epithelial cells. In most instances demonstration of cytokeratin in a tumor can be taken as proof for its epithelial nature.

The cytokeratins are a multigene family of distinct polypeptides. In human tissue they can be divided into two subgroups, the acidic and small (type I) cytokeratins and the basic and large (type II) cytokeratins. Eight type II cytokeratins (CK 1-8) and eleven type I cytokeratins (CK 9-19) have been identified (20, 21).

The electroforetic analysis of normal epithelia has revealed characteristic cytokeratin combinations specific for the type of differentiation of epithelial cells such as squamous or glandular differentiation. Thus most adenocarcinomas (gallbladder, stomach, cervix, ovary, breast and lung) express cytokeratin type 7, 8, 18, 19 and sometimes type 17. Exceptions are hepatocellular carcinoma which shows cytokeratin type 8 and 18 and colon carcinoma, which shows type 8, 18 and 19. Keratinizing squamous cell carcinomas show cytokeratin type 10.

The development of monoclonal antibodies against one type of cytokeratin makes it possible to subtype carcinomas on account of their original cytokeratin pattern. So far only few monoclonal antibodies specific for one type of cytokeratin are commercially available (Eurodiagnostics, Apeldoorn, The Netherlands), among them are RGE 53 (cytokeratin 18) and RKSE 60 (cytokeratin 10). These two monoclonal antibodies allow the distinction between keratinizing and glandular epithelia (table 5).

Table 5. Subdivision of epithelial cells by the presence or absence of cytokeratin 10 and 18 as detected by RKSE 60 and RGE 53, respectively

CK18	CK10	
-	+	squamous cell carcinomas of skin, tongue, oesophagus, cervix and lung (not all cases)
+	-	adenocarcinomas of breast, lung, colon, cervix, ovary, stomach

In the future, the development of monoclonal antibodies against other monotypes of cytokeratins, especially type 5 and 13 will probably allow a subdivision.

Although the above mentioned monoclonal antibodies against cytokeratin components are helpful in the diagnosis of anaplastic carcinomas, the information obtained by analysis of cytokeratin profiles of metastatic carcinomas cannot be used for the prediction of the site of the primary tumor (22).

2.1.4. Differential diagnosis of mesothelioma and adenocarcinoma of the lung

Differentiation of mesothelioma and adenocarcinoma of the lung poses problems for the surgical pathologist because of the limited size of the biopsy specimens available, the variability of histologic patterns within any given area of the tumor and the controversy with regard to the reliability of interpretation of immunohistochemical stainings with heterologous antibodies. More than 50% of the epithelioid and the fibroblastic cells of mesotheliomas express cytokeratins as well as vimentin as detected with the monoclonal antibodies K2080 (broad spectred anti-keratin) and Vim-9 (anti-vimentin). Although coexpression of cytokeratins and vimentin has been described in adenocarcinoma (23, 24) of the lung, it is supposed to be a rare phenomenon. Moreover, the coexpression of vimentin in mesotheliomas is stronger and the orientation is different: in mesotheliomas vimentin is localized in a perinuclear pattern whereas its occasional presence in adenocarcinomas is predominantly near the cell base (24). The proportion of cells with coexpression is also different: when present in adenocarcinomas less than 20% of the cells stain for vimentin.

In addition to the presence of cytokeratins 7, 8, 18 and 19 in adenocarcinoma and mesothelioma, the presence of cytokeratins 5 and 14 has been described in mesotheliomas (22). Especially the presence of cytokeratin 5 in mesotheliomas seems helpful, since it has not been detected yet in adenocarcinomas of the lung.

Most authors (25, 26, 27) agree that the large majority of mesotheliomas do not stain for CEA in contrast to adenocarcinomas of the lung. When mesotheliomas stain for CEA it is weakly and often focally.

Very recently a monoclonal antibody B72.3 has been described that stains at least 10% of the tumor cells in 19 of the 22 adenocarcinomas of the lung tested. None of the 20 mesotheliomas, examined showed this immunoreactivity. This antibody, generated against a membrane-rich fraction of human metastatic breast carcinoma might be a helpful adjunct in this difficult area (28).

Taken together the co-expression of keratin and vimentin, as demonstrated by a double staining technique, the presence of cytokeratin 5, and the absence of CEA and B72.3 in most cases of mesotheliomas are valuable criteria to distinguish mesothelioma from adenocarcinoma of the lung.

2.1.5. Characterization of sarcoma

In general the impact of soft tissue markers in the subclassification of sarcomas is limited. For a review on this subject one is referred to the paper of Roholl et al (14). Some markers however, are worthwile to mention here. Nearly all sarcomas show immunoreactivity for vimentin.

Desmin is a useful marker for tumors with a myogenic differentiation i.e. rhabdomyosarcoma and leiomyosarcoma. Further subtyping of these tumors is possible with skeletal muscle actin, skeletal muscle myosin and myoglobin, all present in rhabdomyosarcomas, and smooth muscle myosin present in leiomyosarcomas. Demonstration of desmin can also easily be performed on cytological preparations.

The endothelial markers factor VIII related antigen and especially Ulex Europaeus agglutinin I are useful in the recognition of angiomatous (vascular) tumors; however, factor VIII related antigen is often not demonstrable in immature endothelial cells. Monoclonal antibodies specific for blood vessel endothelium, but not for lymph vessel endothelium have been described (29). Immunohistochemical studies with these antibodies on a large series of vascular tumors have not yet been published.

The neoplastic cells of haemangiopericytomas do not stain for endothelial markers but stain for smooth muscle myosin (30). So monoclonal antibodies for endothelium and smooth muscle myosin are very useful in distinguishing poorly differentiated forms of haemangiopericytomas and angiosarcomas.

In brain tumors glial fibrillary acidic protein (GFAP) is present in gliomas. For the different degrees of expression of GFAP in gliomas one is referred to the work of Herpers (31). Myelin basic protein (MBP) is a major protein of the myelin sheath in the central and peripheral nervous system (32). It has been demonstrated in malignant schwannoma and in granular cell tumors, but not in other sarcomas.

The usefulness of antibodies directed against S100 proteins is limited. Most heterologous antibodies do not differentiate between the α and ß subunits of the S100 protein. The α and ß subunit of the S100 protein are found in melanomas and chrondrosarcomas, whereas only the ß subunit · is present in malignant schwannomas (33, 34).

2.1.6 Immunotyping of malignant lymphomas

The first step in the classification of lymphomas is the demonstration of Reed-Sternberg cells (RS cells). Such a RS cell in a appropriate environment is indicative for the diagnosis of morbus Hodgkin. Although several monoclonal antibodies reactive with Reed-Sternberg cells have been described, none of them is 100% specific. Thus Ki-I (35) and SR-I (36) are reactive with Sternberg Reed cells and variants, and with some large cell lymphomas and EBV transformed cell lines (Ki-I only). Leu M-1, a granulocyte- specific antibody, which detects the carbohydrate lacto-N-fucopentose III in paraffin and frozen sections, is also clearly reactive with RS cells (37) but also with several epithelial cells. Not all RS cells however are reactive with Leu M-1. Therefore although these antibodies are helpful in detecting RS cells, the contribution of immunohistochemistry to the diagnosis of morbus Hodgkin is limited.

All the lymphomas lacking RS cells are called non Hodgkin's lymphomas. They may be of T cell, B cell or monocyte/macrophage nature. For the surgical pathologist immunophenotyping of lymphomas is useful and sometimes mandatory: 1) to differentiate reactive hyperplasias from malignant lymphomas by demonstrating monoclonality, 2) to differentiate certain types of morbus Hodgkin, especially the lymphocytic predominant type, from small cell lymphomas of B cell type, 3) to recognize the nature of the neoplastic cell-line with respect to prognosis and treatment, 4) to classify reliably and reproducibly NHL, especially diffuse NHL and large cell lymphomas (38, 39). In this respect it has been shown that the reproducibility of classification of NHL increases significantly from 60-70% to nearly 100% when immunophenotyping is used. For more detailed information one is referred to the reviews of Stein et al (40) and Meijer et al (41).

Moreover, recognition of these subtypes of non Hodgkin's lymphoma is important because of the different clinical behaviour. Table 6 shows the markers which we currently use on frozen sections to subtype these lymphomas. We use more than one marker to detect the cell lineage to which the lymphoma cells belong, because some of these markers are not always expressed on lymphoma cells. When only paraplast embedded material is available the monoclonal antibodies LN1, LN2 and LN3 (Clonab laboratories) and MT1, MB1, and MB1 as described by Poppema et al (Chapter.. in this book) are useful, but they do not reach the more accurate results on frozen sections.

Table 6. IMMUNOPHENOTYPING OF MALIGNANT LYMPHOMAS.

1. Reed Sternberg cells present --> M. Hodgkin (if RS cells in appropriate environment)

2. Reed-Sternberg cells not present --> non Hodgkin lymphoma

immunophenotyping				
first level	B cell markers	T cell markers	monocyte/macrophage markers	
	B1 Leu14 surface/cyto-plasmic Ig (κ, λ)	3A1 Leu4 Leu5	OKM1 My7	
second level (subtyping)	B cell lymphoma	T cell lymphoma	true histiocytic lymphoma	no markers of first level present
	cIg,sIg (heavy chains) HLA-DR BA2 CR1 CR2	Leu1 Leu2 Leu3 Leu6 TdT	lysozyme AAT ACT ac ph αNAE	Leu6, Leu3, CRI, CALL, TdT, CR2 lysozyme, AAT, ACT, ac ph, αNAE
				a single lymphoblastic or true histiocytic lymphoma

When in a lymphoma no R-S cells in appropriate environment are present, a non Hodgkin lymphoma is diagnosed. For determination of the nature of the neoplastic cells two levels of immunophenotyping are recognized. In the first level the nature of the neoplastic cell lineage is determined. We find these markers obligatory for the surgical pathologist. In the second level subtyping is performed to classify reproducibly and accurately certain subtypes of lymphomas (for instance centroblastic versus immunoblastic). When in the reticulin stainings the follicular growth pattern is questioned staining for complement receptors (CR1, CR2) or dendritic reticulum cells is very helpful.

Further subtyping of T cell NHL is at the moment of limited value because all patients with T cell NHL that remain after exclusion of mycosis fungoides, Sézary's syndrome and the T cell lymphoma, lymphocytic type, have a poor prognosis (42, 43, 44, 45). However, the introduction of therapy with drugs like α-interferon etc. may require further subtyping since the presence or absence of lymphokine-receptors such as the interleukin 2 receptor may predict the success or failure of such therapeutic strategies.

The presence of monotypic cytoplasmic immunoglobulin (cIg) and absence or weak staining for complement receptors (CRI) differentiate B immunoblastic lymphoma from centroblastic lymphoma. The presence of monotypic cIg in lymphoplasmacytic cells differentiate immunocytoma, lymphoplasmocytoid type, from CLL with reactive plasma cells. BA2 staining in small cell lymphomas support the diagnosis intermediate lymphocytic lymphomas (46). True histiocytic lymphomas are diagnosed by the absence of T cell- (3A1, Leu4, Leu5) and B cell markers (B1, Leu14, surface and cytoplasmic Ig) and the presence of histiocytic markers (OKM1, My7, α-naphtylacetate esterase, acid phosphatase, lysozyme, α1-antitrypsin and α1-antichymotrypsin (47).

3.1. Detection of small numbers of neoplastic cells

The detection of small numbers of neoplastic cells is important in bone marrow and lymph nodes. The use of epithelial markers such as 115D8 and K2080 facilitates the detection of carcinoma cells by the surgical pathologists.

Dearnaley et al (48) have shown that in patients with breast carcinomas small numbers of neoplastic cells could be detected by using these antisera in bone marrow smears, which were not reported by pathologists after examination of Giemsa stained smears. The impact of such a positive bone marrow specimen on therapeutic regimens in patients treated for breast cancer metastases have yet to be defined.

For staging of small cell carcinomas detection of single neoplastic cells in the bone marrow by staining for cytokeratin seems also worthwile, but reports are scarce (18).

Another interesting area is the detection of small numbers of leukaemic cells in bone marrow specimens. In this field increased numbers of cells with terminal deoxynucleotidyl transferase (tdt) or common acute lymphoblastic leukemia (cALL) antigen after treatment points to the recurrence of a leukemia. Their detection seems more reliable than morphologic evaluation alone (49).

4. Assessment of the localization of the primary tumor according to the marker profile of the metastases

Problems in this area are mostly encountered with adenocarcinomas. Squamous cell carcinomas are sensitive to radiotherapy and some cytostatics, but adenocarcinomas especially those from the alimentary tract, kidney and cervix poorly react to these therapeutic regimens. However, treatment for carcinomas of the thyroid, breast, ovary and prostate may yield fair to good results. Therefore, knowledge about the localisation of the primary tumor is important.

Adenocarcinomas of the prostate can be detected by the presence of prostate specific antigen, which is highly specific for this type of carcinoma. It is more sensitive than prostate specific acid phosphatase. The amount of this latter enzyme is inversely related to the morphological differentiation of the carcinoma. The same holds true for thyroglobulin and thyreoid carcinoma. Medullary thyreoid carcinomas have CEA and calcitonin, which is quite specific for this type of carcinoma. More problems are encountered in the more frequent types of cancer, i.e. carcinomas of lung, breast, colon, ovary and endometrium. Here only few markers have been developed that are cell-type or organ specific. In this field especially the development of monoclonal antibodies specific for carcinomas of the ovary seems promising (50, 51, 52).

In table 7 we have depicted a number of monoclonals which seem helpful in the recognition of the origin of the primary tumor. The data have been collected from the literature and our own experience. From these preliminary data it can be seen that the antigen profiles of the tumors do not discriminate clearly between colon- and lungcarcinoma. Differences in antigenic profiles of carcinomas from lung and breast, breast and colon, and colon and ovary seem worthwile for further evaluation. Moreover it has been recognized that the antigenic profile of the primary tumor and its metastasis can differ (54, 66) and thus can negatively influence the finding of the primary tumor. The exact impact of this so-called heterogeneity of tumor cells on the recognition of the site of the primary tumor is not known. As already mentioned the cytokeratin profiles of the metastases do not contribute significantly in the assessment of the localisation of the primary tumors mentioned.

Table 7. Antigen profiles of adenocarcinomas of different origin

	CEA**	CA19-9	OC125*	OV-TL3*
lung	+	+	-(+)	-
breast	+	-	+	-
colon	+	+(-)	-	-
ovary	-(+)	-(+)	+(-)	+
endometrium	-(+)	-	+	-
cervix	-(+)		+	-

* other monoclonal antibodies against ovarial tumors have been described by Fleuren et al (50), Mattes et al (51), and Tsuji et al (52).

** 1) The antibody directed against CEA described here was purified according to Nap et al (53) and described by Van der Linden et al (54).
2) CA19.9 (55)
3) OC125 (56)
4) OVTL3: The staining results given here are derived from immunofluorescence studies (57).

5. Perspectives

In this section we shall briefly mention some perspectives for the application of monoclonal antibodies in tumor pathology.

Recently monoclonal antibodies have been described which

react with cells in certain phases of the cell cycle. Ki67 a monoclonal antibody reacting with nuclei of cells in late G1, S, M and G2 phase is such an example (58, 59).

In this respect the monoclonal antibodies against the transferrin receptor, involved in mitoses, are also of value. The stained cells can be evaluated by quantitative morphologic methods and thus accurate information about the dividing tumor cells can be obtained. These results seem superior and more reproducible than classical counting of mitoses.

The detection of function associated receptors i.e. lymphokine receptors such as interleukin 2 receptor, and growth factor receptors such as the epidermal growth factor receptor and platelet derived growth factor receptor are likely to be important in the future. The discovery of biologically active products such as the interferons and the development of factors which can block their receptors may stimulate future studies on characterisation of these receptors on certain tumors.

In this respect the observation that certain growth factors such as platelet derived growth factor, a potent mitogen for connective tissue cells and onc gene products such as the v-sis protein represent the same cellular gene is of importance (60). This stresses the need for analysis of onc gene products, lymphokine- and growth receptors in relation to the response of tumors to biologically active products.

Another interesting observation is the detection of certain classes of receptors present on the surface of tumor cells which influence the attachment of the cell to basement membrane substances such as laminin (61, 62). These receptors may play an important role in the metastatic potential of tumor cells. Moreover in rodent and human lymphoid cells a class of receptors has been described which interact with high endothelial venules (63, 64). These so-called homing receptors are presumed to play a role in the migration and homing pattern of lymphoid cells in normal and pathologic conditions. The influence of certain lymphokines on the phenotypic expression of endothelial cell markers makes analysis of these receptors by immunohistochemistry useful.

Important constituents of the basement membrane are laminin and collagen type II and type IV. Analysis of these substances seems important in the detection of early infiltration through the basement membrane of in situ carcinomas of the cervix, larynx, breast and prostate. Analysis of basement membrane substances in laryngeal dysplasia and carcinoma casts some doubt on the value of this technique since the presence of inflammation is often associated with loss of the structural integrity of the basement membrane (65). The scarcity of inflammatory infiltrate in early neoplastic lesions of breast and prostate makes analysis of laminin and collagen type II and IV in these organs more worthwhile.

6. Conclusions

In conclusion, monoclonal antibodies specific for one tumor type are very rare. Therefore we have chosen for the use of small panels of monoclonal antibodies in certain problematic areas of diagnostic tumor pathology. The use of monoclonal antibodies for the detection of small numbers of tumor cells in bone marrow and lymph nodes is briefly discussed. Moreover the (im)possibilities to predict the localisation of the primary tumor on the antigenic profile of its metastases have been described. Finally some perspectives for the future role of immunohistochemistry in diagnostic tumor pathology are given.

Acknowledgement

We thank Mrs. Désirée de Jong and Mrs. Carla van Rijn for typing the manuscript carefully as always.

References

1. Kersey JH, LeBien TW, Abramson LS, Newman R, Sutherland R, Greaves M: P24: A human leukemin associated and lymphohemopoietic progenitor cell surface structure identification with monoclonal antibody. J Exp Med 153: 726-731, 1981.

2. Dvoretski Ph, Wood GS, Levy R, Warnke RA: T lymphocyte subsets in follicular lymphomas compared with those in non-neoplastic lymph nodes and tonsils. Human Pathology 13: 618-623, 1982.

3. Brandtzaeg P: Tissue preparation methods for immunohistochemistry. In: Techniques in immunohistochemistry, Vol 1. Edited by GR Bullock and P Tetrus. Academic Press, London, New York, pp 1-75, 1985.

4. Polak JM, Van Noorden S: Immunocytochemistry. Practical applications in pathology and biology. Chapter 2, pp 11-42. Publ. John Wright 1 Sons Ltd. Stonebridge press, Bristol BS45MU, England, 1983.

5. Gatter KC, Alcock C, Heryet A, Pulford KA, Taylor-Papadimitriou J, Stein H, Mason DY. The differential diagnosis of routinely processed anaplastic tumors using monoclonal antibodies. Am J Clin Pathol 82: 33-43, 1984.

6. Meijer CJLM, Willemze R, Henzen-Logmans SC, Van der Valk P: Monoclonal antibodies in the histopathological diagnosis of non- Hodgkin's lymphomas. Neth J Med 38, 138-141, 1985.

7. Gown AM, Vogel AM: Monoclonal antibodies to human intermediate filament proteins. III. Analysis of tumors. Am J Clin Pathol 84: 413-424, 1985.

8. Van Duinen SG, Ruiter DJ, Hageman Ph, Vennegoor C, Dickersin GR, Scheffer E, Rümke Ph: Immunohistochemical and histochemical tools in the diagnosis of amelanotic melanoma. Cancer 53: 1566-1573, 1984.

9. Vennegoor C, Calafat J, Hageman Ph, Van Buitenen F, Janssen H, Kolk A, Rümke Ph: Biochemical characterization and cellular localization of a formalin resistant melanoma-associated antigen reacting with monoclonal antibody NKI/C3. Int J Cancer 35: 287-295, 1985.

10. Natali PG, Imai K, Wilson BS, Bigotti A, Cavaliere R, Pellegrino MA, Ferrone S: Structural properties and time distribution of the antigen reorganized by the monoclonal antibody 653.40.S to human melanoma cells. J Natl Cancer Inst 67: 591-595, 1981.

11. Suter L, Bröcker EB, Brüggen J, Ruiter DJ, Sorg C: Heterogeneity of primary and metastatic human malignant melanoma as detected with monoclonal antibodies in cryostat sections of biopsies. Cancer Immunol Immunother 7: 405-413, 1983.

12. Vennegoor C: Personal communication, 1986.

13. Ruiter DJ, Broecker EB, Vennegoor C, Ferrone S: Monoclonal antibodies recognizing melanoma associated antigens. Chapter 8 in this volume.

14. Roholl PJM, De Jong ASH, Ramaekers FCS. Application of markers in the diagnosis of soft tissue tumours. Histopathology 9, 1019-1035, 1985.

15. Osborn M, Dirk T, Käser H, Weber K, Altmannsberger M: Immunohistochemical localization of neurofilaments and neuron-specific enolase in 29 cases of neuroblastoma. Am J Pathol 122: 433-442, 1986

16. Osborn M, Weber K: Tumor diagnosis by intermediate filament typing. Lab Invest 48: 372-394, 1983.

17. Osborn M, Altmannsberger M, Shaw G, Schauer A, Weber K: Various sympathetic derived human tumors differ in neurofilament expression. Use in diagnosis of neuroblastoma, ganglio-neuroblastoma and pheochromocytoma. Virchows Arch B (Cell Path) 40: 141-156, 1982.

18. De Ley L et al, Chapter 10 in this volume.

19. De Jong ASH, van Vark M, Albus-Lutter ChE, van Raamsdonk W, Voûte PA: Myosin and myoglobin as tumor markers in the diagnosis of rhabdomyosarcoma: a comparative study. Am J Surg Pathol 8: 512-528, 1984.

20. Sun TI, Eichner R, Schermer A, Cooper D, Nelson WG, Weiss RA: In: Cancer Cells 1, The transformed phenotype (Eds. AJ Levine, GF Vande Woude, WC Topp, JD Watson), Cold Spring Harbor Symp. Cold Spring Harbor, pp 169-176, 1984.

21. Moll R, Franke WW, Schiller DL, Geiger B, Krepler R: The catalog of human cytokeratins: patterns of expression in normal epithelial tumors and cultures cells. Cell 31: 11-24, 1982

22. Moll R, Franke WW: Cytochemical cell typing of metastatic tumors according to their cytoskeletal proteins. In: Biochemistry and molecular genetics of cancer metastasis. K Lagris, LA Liobta and AS Rabion (eds). Martinus Nijhoff Publishing, Boston, Dordrecht, Lancaster, pp 101-113, 1986.

23. Jasani B, Edwards RE, Thomas ND, Gibbs AR: The use of vimentin antibodies in the diagnosis of malignant mesotheliomas. Virchows Arch (Pathol Anat) 406: 444-448, 1985.

24. Mullink H, Henzen-Logmans SC, Alons-van Kordelaar JJM, Tadema TM, Meijer CJLM: Simultaneous immunoenzyme staining of vimentin and cytokeratins with monoclonal antibodies as an aid in the differential diagnosis: malignant mesothelioma - pulmonary adenocarcinoma. Virchow's Arch B (Cell Path), 1986 (in press).

25. Corson JM, Pinkus GS: Mesothelioma: profile of keratin proteins and CEA. An immunoperoxidase study of 20 cases and comparison with pulmonary adenocarcinoma. Am J Pathol 108: 80-87, 1982.

26. Gibbs AR, Harach NR, Wagner JC, Jasani B: Comparison of tumour markers in malignant mesothelioma and pulmonary adenocarcinoma. Thorax 40: 91-95, 1985.

27. Kwee WS, Veldhuizen RW, Golding RP, Mullink H, Stam J, Donner R, Boon ME: Histologic distinction between malignant mesotheliomas, benign pleural lesions and carcinoma metastasis. Virchows Arch A (Pathol Anat) 397: 287-299, 1982.

28. Szpak CA, Johnston WW, Roggli V, Kolbeck J, Lottich C, Vollmer R, Thor A, Schlom J: The diagnostic distinction between malignant mesothelioma of the pleura and adenocarcinoma of the lung as defined by a monoclonal antibody (B72.3). Am J Pathol 122: 252-260, 1986.

29. Schlingemann RO, Dingjan GM, Emeis JJ, Warnaar SO, Ruiter DJ: Monoclonal antibody PAL-E specific for endothelium. Lab Invest 52: 71-77, 1985.

30. Donner L, de Lanerolle P, Costa J: Immunoreactivity of paraffin-embedded normal tissue and mesenchymal tumors for smooth muscle myosin. Am J Clin Pathol 80: 677-681, 1983.

31. Herpers MJHM: Intermediate filament expression in human neuro- ectodermal brain tumors. Academic thesis, State University Limburg. Schrijen-Lippertz BV Voerendaal 1986.

32. Bonnin JR, Rubinstein LJ: Immunohistochemistry of central nervous system tumours. Its constitution to neurosurgical diagnosis. J Neurosurgery 60: 1121-1131, 1984.

33. Isobe T, Ichimosi K, Nakajima T, Okuyema T. The alpha-subunit of S100 proteins present in tumor cells of human malignant melanomas, but not in schwannomas. Brain Res 294: 381-384, 1984.

34. Takahashi J, Isobe T, Ohtsuki Y, Akahji T, Sonobe H, Okuyama T: Immunohistochemical study on the distribution of alpha and beta subunits of S-100 protein in human neoplasm and normal tissue. Virchows Arch B (Cell Path) 45: 384-396, 1984.

35. Schwab U, Stein H, Gerdes J, Lemke H, Kirchner H, Schaadt M, Diehl V: Production of a monoclonal antibody specific for Hodgkin and Reed-Sternberg cells of Hodgkin's disease and a subset of normal lymphoid cells. Nature 294: 65-67, 1982.

36. Poppema S, Brinker M, Buys CHCM, Timens W, Osinga J, Visser L: On the origin of Reed Sternberg cells. Immunoglobulin gene rearrangements in Hodgkin's disease cell lines and in tissues from patients with Hodskin's disease. Submitted for publication.

37. Hsu SM, Jaffe ES: LeuM1 and peanut agglutinin stain the neoplastic cells of Hodgkin's disease. Am J Pathol 82: 29-32, 1984.

38. Jaffe ES, Strauchen JA, Berard CW: Predictability of immunologic phenotype by morphologic criteria in diffuse aggressive non-Hodgkin's lymphomas. Am J Clin Pathol 77: 46, 1982.

39. Nathwani BN, Winberg CD: Non-Hodgkin's lymphomas: an appraisal of the 'working formulation of non-Hodgkin's lymphomas for clinical usage'. In: Malignant lymphomas, Pathology Annual Monograph. Eds S Sommers and PP Rosen. Appleton-Century-Crofts, Norwalk, Connecticut, pp 1-63, 1983.

40. Stein H, Lennert K, Feller AC, Mason DY: Immunohistological analysis of human lymphoma: Correlation of histological and immunological categories. Adv Cancer Res 42: 67-147, 1984.

41. Meijer CJLM, Van der Valk P, Poppema S: Marker studies in lymphomas. In: Monographs in immunology. Eds W den Otter and E Ruitenberg. Elsevier, Amsterdam, 1986 (in press).

42. Van den Oord JJ, de Wolf-Peeters C, Frizzera G, Desmet VJ, Tricot G, Thomas J, Marien K, Gatter KC, Mason DY: T-helper cell lymphoma involving the lymph nodes and skin. A clinical, morphologic and immunohistochemical analysis of 5 cases. Cancer 55, 1714-1721, 1985.

43. Van der Valk P, Willemze, R, Meijer CJLM: Peripheral T cell lymphomas. A clinicopathological and immunologic study of 10 cases. Histopathology 10: 235-249, 1986.

44. Waldron JA, Leech JH, Glick AD, Flexner JM, Collins RD: Malignant lymphomas of periphernal T-lymphocyte orgin. Immunologic, pathologic and clinical features in 6 patients. Cancer 40, 1604-1617, 1977.

45. Watanabe S, Shimosato Y, Shimoyama M: Lymphoma and leukemia of T-lymphocytes. Pathology Annual 16, 155-203, 1981.

46. Weisenburger DD, Nathwani BN, Diamond LW, Winberg CD, Rappaport H: Malignant lymphoma, intermediate lymphocytic type. A clinico- pathologic study of 42 cases. Cancer 48: 1415-1425, 1981.

47. Van der Valk P, Meijer CJLM: Histiocytic sarcoma. Path Annu (2) 1-14. Appleton-Century Croft, New Castle, Connecticut, 1985.

48. Dearnaley DP, Sloan JP, Ormerod MG et al: Increased detection of mammary carcinoma cells in marrow smears using antisera to epithelial membrane antigen. Brit J Cancer 44: 85-89, 1981.

49. Van Dongen JJM, Adriaansen HJ, Hooijkaas H: Immunological characterization of cells in the various hematopoietic differentiation stages and their malignant counterparts. Chapter 6 in this volume.

50. Fleuren GJ: Monoclonal antibodies against ovarian cancer. Chapter 13 in this volume.

51. Mattes MJ, Cordon-Cardo C, Lewis JL, Old JL, Lloyd KO: Cell surface antigens of human ovarian and endometrial carcinoma defined by mouse monoclonal antibodies. Proc Natl Acad Sci USA 81: 568-572, 1984.

52. Tsuji Y, Suzuki T, Nishiura H, Takemura T, Osojima S: Identification of two different surface epitopes of human ovarian epithelial carcinomas by monoclonal antibodies. Cancer Res 45: 2358-2362, 1985.

53. Nap M, ten Hoor KA, Fleuren GJ: Cross reactivity with normal antigens in commercial anti CEA sera, used for immunohistology. The need for tissue controls and absorptions. Am J Clin Pathol 79: 25-31, 1983.

54. Van der Linden JC, Baak JPA, Lindeman J, Smeulders AWM, Meijer CJLM: Carcinoembryonic antigen expression and peanut agglutinin binding in primary breast cancer and lymph node metastases; lack of correlation with clinical, histopathological, biochemical and morphometric features. Histopathology 9: 1051-1059, 1985.

55. Koprowsky H, Herlijn M, Steplewsky HH, Sears HF: Specific antigen in serum of patients with colon carcinoma. Science 212: 53-55, 1981.

56. Bast RC, Feeney M, Lazarus H, Nadler LM: Reactivity of a monoclonal antibody with human ovarian carcinoma. J Clin Invest 68: 1331-1337, 1981.

57. Poels L, Peters O, Van Megen Y, Vooys GP, Verheyen R, Willemsen A, Van Niekerk C, Jap P, Mungyer G, Kenemans P: Monoclonal antibody against human ovarian tumor associated surface antigens. J Natl Cancer Inst.: in press, 1986.

58. Gerdes J, Schwab U, Lemke H, Stein H: Production of a mouse monoclonal antibody reactive with a human nuclear antigen associated with cell proliferation. Int J Cancer 31: 13-20, 1983.

59. Gerdes J, Lemke H, Batch H, Waeker H, Schwab U, Stein H: Cell cycle analysis of a cell proliferation-associated human nuclear antigen defined by the monoclonal antibody Ki-67. J Immunol 133: 1710-1715, 1984.

60. Doolittle RF, Hunkapiller MW, Hood LE, Devare SG, Robbins KC, Aaronson KSA, Antoniades HN: Simian sarcoma virus onc gene, v-sis, is derived from the gene (or genes) encoding a platelet-derived growth factor. Science 221: 275-277, 1983.

61. Kramer RH, Nicolson GL: Invasion of vascular endothelial cell monolayers and underlying matrix by metastatic human cancer cells. In Schweiger GH (ed): International Cell Biology, p 794, Berlin, Springer Verlag, 1981.

62. Rao CN, Margulies IMK, Tralka TS, Madri J, Liotta LA Isolation of a subunit of laminin and its role in tumor cel attachment. J Biol Chem 257: 9740, 1982.

63. Jalkanen ST, Butcher EC: In vitro analysis of the homin properties of human lymphocytes: Developmental regulation c functional receptors for high endothelial venules. Blood 66 577-584, 1985.

64. Pals ST, Kraal G, Horst E, Groot A de, Scheper RJ, Meije CJLM: Human lymphocyte - high endothelial venul interactions: organ selective binding of T- and B-lymphocyt populations to high endothelium. J Immunol 1986 (in press).

65. Visser R, Van der Beek JMH, Havenith MG, Cleutjens JPM Bosman FT: Immunocytochemical detection of basement membran antigens in the histopathological evaluation of laryngea dysplasia and neoplasia. Histopathology 10: 171-180, 1986.

66. Skipper HE, Simpson-Herren L: Relationship between tumor ste cell heterogeneity and responsiveness to chemotherapy. In Important advances in oncology 1985, pp 63-77, eds VT d Vita, S Hellman, SA Rosenberg. JB Lippincot Company Philadelphia, 1985.

PRACT.MAN/MEIJER3

CASE PRESENTATIONS.

18. CASE 1: CARCINOMA OR LARGE-CELL LYMPHOMA? IMMUNOHISTOCHEMICAL APPROACH OF UNDIFFERENTIATED TUMORS IN THE SKIN.

C.J.L.M. MEIJER, R. WILLEMZE, S.C. HENZEN-LOGMANS, H. MULLINK

CLINICAL FINDINGS

A 53 year-old man was admitted to our hospital because of a small subcutaneous tumor localized in the subareolar area of the left breast. Physical examination did not reveal any abnormalities; no enlarged axillar lymph nodes were found. Because a breast carcinoma was suspected, a biopsy was performed.

PATHOLOGICAL FINDINGS

The biopsy measured 2x1x1 cm. Representative tissue specimens were fixed in buffered formalin and embedded in paraplast or frozen in liquid nitrogen. Two circumscript nodules (fig. 1a) localized in the dermis and subcutis were observed. They consisted of large cells with a moderate amount of cytoplasm and large nuclei with sometimes irregular outline and 1 or two small nucleoli (fig. 1b). Two mitoses per high power field were found. The reticulin staining (fig. 1c) and PAS staining were not helpful in the differential diagnosis between large cell lymphoma and carcinoma. To differentiate between large cell lymphoma and undifferentiated carcinoma the "large cell tumor panel" was used (table 1). This panel consists of 5 antibodies of which the positive and negative staining results reinforce each other. It can be used on buffered formalin fixed paraplast embedded material (1). This panel is in use in our laboratory for surgical pathology specimens since June 1984. The immunohistochemical results keratin -, vimentin + (fig. 1 d), NKI/C-3 -, 115D8 -, common leucocyte antigen + (fig. 1e) pointed to the diagnosis of a large-cell non-Hodgkin lymphoma (table 1). Additional marker studies to characterize this lymphoma (table 1) were performed on frozen tissue sections (table 2).
The immunohistochemical results revealed a B cell lymphoma (leu14+, Leu4-). The neoplastic cells had weak monotopic surface Ig (IgM,K) on their surface membrane and showed c3bi receptors. In conjunction with histology the diagnosis of a diffuse growing non-Hodgkin lymphoma large cell non cleaved/cleaved according to the working formulation was made (centroblastic lymphoma in the Kiel classification).

Table I. Immunihistochemical results with the "large cell tumor panel".

Antibody	Source	Determinant	Main cell specifity	Staining results
anti keratin	Dako	cytokeratin (broad spectred) MW 45-68 KD	epithelial cells	-
anti-vimentin	Euro diagnostics	vimentin MW 57 KD	mesenchymal cells	+
115D8	Hilkens*	MAM-6 antigen MW 25-110 KD	epithelial cells	-
NKI/C-3	Vennegoor*	melanoma associated antigen MW 25-110 KD	melanocytic cells	-
anti-common leucocyte antigen (2B11, PD7/26)	Dako	common leucocyte antigen MW 200 KD	leucocyte	+

* Nederlands Kanker Instituut, Amsterdam (see appendix)
** Staining results obtained on formalin fixed paraplast embedded sections.
MW = molecular weight.

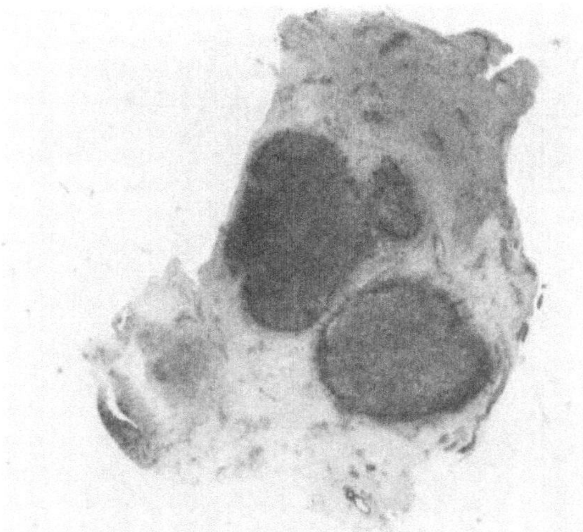

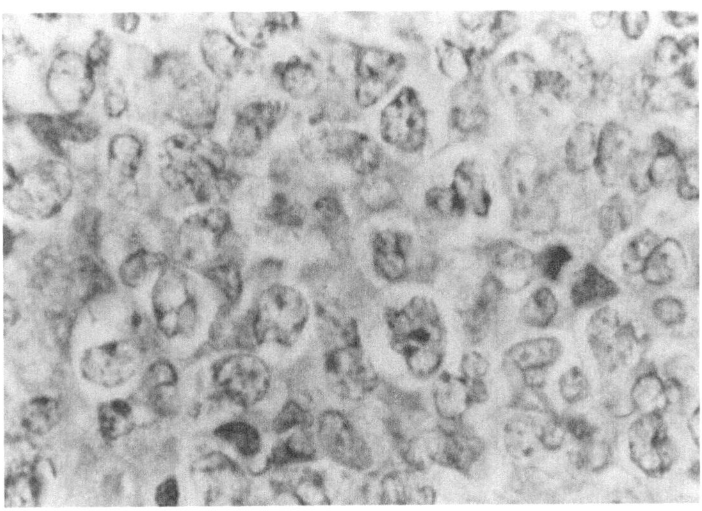

Fig. 1a: Low magnification of the biopsy specimen. Two nodules of tumor tissue between pre-existent breast tissue.

Fig. 1b: High magnification of the tumor (x 500). The neoplastic cells have large nulce; with sometimes irregular outlines and 1 or 2 small nucleoli.

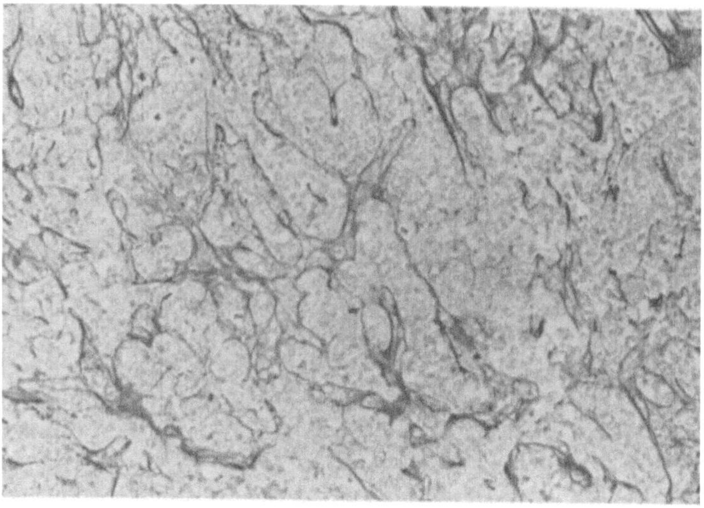

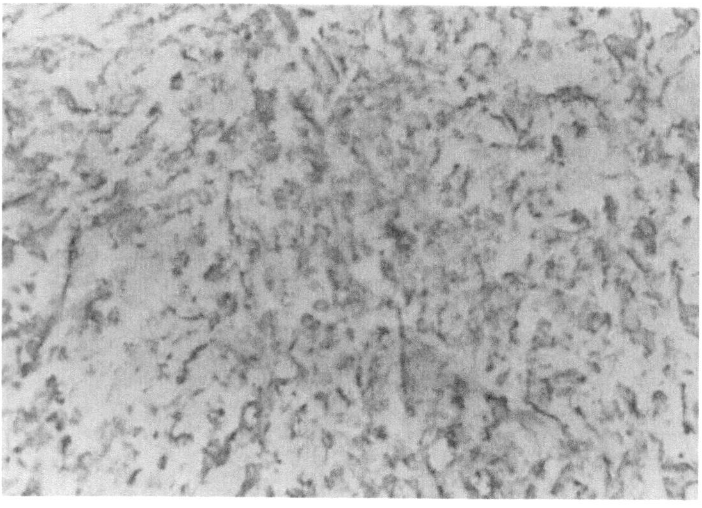

Fig. 1c: Reticulin staining of the tumor (x125). This pattern is not helpful to differentiate between carcinoma and lymphoma.

Fig. 1d: Vimentin staining of the tumor (x125). Notice that not all tumor cells stain positive for vimentin. The tumor cells did not stain for cytokeratin (formalin fixed, paraplast embedded material pretreated with pronase, no counterstaining x 75).

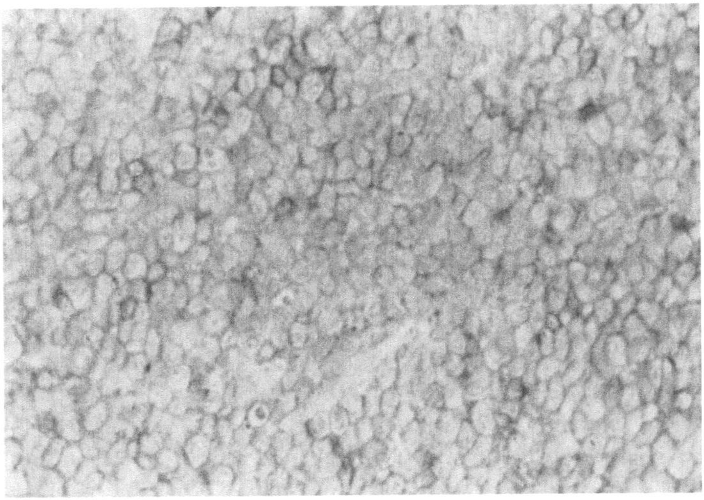

Fig. le: Common leucocyte antigen is present on the surface of the tumor cells (formalin fixed, paraplast embedded material, x 125).

CLINICAl COURSE

Since the staging procedure including bone marrow biopsy, differential blood count, X-thorax and CT scan of the abdomen did not reveal extracutanerus localizations, a primary cutaneous non Hodgkin lymphoma was diagnosed. During the staging procedure the patient developed red to violaceous cutanerus nodules or tumors on the back, thorax and abdomen. After 3 courses of cytostatic treatment (CHOP: cyclosphosphamid adriamycin, oncovin and prednisone), a complete remission was reached. Two years later he is still in complete remission.

DISCUSSION

The differential diagnosis of anaplastic large cell tumors, localized in the skin includes carcinoma, Merkel cell tumor, amelanotic melanoma, large cell lymphoma and undifferentiated sarcoma. This last tumor is very rare in the skin.
When the surgical pathologist is unable to classify these tumors on light microscopical grounds, immunohistochemistry can be helpful (2, 3).
Since most antibodies are not specific for one tumor type, we are using a panel of 5 antibodies to differentiate large cell tumors. The panel is composed in such a way that the positive and negative staining results reinforce each other to achieve a definite diagnosis. (see chapter of Meijer et al.).
The results obtained with this panel on this tumor indicate a large cell lymphoma (cytokeratins -, vimentin +, 115D8 -, NKI/C3 -, common leucocyte antigen +). Interestingly not all the tumor cells stained positive for vimentin (fig. 1d.), a phenomenon well-known for lymphomas.

Table 2: Immunohistochemical characterization of the large cell non-Hodgkin lymphoma

Monoclonal antibody	Specificity	Main cell type	Staining results
pan T cell antibodies			
CD7 (3 A1)	T cell antigen (p41)	all T cells, 5% of AML	-
CD2 (Leu11)	T11 antigen (p50)	all T cells	-
CD (Leu4)	T3 antigen (19-9)	mature T cells	-
pan B cell antibodies			
CD22 (Leu4)	B cell antigen (p135)	nearly all B cells	+
CD20 (B1)	B cell antigen (p35)	all B cells	+
Monocyte/macrophages			
CDW13 (My7)	myelomonocytic antigen (p169)	all myeloid and monocytic cells	-
Others			
Immunoglobulins	immunoglobulin	B cells	weak membr staining f IgM, K
HLA-DR	HLJA-DR, non polymorphic antigen (p29-34)	haemopoietic precursor cells, B cells, activated T cells, monocytes, macrophages	+
CR1	C3b1 receptor (p95-150)	myeloid, monocytic and some B cells	+
T9	transferrin receptor	proliferating activated cells	+

When a large cell lymphoma is present it is important to recognize subtypes, i.e. centroblastic-, large centrocytic-, T- and B-immunoblastic- and true histiocytic lymphomas since these node based large cell lymphomas have a different clinical behaviour (4, 5).
For recognition of subtypes of large cell lymphomas immunophenotyping is necessary to achieve a reliable and reproducible classification. Jaffe et al. (6) have shown that in a series of large cell lymphoma the phenotype was correctly predicted on morphological features in only 61%, even when high quality sections were used. For further classification of large cell lymphomas we used 3 T cell antibodies (3A1, Leu5 and Leu4), 2 B cell antibodies (B1 and Leu14) and 1 monocyte/macrophage antibody (My7). More than one antibody per cell type seems necessary, since some large cell lymphomas do not reveal all T or B cell antigens.
In our case the positive staining for Leu14 and B1 and the negative staining for 3A1, Leu4 and Leu5 and My7 were compatible with a B cell lymphoma. The absence of cytoplasmic staining for monotypic Ig, the presence of surface IgM, K and the presence of C3b1 receptors indicate a follicle center cell origin and support the diagnosis suspected on morphological grounds: diffuse growing non Hodgkin lymphoma, large cell, non cleaved/cleaved according to the working formulation (centroblastic lymphoma in the Kiel classification), and excluded a B-immunoblastic lymphoma.

In addition to the cutaneous epidermotropic cutaneous T cell lymphomas mycosis fungoides and Sezary's syndrome it is not uncommon to find the diffuse large cellular follicular center cell lymphomas in the skin.
Recently we have described 16 patients with this histologic subtype of malignant lymphoma who had only skin lesions at presentation. These patients presented with multiple red to violaceous nodules or tumors (7). Histologically these lymphomas showed non epidermotropic diffuse dermal infiltrates, mainly consisting of large follicular center cells, with a variable admixture of small cleaved cells, and small numbers of immunoblasts, T lymphocytes and macrophages.
In 10 cases the skin lesions were confined to a rather circumscribed area on the trunk. In 8 of these cases the tumors has been preceded for one to twenty years by the presence of slowly progressing papular and plaque like lesions, clinically suspected of lymphocytic infiltration of the skin (Jessner) or lymphocytoma cutis.
The original biopsies in the three cases of the preceeding lesions in retrospect raised suspicion on a mixed cell follicular lymphoma, but since only paraplast embedded material was available, no definite proof for malignancy by demonstration of monotypic light chain immunoglobulin was obtained.
Radiotherapy and/or polychemotherapy resulted in complete remission in 14 of 16 patients. Two elderly female patients died before radiotherapy had been instituted. Three patients had a cutaneous relapse which was successfully treated with additional radiotherapy. Only two patients developed

extracutaneous disease during the follow-up period. Follow-up data showed sustained complete remission in 13 of 16 patients with a median survival of 40 months. These data indicate that these cutaneous B cell lymphomas of follicle center origin have a rather favorable prognosis.

REFERENCES

1. Henzen-Logmans SC, Mullink H, Vennegoor C, Hilgers J, Oort J, Meijer CJLM: Anaplastic large cell tumors: Differentiation by means of monoclonal antibodies. Virchows Archiv A in press.

2. Gatter KC, Alcock C, Heryet A, Pulford KA, Heyderman E, Taylor-Papadimitrious J, Stein H, Mason DY: The differential diagnosis of routinely processed anaplastic tumors using monoclonal antibodies. Am J Clin Pathol 82: 33-43, 1984.

3. Meijer CJLM, Willemze R, Mullink H, Henzen-Logmans SC, Valk P van der: Monoclonal antibodies in the histopathological diagnosis of non-Hodgkin's lymphoma. Neth J Med 28: 138-141, 1985.

4. Strauchen JA, Young RC, De Vita VT et al.: Clinical relevance of the histopathologic subclassification of diffuse "histiocytic" lymphoma. N Engl J Med 299: 1382-1386, 1978.

5. Berard CW, Isaacson PG, Neiman RS, Peiper SC, Watanabe S, Wolf BC, Wright DH: Symposium on histiocytic or large cell lymphomas. In: "Malignant lymphomas. A pathology annual monograph". ShC Sommers and PS Rosen (eds), pp 109-168, Appleton Century Croft, Norwalk, Connecticut, 1983.

6. Jaffe ES, Strauchen JA, Berard CW: Predictability of immunologic phenotype by morphologic criteria in diffuse aggressive non-Hodgkin's lymphomas. Am J Clin Pathol 77: 46-50, 1982.

7. Willemze R, Meijer CJLM, Scheffer E, Kluin Ph, Vloten WA van, Toonstra J, Putte SCJ van der: Diffuse large celular follicular center cell lymphomas of the skin. A clinicopathologic and immunologic study of 16 patients. Am J Path in press.

CASE PRESENTATIONS.

19. CASE 2: CARCINOMA OR SARCOMA?

S.C. HENZEN-LOGMANS, C.J.L.M. MEIJER

CLINICAL FINDINGS

A 63 year old woman presented with rectal bleeding. During clinical examination a rectal tumor was found from which a biopsy was taken. The pathologists were unable to make a definite diagnosis on conventional histology. A differential diagnosis of undifferentiated carcinoma or histiocytic sarcoma was made.

PATHOLOGICAL FINDINGS I.

Histological examination of the slides, made from formalin fixed, paraffin embedded tissue blocks, showed cellular solid tumor tissue, mainly localized in the submucosal area of the rectal wall. No clear relationship with the mucosa was seen. The overlying mucosa showed ulceration. The solid tumor fields were composed of large uniform spindle cells, with ill-defined cell boundaries, acidophilic occasionally vacuolated cytoplasm and vesicular nuclei. Frequent mitotic figures, but no bizarre mitoses were found. In between these tumor cells a mononuclear infiltrate was present. No duct-like structures were seen (see Figures 1a and b). Histochemical stains for mucin were negative. Although an undifferentiated carcinoma was most likely, a sarcoma could not be excluded.
Additional immunohistochemical examination was done with a panel of antibodies, routinely in use in our laboratory to differentiate anaplastic large cell tumors (Ace Table I of case 1) (1). The immunohistochemical results (keralint, 115D8-, Vimentin-, NKI/C3 -common leucocyte antigen-) strongly supports the epithelial nature of the tumor cells. In Figure 1c the staining with anti-cytokeratins is shown. Based on these immunohistochemical findings a diagnosis of carcinoma was made.

CLINICAL COURSE I

Four years after diagnosis, the patient was admitted to our hospital with localized liver metastases, found on routine screening. The metastases were resected from the liver. During the operation, the patient showed a "flushing" phenomenon.

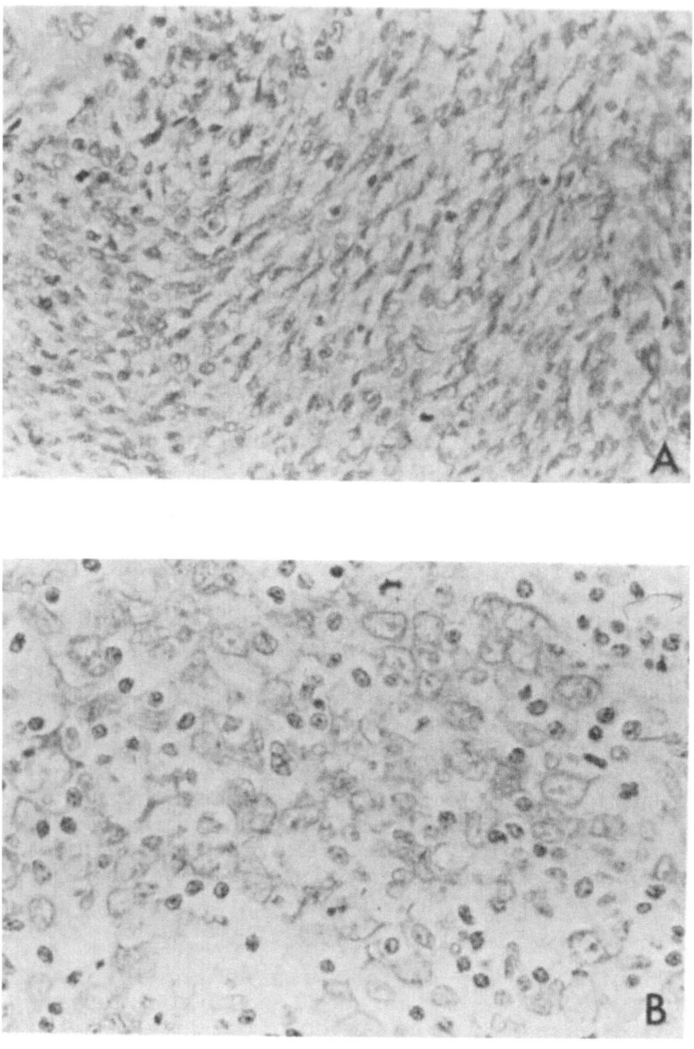

Fig. 1.
Histological and immunohistochemical findings in the primary tumor.

a) The solid tumor fields are composed of large uniform spindle cells, with ill-defined cell boundaries, acidophilic, sometimes vacuolated cytoplasm, vesicular nuclei and frequent mitotic figures. Haematoxylin-eosin (x 330).

b) High-power view of the vesicular nuclei. Haematoxylin-eosin (x 528).

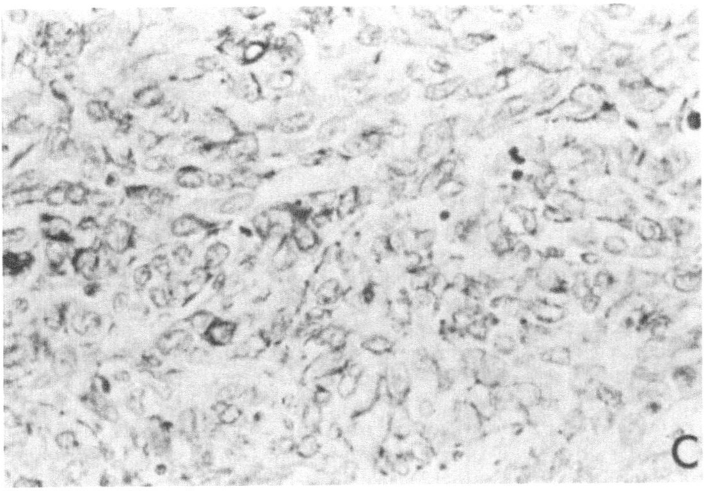

Fig. 1.
c) The tumor cells stained positive for cytokeratins in the indirect immunoperoxidase technique (x 330).

PATHOLOGICAL FINDINGS II

Fresh liver tissue was received, containing several solid white lesions measuring 5 to 7 cm in diameter. Representative slices were taken for conventional histology. In addition tissue was a) snap frozen in liquid nitrogen for immunohistochemistry, b) fixed in 2% phosphate buffered glutaraldehyde (pH 7.4) for electron microscopy (EM).
Histological examination showed the same morphological and immunohistochemical pattern as shown in the rectal tumor. Additional histochemical stainings revealed a few argyrophilic tumor cells. Additional immunohistochemistry with markers known to be associated with neuro-endocrine differentiation such as neuron specific enolase, S100-protein, serotonin, and neurofilament were completely negative.
Additional EM examination revealed cells with desmosomes, mucin granules, inter- and intracellular lumina with microvilli; some cells contained a few neuro-secretory granules.
Based on histology, immunohistochemistry and electron microscopy, which showed adeno- and neuroendocrine differentiation the final diagnosis was: liver metastases of the undifferentiated large-cell rectal carcinoma as defined by Gibbs et al. (2).

TREATMENT AND CLINICAL COURSE II

Eighteen months after metastasectomy, recurrent metastases in the liver were found.
Therapy consisted of 5-Fluorouracyl, which resulted in partial tumor regression. Six months after chemotherapy the patient is still alive.

DISCUSSION

Small panels of antibodies have been developed for use in surgical pathology. These panels are composed in such a way that the positive and negative staining results reinforce each other. To differentiate anaplastic large cell carcinoma from lymphoma, sarcoma or melanoma several panels have been described (1, 3). The panel we routinely use in our laboratory consists of anti-cytokeratins, anti-vimentin, anti-common leucocyte antigen, 115D8 (directed against milk fat globule membrane antigen MAM-6) and NKI/C3 (directed against a melanoma associated antigen).
In the primary tumor of our patient the epithelial nature is proven by the positive staining with the anti-cytokeratin antibody, especially in combination with the negative staining with anti-vimentin.
A combined expression of cytokeratins and vimentin in tumor cells has been described in some carcinomas and in synovial sarcomas, epitheloid sarcomas and mesotheliomas (4, 5, 6, 7). The term undifferentiated carcinoma of the large intestine was used by Gibbs (2) to describe a carcinoma which does not show tubule formation on the light microscopic level. This particular tumor differs from other anaplastic carcinomas by its uniform cell pattern, its lack of nuclear pleiomorphism and the absence of bizarr mitoses.
Although the tumor tends to grow to a large size before symptoms are produced, the patients have a relatively favorable prognosis, when the tumor is locally resectable. Thus, recognition of this tumor type is relevant for clinical management.
Argyrophilic cells were found in small numbers in the liver metastases of our patient. They were also found in 6 out of the 8 cases of undifferentiated carcinoma described by Gibbs (2). This does not imply, that these tumors merely represent morphological variants from the malignant non-argentaphinic carcinoids. Some apparently non neuro-endocrine tumors (such as squamous carcinomas) may contain membrane bound granules indistinguishable from neuro-secretory granules (8) and mixed patterns of differentiation are found in 2-3% of the gastro-intestinal tumours, suggestive of pluripotential differentiation (9, 10). Whether these tumors should be termed carcinoma with neuro-endocrine differentiation, neuro-endocrine carcinoma, or poorly differentiated carcinoid is still a matter of debate. We prefer to call this neoplasm carcinoma with adeno- and neuro-endocrine differentiation at the electronmicroscopical level.

REFERENCES

1. Meijer CJLM, Willemze R, Mullink H, Henzen-Logmans SC, Valk P van der: Monoclonal antibodies in the histopathological diagnosis of non Hodgkins' lymphoma. Neth J Med 28: 138-131, 1985.

2. Gibbs NM: Undifferentiated carcinoma of the large intestine. Histopathology 1: 77-84, 1977.

3. Gatter KC, Alcock C, Heryet A, Pulford KA, Heyderman E, Taylor-Papadimitriou J, Stein H, Mason DY: The differential diagnosis of routinely processed anaplastic tumors using monoclonal antibodies. Am J CLin Pathol 82: 33-43, 1984.

4. Chase DR, Enzinger FM, Weiss SH, Langloss JM: Keratin in epitheloid sarcoma. An immunohistochemical study. Am J Surg Pathol 8: 435-441, 1985.

5. Corson JM, Weiss LM, Banks-Schlegel SP, Pinkus GS: Keratin proteins and carcino-embryonic antigen in synovial sarcomas: An immunohistochemical study of 24 cases. Human Pathol 15: 615-621, 1984.

6. Mullink H, Henzen-Logmans SC, Alons-Van Kordelaar JJM, Tadema T, Meijer CJLM: Diagnosis of malignant mesothelioma by simultaneous immunoenzyme staining of vimentin and keratin with two monoclonal antibodies Virchow's Archiv B. (Cell.Pathol)., in press.

7. Miettinen M, Fransilla K, Letho V, Paasivo R, Virtanen I: expression of intermediate filament protein in thyroid gland and thyroid tumors. Lab Invest 50: 262-269, 1984.

8. Churg A, Johnston WH, Stulbarg M: Small cell squamous and mixed cell squamous - small cell anaplastic carcinomas of the lung. Am J Surg Pathol 4: 255-263, 1980.

9. Shousha S: Paneth cell-rich papillary adenocarcinoma and a mucoid adenocarcinoma occuring synchronously in colon: a light and electron microscopic study. Histopathology 3: 489-501, 1979.

10. Kubo T, Watanabe H: Neoplastic argentaphin cells in gastric and intestinal carcinomas. Cancer 27: 447-454, 1971.

CASE PRESENTATIONS.

20. CASE 3: TYPE OF SARCOMA?

D.J. RUITER, A.H.M. TAMINIAU

CLINICAL FINDINGS

A 18-year-old woman was admitted to the hospital because of pain in the left upper leg. X-ray examination revealed an irregular osteolytic defect in the distal femur with extraosseal extension. A differential diagnosis of Ewing sarcoma, osteosarcoma and osteomyelitis was made.An open biopsy was taken, both from the intra- and extraosseal parts of the lesion.

PATHOLOGICAL FINDINGS

Two unfixed pieces of solid white tissue with a maximal dimension of 2 and 3 cm, respectively were received for pathological examination. Representative slices were taken for conventional histology. In addition, tissue was snap-frozen and stored at -70˜C for immunohistochemistry, and fixed in McDowell-Trump fixative (a 1:4 mixture of 1% glutaraldehyde and 4% formaldehyde in phosphate buffer) for transmission electron microscopy. Histological examination showed cellular solid tumor tissue arranged in nests and cords consisting of epitheloid cells having a compact eosinophilic cytoplasm. Scattered groups of tumor cells showed a clear cytoplasm, containing much glycogen (Fig. 1). The nuclei were pleomorphic, vesicular with a prominent nucleolus. Scattered mitotic figures were found. No osteoid or chondroid intercellular substance were encountered. Staining for melanin was negative.

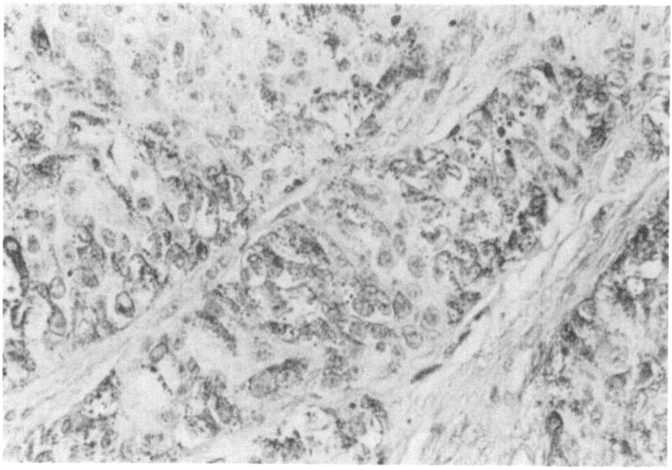

Fig. 1. Clear cell tumor of bone showing the presence of glycogen in the tumor cells (x 400, PAS stain).

Tumor tissue showed marked invasive growth into striated muscle. No differences in histological appearance were found between the extraosseal and intraosseal compartments. It was concluded that the histological appearance was unusual for a primary bone tumor. The relatively large cell size and vesicular nuclei with prominent nucleolus strongly argued against Ewing sarcoma. Because of lack of intercellular substance a diagnosis of osteosarcoma or chondrosarcoma could not be made. A diagnosis of clear cell sarcoma of bone was considered, because of the growth pattern in nests, the clear cell aspect, the abundance of glycogen and the vesicular nuclear appearance with prominent nucleolus. Clinically no evidence for an extraskeletal primary tumor was found. Additional immunohistochemical and electronmicroscopical examination was done in order to confirm the diagnosis.
The immunohistochemical results can be summarized in a Table.

Table. Immunohistochemical results.

Monoclonal antibody	Source*	Specificity	Tissue preparation	Staining result
anti-cytokeratin (2080)	SANBIO	Epithelial cells	Frozen section	Negative
anti-vimentin (V9)	SANBIO EURODIAGN.	Connective tissue, melacytes	Frozen section	Markedly positive, diffuse
anti-desmin (D33)	SANBIO	Muscular cells	Frozen sections	Negative
anti-neurofilament (2F11)	SANBIO	Neuronal cells	Frozen section	Negative
anti-leukocyte antigen (2B11, PD7/26)	DAKO	Leucocytes	Frozen section	Negative
anti-high molecular weight antigen	Dr. S. Ferrone NY Med. Coll. Valhalla, NY, USA	Melanocytic tumors	Frozen section	Positive, local
M.2.2.4	Dr. C. Sorg Wilhelms Univ. Münster, FRG	Melanocytic tumors	Frozen section	Positive, local
NKI/C3	Dr. C. Vennegoor Neth. Cancer Inst. Amsterdam, The Netherlands	Melanocytic tumors	Paraffin section	Markedly positive, diffuse
Anti-S100 (polyvalent antiserum)	DAKO	Melanocytic tumors, Schwann cell tumors	Paraffin section	Markedly positive, diffuse

*For further details on the source of the antibodies with list of available monoclonal antibodies and manufacturers. see APPENDIX .

The staining for vimentin and for melanoma-associated antigens strongly supports the diagnosis of clear cell sarcoma. In Fig. 2. the staining with NKI/C3 is shown.

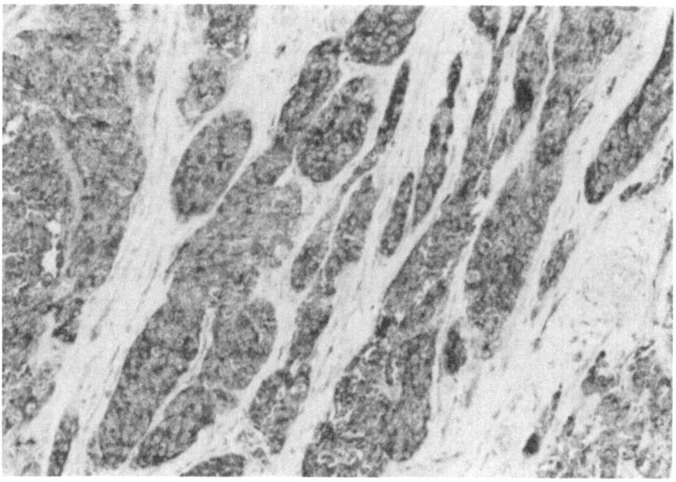

Fig. 2. Clear cell sarcoma of bone showing marked staining with the monoclonal antibody NKI|C3 (x 160, with hematoxylin counterstaining).

Electronmicroscopical examination revealed premelanosomes in occasional tumor cells, giving further evidence for melanocytic differentiation. Therefore, a diagnosis of clear cell sarcoma of bone was made.

TREATMENT AND CLINICAL COURSE

During further clinical investigation an enlarged lymph node was found in the left inguinal region and excised. Pathological examination showed a lymph node metastasis of clear cell sarcoma. Local radiotherapy was given and in addition chemotherapy, consisting of doxorubicin and ifosfamide. During treatment signs of lymphangitis carcinomatosa developed in both lungs.
Seven months after biopsy the patient died of massive intrathoracal and intraabdominal tumor metastases. Autopsy was not performed.

DISCUSSION

Clear cell sarcoma of soft tissues is a relatively rare tumor, only 141 cases have been reported (1). It represents approximately 1% of the total number of soft tissue sarcomas (2). Because in two-third of the cases melanin granules and/or premelanosomes are found (1) this tumor is considered by Enzinger and Weiss as melanoma of soft parts (3). Van Duinen et al. (4) reported staining of 1 out of 3 cases of clear cell sarcoma with the monoclonal antibody NKI/C3, giving further support for this designation. A neural crest origin was also suggested by Kindblom et al. (5) and Mukai et al. (6), who reported staining with anti-S100. Primary clear cell sarcoma of bone is much rarer than that of soft tissues. In the Registry of the Netherlands Committee on Bone Tumors comprising 1970 malignant cases only 2 cases of primary clear cell sarcoma of bone have been collected (Th.G. van Rijssel, personal communication).

The diagnosis of poorly differentiated melanocytic tumors remains difficult despite the use of additional immunohistochemical and electronmicroscopical techniques (4). Sufficient sampling of tumor tissue for histological examination in our experience is important for identification of areas with evidence of melanin production by tumor cells. The most sensitive and specific staining procedure for melanin is the modified Warthin-Starry technique (7), that can be applied even on semithin and ultrathin epoxy resin sections (8). If no melanin can be demonstrated the diagnosis amelanotic melanoma can be assessed by a combination of immunohistochemistry and electron microscopy (4). Immunohistochemistry for melanoma-associated antigens has a much higher sensitivity than electron microscopy for premelanosomes or enzyme histochemistry for tyrosinase, but currently its specifity is less.

REFERENCES

1. Enzinger FM, Weiss SW: Soft Tissue Tumors. St. Louis: The CV Mosby Cy, USA, 1983.

2. Plavidis NA, Fisher C, Wiltshaw E: Clear-cell sarcoma of tendons and aponeuroses: a clinicopathologic study. Cancer 54: 1412-1417, 1984.

3. Chung EB, Enzinger FM: Malignant melanoma of soft parts. A reassessment of clear cell sarcoma. Am. J. Surg. Pathol. 7: 405-413, 1983.

4. Van Duinen SG, Ruiter DJ, Hageman P, Vennegoor C, Dickersin GR, Scheffer E, Rümke Ph: Immunohistochemical and histochemical tools in the diagnosis of amelanotic melanoma. Cancer 53: 1566-1573, 1984.

5. Kindblom LG, Lodding P, Angervall L: Clear cell sarcoma of tendons and aponeuroses; an immunohistochemical and electronmicroscopic analysis indicating neural crest origin. Virch. Arch (Path. Anat) 401: 109-128, 1983.

6. Mukai M, Torikata C, Iri H, Mikata A, Kawai T, Hanaoka H, Yakumaru K, Kageyama K.: Histogenesis of clear cell sarcoma of tendons and aponeuroses. Am. J. Pathol. 114: 264-272, 1984.

7. Warkel RL, Luna LG, Helwig EB: A modified Warthin-Starry procedure at low pH for melanin. Am. J. Clin. Pathol. 73: 812-815, 1980.

8. Van Duinen SG, Ruiter DJ, Scheffer E: A staining procedure for melanin in semithin and ultrathin epoxy sections. Histopathology 7: 35-48, 1983.

CASE PRESENTATIONS.

21. CASE 4: TYPE OF SMALL-CELL UNDIFFERENTIATED CANCER?

D.J. RUITER, W.V. DOLSMA

CLINICAL FINDINGS

A 34-year old woman was admitted to an outside hospital because of acute loss of vision of the right eye. Conventional X-ray examination revealed an irregular osteolytic defect of the right maxilla with marked destruction and extension into the maxillar sinus and orbita and the base of the skull. CT scanning showed a large mass in the pterygoid fossa with extensive bone involvement. A small trans-nasal biopsy was taken. Frozen section examination revealed a small-cell undifferentiated tumor, probably sarcoma.

The patient was referred to our hospital for further diagnosis and treatment. Here, a second biopsy for further typing of the tumor was taken.

PATHOLOGICAL FINDINGS

Unfixed tissue fragments with a maximal dimension of 0.5 cm were received for pathological examination. Representative fragments were taken for conventional histology. In addition, tissue was snap-frozen for immunohistochemistry and fixed for electron-microscopy. Histological examination showed partly edematous, partly cellular and compact tumor tissue, consisting of small undifferentiated cells (Fig. 1). The tumor cells were occasionally star or spindle shaped. The nuclei were relatively monomorphic, oval, but hyperchromatic. Scattered mitotic figures were found. Locally large epitheloid cells with abundant eosinophilic cytoplasm were observed. However, clear cross-striation could not be demonstrated. No glycogen was found.

Locally fine fibrillar intercellular material was seen; no osteoid or chondroid substance could be demonstrated.

Based on this histological appearance a differential diagnosis of embryonal rhabdomyosarcoma or esthesioneuroblastoma was made. Additional immunohistochemical and electronmicroscopical examination was performed in order to discriminate between these possibilities, and to exclude other diagnoses. The tissue processed for electronmicroscopy was not representative. The immunohistochemical results can be summarized in Table 1.

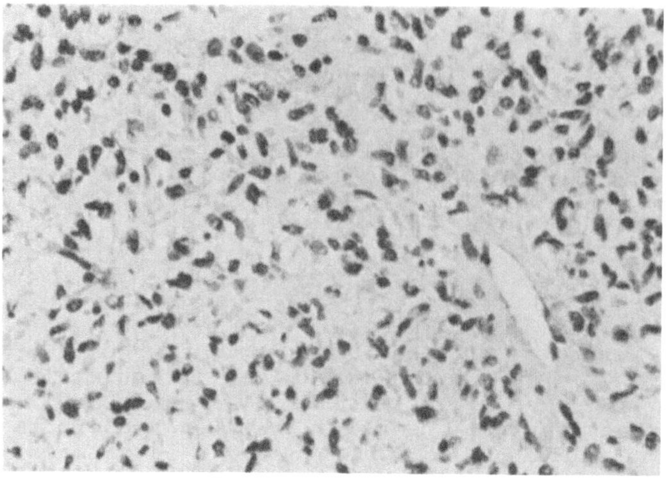

Figure 1. Poorly differentiated malignant small-cell tumor of the maxillary sinus (x400, H and E staining).

Table 1. Immunohistochemical results.

Monoclonal antibody	Source*	Specificity	Tissue preparation	Staining result
anti-cytokeratin (2080)	SANBIO	Epithelial cells	Frozen section	Negative
anti-vimentin (V9)	SANBIO	Connective tissue	Frozen	Positive, diffuse
anti-desmin (D33)	SANBIO	Muscular cells	Frozen section	Large cells markedly positive, small cells weakly positive
anti-neurofilament (2F11)	SANBIO	Neuronal cells	Frozen section	Negative
anti-GFAP (GFAP)	SANBIO	Glial cells	Frozen section	Negative
anti-common leukocyte antigen (2B11, PD7/26)	DAKO	Leukocytes	Frozen section	Negative

*For further details on the source of the antibodies with list of available monoclonal antibodies and manufacturers. see APPENDIX.

The staining for desmin strongly supports the diagnosis embryonal rhabdomyosarcoma, and argues against esthesioneuroblastoma. In Fig. 2 the staining with a monoclonal antibody recognizing desmin is shown.

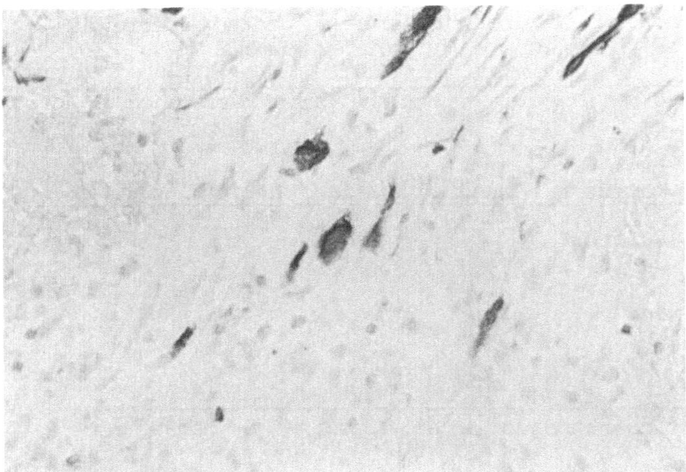

Fig.2. embryonal rhabdomyosarcoma of the maxilla showing marked staining with an anti-desmin monoclonal antibody. Note staining preference for large epitheloid cells (x 400, with hematoxylin counterstaining).

TREATMENT AND CLINICAL COURSE

The patient was treated with ifosfamide, vincristine and actinomycin-D. Because no response was observed after three courses the chemotherapy was changed into cis-platinum and doxorubicin, which resulted in partial response. Because of chemotherapy-induced leukopenia the tumor was irradiated with the linear accelerator, energy 8 MeV. Eight months after diagnosis the patient is alive with local tumor; no evidence of metastasis.

DISCUSSION

The diagnosis of small-cell malignant undifferentiated tumors of childhood (that also may occur in young adults, as is illustrated by this case) has been improved by the application of immunohistochemistry and electron microscopy (1-3). The contribution of immunohistochemistry to the diagnosis of small-cell malignant undifferentiated tumors (derived from (4) and our own experience) is summarized in Table 2.

From this Table it can be concluded that the use of (monoclonal) antibodies recognizing intermediate-sized filaments has proven valuable especially for identification of rhabdomyosarcoma, neuroblastoma and undifferentiated carcinoma.

Table 2. Contribution of immunohistochemistry to the differential diagnosis of small-cell malignant undifferentiatied tumors.

	Staining results* with monoclonal antibodies recognizing				
Tumor type	Cytokeratin	Vimentin	Desmin	Neurofil.	Leukocyte common antigen
Ewing sarcoma	-	+	-	-	-
Lymphoma	-	+	-	-	+
Neuroblastoma	-	-	-	-/+	-
Rhabdomyosarcoma	-	-/+	+	-	-
Carcinoma	+	-/+	-	-	-
Nephroblastoma	-/+	+	-	-	-

*+: positive; -|+ occasionally or locally positive, -: negative.

Further immunohistochemical or electronmicroscopical examination is then needed to type lymphoma or carcinoma, and to confirm the diagnosis of neuroblastoma if only local staining for neurofilament is found. In neuroblastoma, neuroendocrine granules can be demonstrated, or positive staining with antibodies against neuroendocrine markers (5). The diagnosis of Ewing sarcoma can be made with confidence if the radiological appearance is compatible, glycogen is demonstrable in the cytoplasm of the tumor cells, vimentin in the only filament type present and abortive intercellular junctions are found electronmicroscopically.

Staining for desmin in large-cell or spindle cell sarcomas is found not only in case of rhabdomyosarcoma, but also in leiomyosarcoma (1,2,4). The diagnosis rhabdomyosarcoma can be established if the tumor also contains myoglobin or skeletal muscle actin as demonstrated by immunohistochemistry (6,7) or if Z-bands can be demonstrated by electronmicroscopy.

REFERENCES

1. Brooks JJ: Immunohistochemistry of soft tissue tumors: Progress and prospects. Hum. Pathol. 13: 969-974, 1982.
2. Miettinen M, Lehto V-P, Badley RA, Virtanen I: Expression of intermediate filaments in soft tissue sarcomas. Int. J. Cancer 29: 541-547, 1982.
3. Kahn HJ, Yeger H, Kassim O, Jorgensen AO, MacLennan DH, Baumal R, Smith CR, Phillips MJ: Immunohistochemical and electronmicroscopical assessment of childhood rhabdomyosarcoma. Cancer 51: 1897-1903, 1983.

4. Osborn M, Altmannsberger M, Debus E, Weber K: Differentiation of the major human tumor groups using conventional and monoclonal antibodies specific for individual intermediate filament proteins. Annals New York Acad. Sci. 455: 649-668, 1985.
5. Sappino AP, McIlhinney RAJ, Ellison M, Monaghan P, Munro Neville A: A monoclonal antibody detecting neural and neuroendocrine differentiation. J. Histochem. Cytochem. 32: 1041-1047, 1984.
6. Mukai K, Rosai J, Hallaway BE: Localization of myoglobin in normal and neoplastic skeletal muscle cells using an immunoperoxidase method. Am. J. Surg. Pathol. 3: 373-376, 1979.
7. Corson JM, Pinkus GS: Intracellular myoglobin - a specific marker for skeletal muscle differentiation in soft tissue sarcomas. An immunoperoxidase study. Am. J. Pathol. 103: 384-390, 1981.

CASE PRESENTATIONS.

22. CASE 5: TYPE OF EPITHELOID AND CLEAR CELL CANCER?

D.J. RUITER, A.H.M. TAMINIAU.

CLINICAL FINDINGS

A 80-year old woman was admitted to the hospital because of pain in the left hip. X-ray examination revealed an irregular osteolytic defect in the acetabulum with marked extraosseal extension. A differential diagnosis of metastatic carcinoma or primary malignant bone tumor was made. An open biopsy was taken.

PATHOLOGICAL FINDINGS

An unfixed irregular piece of solid grey-brown tissue with maximal dimensions of 4x3x1 cm was received for pathological examination. Representative slices were taken for conventional histology. In addition, tissue was snap-frozen for immunohistochemistry and fixed for electronmicroscopy. Histological examination showed cellular, partly epitheloid, partly spindle shaped tumor tissue, in a diffuse pattern (Fig. 1). The tumor cells showed a compact amphophylic cytoplasm; no demonstrable glycogen. Marked nuclear pleomorphism and hyperchromasia were seen and many mitotic figures observed. Locally giant tumor cells with large bizarr nuclei were found. No glandular formations were seen. Between the tumor cells slender bands of hyalinized collagen were found, no osteoid could be demonstrated. Marked invasion into striated muscle was present.
Based on this histological appearance a differential diagnosis of metastatic carcinoma or sarcoma, probably malignant fibrous histocytoma was considered. Additional immunohistochemical and electronmicroscopical examination was done in order to discriminate between these possibilities, and to exclude other diagnoses.
The immunohistochemical results can be summarized in a Table*.

*For further details on the source of the antibodies with list of available monoclonal antibodies and manufacturers see APPENDIX.

Table. Immunohistochemical results.

Monoclonal antibody	Source*	Specificity	Tissue preparation	Staining result
anti-cytokeratin (2080)	SANBIO	Epithelial cells	Frozen section	Markedly positive, majority of tumor cells
anti-vimentin (V9)	SANBIO	Connective tissue,	Frozen section	Markedly positive, all tumor cells
anti-desmin (D33)	SANBIO	Muscular cells	Frozen sections	Negative
anti-neurofilament (2F11)	SANBIO	Neuronal cells	Frozen section	Negative
anti-leukocyte antigen (2B11, PD7/26)	DAKO	Leucocytes	Frozen section	Negative
OV632	Dr.G.J.Fleuren	Ovarian carcinoma	Frozen section	Negative
G 250	Dr.S.O.Warnaar	Renal cell carcinoma	Frozen section	Markedly positive, minority of tumor cells
RC 38	Dr.S.O.Warnaar	Renal cell carcinoma	Frozen section	Negative
anti-thyreoglobulin	Dr.G.J.Fleuren	Thyroid epithelial cells	Paraffin section	Negative
anti-CEA	Dr. M. Nap	Malignant epithelial tumor cells of colon, lung breast	Paraffin section	Negative
Anti-S100 (polyvalent antiserum)	DAKO	Melanocytic tumors, Schwann cell tumors	Paraffin section	Negative

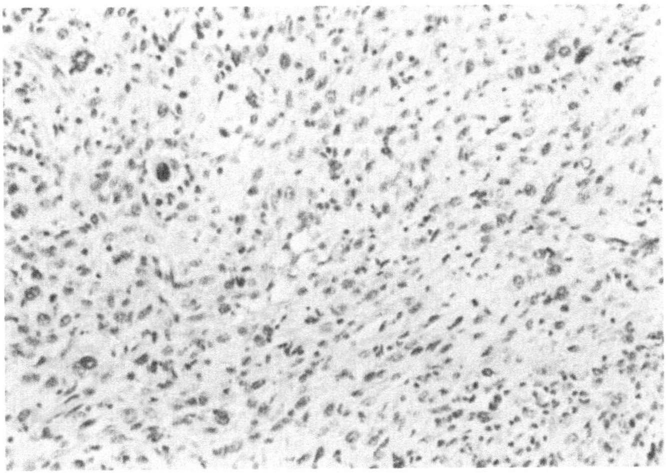

Fig. 1. Poorly differentiated malignant tumor of bone with epitheloid and spindle cell appearance (x 160, H and E staining).

Co-expression of vimentin and cytokeratin can be found in occasional carcinomas (e.g. renal cell carcinoma, thyroid carcinoma), mesothelioma and in some sarcomas (i.e. synovial sarcoma, epitheloid sarcoma). Because of the staining with G 250 and the absence of staining with antibodies recognizing other tumor types the diagnosis of metastatic renal carcinoma was considered most likely. In Fig. 2 the staining results with anti-vimentin, anti-cytokeratin and G250 are shown. Electronmicroscopical examination showed complex cellular interdigitations and abortive intercellular junctions. No evidence for histiocytic differentiation was found. It was concluded, that the electronmicroscopical appearance did not allow discrimination between poorly differentiated carcinoma and poorly differentiated sarcoma.

Fig. 2. (A, B, and C). Metastatic renal carcinoma of bone showing marked staining with the monoclonal antibodies recognizing vimentin (A), cytokeratin (B) and a renal cell carcinoma-associated antigen (C). Note that the staining pattern is diffuse in A, less diffuse in B and focal in C. (x 160, with hematoxylin counterstaining).
(See following page).

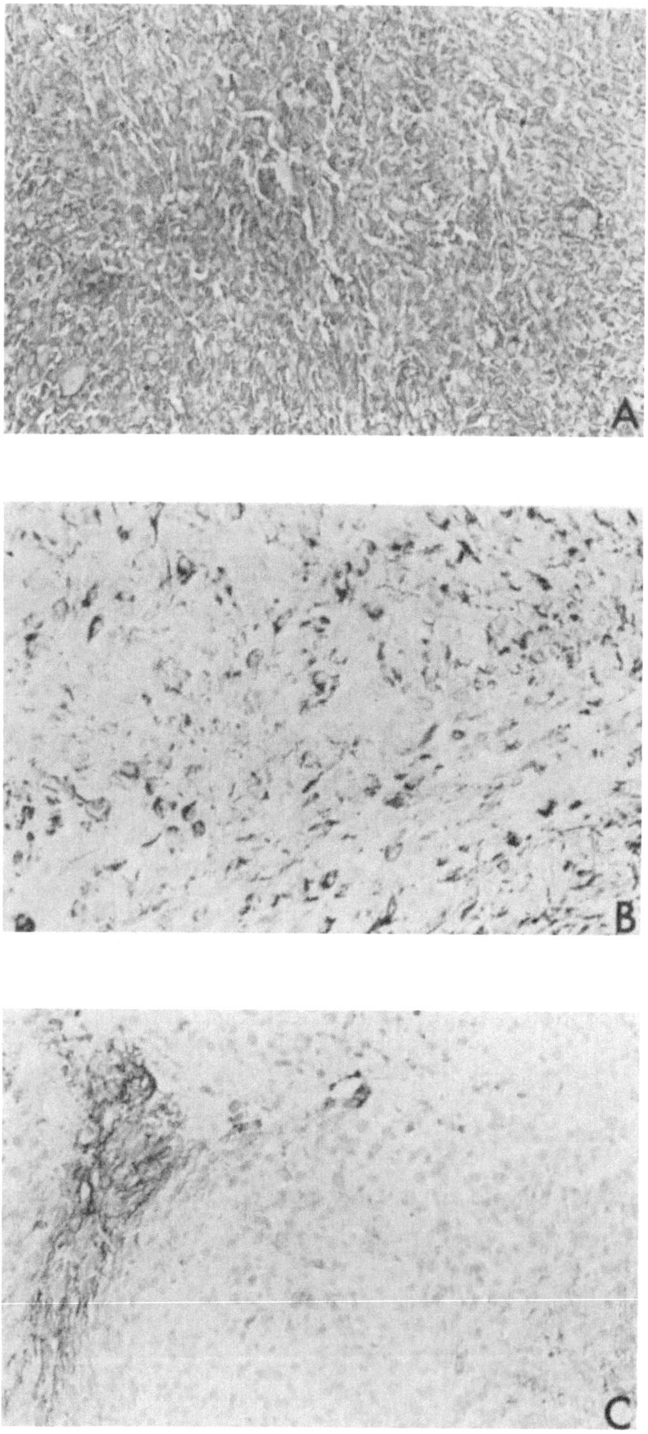

TREATMENT AND CLINICAL COURSE.
Clinically no evidence for a primary extraossal tumor could be found. The patient was treated with local radiotherapy. During follow-up hematuria developed, and a tumor could be palpated in the left flank. A needle biopsy taken from this tumor revealed a histopathological diagnosis of adenocarcinoma compatible with renal carcinoma. The patient died six months after the initial biopsy. Autopsy was not performed.

DISCUSSION
The differential diagnosis of poorly differentiated epitheloid and spindle cell malignant tumors comprizes sarcomatoid carcinoma, malignant melanoma, malignant mesothelioma and sarcoma, especially synovial sarcoma, epitheloid sarcoma, malignant fibrous histiocytoma and malignant epitheloid Schwannoma. Because of the co-expression of vimentin and cytokeratin in this case the possibilities of malignant melanoma, malignant fibrous histiocytoma and malignant Schwannoma are highly unlikely (1). Malignant mesothelioma is not likely either because of the localization in the pelvis. Epitheloid sarcoma is also not likely because of the absence of guirlande-like necrosis and the presence of marked nuclear atypia. Synovial sarcoma is less likely than metastatic sarcomatoid carcinoma because of the localization in bone and the absence of glandular formations in the epitheloid cell areas. Therefore, metastatic carcinoma is the most probable diagnosis. Because of the localization in bone in this female patient metastasis of breast carcinoma, thyroid carcinoma, renal cell carcinoma and lung carcinoma have to be considered as origin of the pelvic metastasis. The staining with the monoclonal antibody RC 250 supports the possibility of renal cell carcinoma (2). Furthermore, in renal cell carcinoma the expression of vimentin often exceeds that of cytokeratin (3, 4).

REFERENCES
1. Ruiter DJ, Van Muijen GNP, Warnaar SO. Monoclonal antibodies in diagnostic tumor pathology. Koprowski H, Ferrone S, Albertini S (eds.): Biotechnology in diagnostics. Amsterdam/New York/Oxford: Elsevier Sciene Publ., pp. 31-43, 1985.

2. Oosterwijk E, Ruiter DJ, Wakka JC, Huiskens-Van der Meij JW, Jonas U, Fleuren GJ, Zwartendijk J, Hoedemaeker Ph, Warnaar SO. Immunohistochemical analysis of monoclonal antibodies to renal antigens: application in the diagnosis of renal cell carcinoma. Am. J. Pathol. (in press).

3. Herman CJ, Moesker O, Kant A, Huysmans A, Vooys GP, Ramaekers FCS. Is renal (Grawitz) tumor a carcino-sarcoma? Evidence from analysis of intermediate

filament types. Virchow's Arch. (Cell Pathol) 44: 73-83, 1983.

4. Holthöfer, Miettinen A, Paasivuo R, Lehto V-P, Linder E, Alfthau O, Virtanen I. Cellular origin and differentiation of renal carcinomas. A fluorescence microscopic study with kidney specific antibodies, anti-intermediate filament antibodies and lectins. Lab. Invest. 49: 317-326, 1983.

CASE PRESENTATIONS.

23. CASE 6: MESOTHELIOMA OR ADENOCARCINOMA?

S.C. HENZEN-LOGMANS, W.F.M. STRANKINGA, H. MULLINK, C.J.L.M. MEIJER

CLINICAL FINDINGS

A 60-year old man was admitted to the hospital because of pain in the right thorax with dyspnea. Anamnestically no asbest contact was known. X-ray examination revealed only pleural effusion, no further characteristics. Cytological examination of the pleural effusion showed malignant cell groups on which a distinction between adenocarcinoma or mesothelioma was not possible. Thoracoscopy revealed a thickened parietal pleural wall. Biopsies showed only chronic inflammation with fibrosis. Surgical biopsies were taken to achieve a histological diagnosis.

PATHOLOGICAL FINDINGS

Three unfixed pieces of fibrous tissue measuring 2 x 1 x 1 and 1 x 1 x 2.5 cm, respectively. Representative tissue specimens were embedded in paraffin for conventional histology. In addition tissue was snap frozen in liquid nitrogen for immmunohistochemistry or fixed in 2% phosphate buffered glutaraldehyde (pH 7.4) for electron microscopy (EM). Histological examination revealed collagen rich stroma with a varying cellularity. Cellular areas showed epithelioid cells arranged partly in solid sheets, partly in duct-like structures and spindle cells. Epithelioid cells showed acidophilic sometimes vacuolated cytoplasm, and rounded vesicular nuclei. Mitoses were rare (see Figures 1 a, b and c).

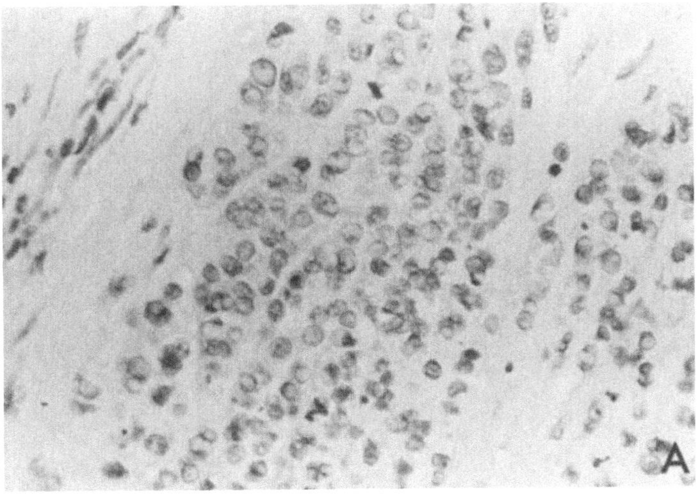

Fig. 1a

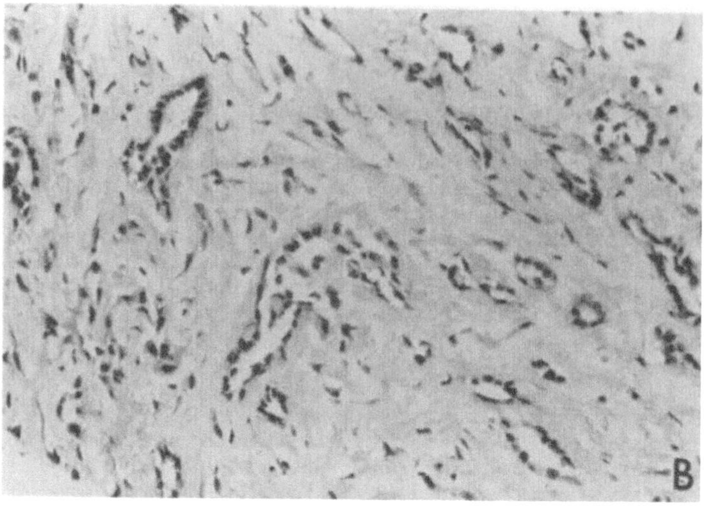

Fig. 1b

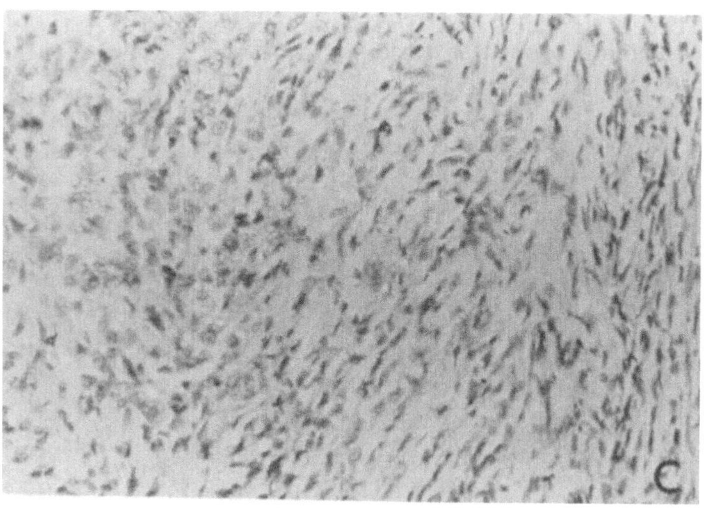

Fig. 1c

Fig. 1. Histological findings in the surgical biopsy of the parietal pleural wall. Collagen rich stroma with varying cellularity: solid sheets of epithelioid cells, with acidophilic sometimes vacuolated cytoplasm, rounded vesicular neclei, rare mitoses (a); other areas showed duct-like structures (b) and spindle cells (c). Haematoxylin-eosin (x 330).

Staining for mucin revealed a few cells with PAS-diastase resistent material in their cytoplasm. The Alcian blue staining showed an apical rim of positivity in the duct-like structures. This positivity disappeared after treatment with hyaluronidase. Although histologically a mesothelioma was most likely, a poorly differentiated adenocarcinoma could not be excluded.
Additional immunohistochemistry (IH) and EM was performed in order to establish the diagnosis.

The immunohistochemical results are summarized in a Table.

TABLE WITH IMMUNOHISTOCHEMICAL RESULTS

MoAb	Specificity	Tissue preparation	Staining results
Anti-cytokeratins (2080)	cytokeratins (broad spectrum). Nearly all epithelial cells react	frozen/formalin* fixed sections	positive
Anti-vimentin Vim-9	Vimentin mesenchymal cells react	frozen/formalin* fixed sections	positive
Anti-CEA (parlam 1)	epithelial cells react	formalin fixed sections	negative

* preincubation with pronase is necessary to restore antigenecity.

For details of the source of monoclonal antibodies see APPENDIX with list of available monoclonal antibodies and manufacturers.

A special double immunoenzyme staining technique was used to study the co-expression of cytokeratins and vimentin in the same cell (1). Cytokeratins showed a more peripheral and vimentin a cytoplasmic perinuclear distribution pattern (see fig. 2).
The co-expression of cytokeratins and vimentin within the same cell, its distribution pattern and the negative staining with anti-CEA strongly supports the diagnosis of mesothelioma (2,3).
EM revealed cells with "bushy" microvilli at the cell surface, giving further evidence.
The immunohistochemical and EM findings lead us to a diagnosis of mesothelioma.

figure 2

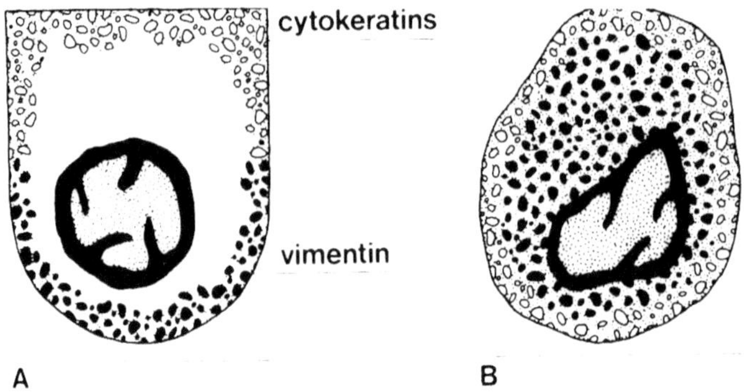

Fig. 2. Schematic drawing of the possible distribution pattern of cytokeratins and vimentin. The figure shows the distribution pattern of cytokeratins and vimentin as detected by the double immunoenzyme staining technique using K 2080 and Vim-9.
Cell type A shows vimentin orientated near the basal end and cytokeratins near the apical end of the cells. This pattern can be observed in some well differentiated adenocarcinomas.
Cell type B shows vimentin in a perinuclear and cytokeratin in a peripheral orientation. This pattern is observed in mesotheliomas, also in the duct-like structures, and can also be found in part of the undifferentiated carcinomas.

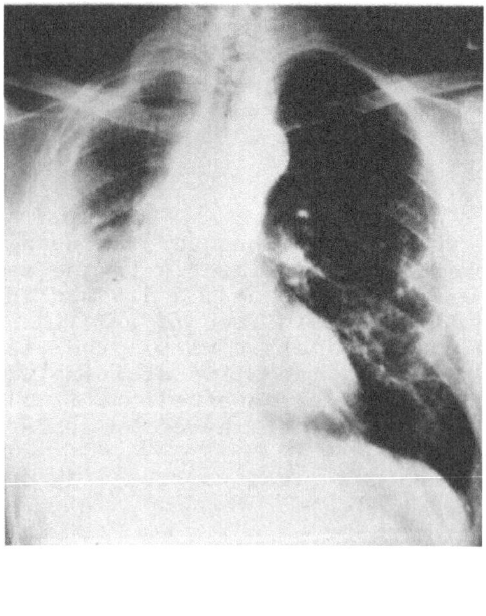

Fig. 3. X-ray made after several months: The pleural wall of the right thorax cavity is thickened with obscuring of the diaphragma, retraction of the lung and a shift of the heart and trachea to the right.

CLINICAL COURSE

The patient developed progressive dyspnoe and thoracic pain. An X-ray made after several months showed a picture compatible with mesothelioma (see Figure 3).
The patient died after 17 months.

DISCUSSION

Separating mesotheliomas from carcinomas on a histological picture can be notoriously difficult. Early diagnosis is important because of prognostic, therapeutic, financial consequences. Many groups have looked for additional means to make a definite diagnosis, such as histochemistry and EM but both are not always satisfactory.
Immunohistochemistry has also been used with a variety of markers, amongst them CEA (3). So far, to the best of our knowledge, no marker is 100% specific for mesothelioma. Therefore a small panel of antibodies was used in order to obtain more information.
For mesotheliomas, promising results can be obtained by the use of MoAbs directed against cytokeratins, vimentin and CEA. Mesotheliomas do co-express cytokeratins and vimentin within the same cell. Most adenocarcinomas, especially the well differentiated ones, do not. Most adenocarcinomas from the lung and gastro-intestinal tract do contain CEA, and most mesotheliomas do not (3).
However, there are some pitfalls: 1) co-expression of cytokeratins and vimentin have been found in adenocarcinomas of the thyroid gland, kidney, salivary gland and lung (4,5,6). Undifferentiated carcinomas may also show this co-expression (personal observation). Most adenocarcinomas of the lung, especially the well differentiated ones do not show this co-expression or only in a small number of cells (2); 2) on the presence of CEA in mesotheliomas conflicting reports have been published (3,7). Part of these can be explained by the different antibodies used. In our experience most mesotheliomas do not stain for CEA, or only locally and weak.
With the pitfalls described above in mind, it is possible to achieve a definite diagnosis after careful evaluation of the clinical, histological and immunohistochemical findings obtained with this panel.
The co-expression of cytokeratins and vimentin within the same cell, with a distribution pattern in the duct-like structures (peripheral cytokeratins, peri-nuclear vimentin) found to be present in mesotheliomas, and not in the more differentiated adenocarcinomas; in combination with the negative staining results with anti-CEA this strongly supports the final diagnosis of mesothelioma in this case.

REFERENCES

1. Mullink H, Boorsma DM, Henzen-Logmans SC, Meijer CJLM: Double immunoenzyme staining methods with special reference to monoclonal antibodies. See Chapter 3.

2. Mullink H, Henzen-Logmans SC, Alons van Kordelaar JJM, Tadema T, Meyer CJLM: Diagnosis of malignant mesothelioma by simultaneous immunoenzyme staining of vimentin and keratin with two monoclonal antibodies. Virchows Arch B (Cell Path), in press, 1986.

3. Kwee WS, Veldhuizen RW, Golding RP, Mullink H, Stam J, Donner R, Boon ME: Histologic distinction between malignant mesothelioma, benign pleural lesion and carcinoma metastasis Virchows Arch A, 397: 287-299 - 1982.

4. Henzen-Logmans SC, Mullink H, Ramaekers FCS, Tadema T, Meyer CJLM : Expression of cytokeratins and vimentin in epithelial cells of normal and pathologic thyroid tissue (submitted, 1986).

5. Miettinen M, Franssila,F, Lehto VP, Paasviuo, R, Virtanen,I: Expression of intermediate filament proteins in thyroid gland and thyroid tumors. Lab Invest 50: 262-270, 1984.

6. Miettinen M, Lehto V, Virtanen I: Antibodies to intermediate filament proteins in the diagnosis and classification of human tumors. Ultrastructural pathology 7: 83-107, 1984.

7. Holden J., Churg A : immunohistochemical staining for keratin and carcinoembryonic antigen in the diagnosis of malignant mesothelioma. Am J Surg Pathol 8: 277-279, 1984.

CASE6.MAN/HENZEN1

24. CASE 7: ORIGIN OF METASTATIC CARCINOMA?

G.J. FLEUREN, C. V.D. BERG, O.A.M. LANGEZAAL

CLINICAL FINDINGS

A 73-year old woman was admitted to the hospital because of herniation of an old appendectomy scar. At operation a hernial sac with a diam. of 4 cm was found, which was resected.

PATHOLOGICAL FINDINGS:

The hernial sac consisted of a thick fibrous wall,representative fragments were prepared for conventional histology. Histological examination showed collagenous fibrous and fatty tissue partially covered by a mesothelial lining. Locally cellular areas consisting of solid nests and duct-like structures with high cylindrical cells were present. Nuclear pleomorphism, hyperchromasia and many mitotic figures were observed in these areas. Staining for mucin revealed PAS-Diastase resistent and Alcian blue positive material in vacuoles in the cytoplasm of the duct-like structures,the solid nests being negative. Based on the histological appearance a diagnosis of metastatic adenocarcinoma combined with active mesothelial proliferation and fibrosis was considered.
Additional immunohistochemical examinations were done in order to confirm this diagnosis and to establish the nature of the metastastic carcinoma.
Because consultation of the surgeon made a metastic process derived from colon or ovarian carcinoma most likely, we started with a panel of antibodies discriminative for these tumortypes. The immunohistochemical results are summarized in a table.
Anti-vimentin antibodies are staining both fibrous tissue and mesothelial cells (fig.1.)
The staining for CEA (fig.2) strongly supports the possibility of a tumor of the gastrointestinal tract. The negative staining with OV632 makes an ovarian cancer rather unlikely.
It has to be noticed that OC125 reacts with (reactive) mesothelial cells (fig.3).

TABLE. Immunohistochemical results.

Monoclonal antibody	Specificity	Tissue preparation	Staining result
anti-cytokeratin (2080)	epithelial cells	frozen section	markedly positive, majority of tumor c and mesoth cells
anti-vimentin (Vg)	connective tissue	frozen section tissue	markedly positive c fibrous tissue and mesoth cells
OV632	ovarian carcinoma	frozen section	negative
anti-CEA (F-6)	majority of colon,lung and breast cancers	paraffin section	positive c tumor cel
OC125	ovarian carcinoma (moderately specific)	frozen section	positive c mesothelia cells

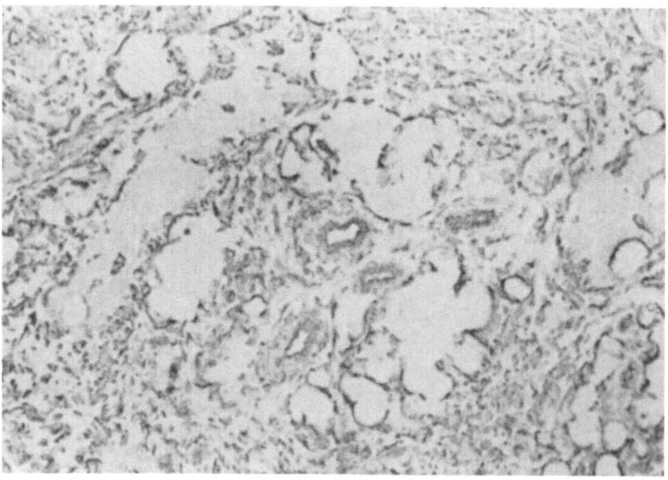

Fig.1 Fibrous cells and mesothelial cells showing abundant positive immunostaining for vimentin. Note negative areas, which consist of epithelial cells (Frozen section, x 200).

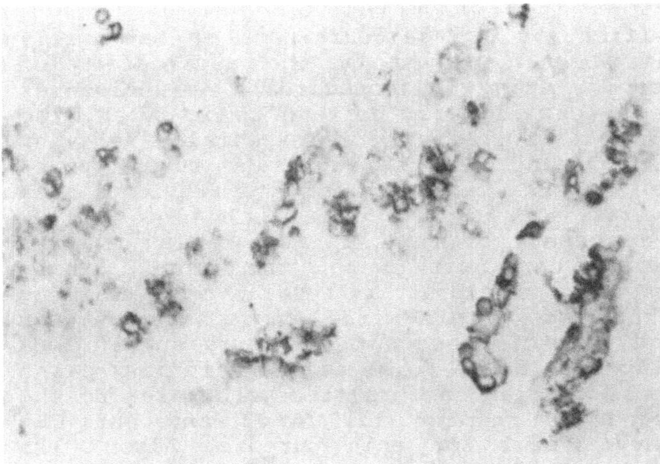

Fig.2 Cytoplasmic staining for CEA. Small lumina are present (Paraffin section, x 500).

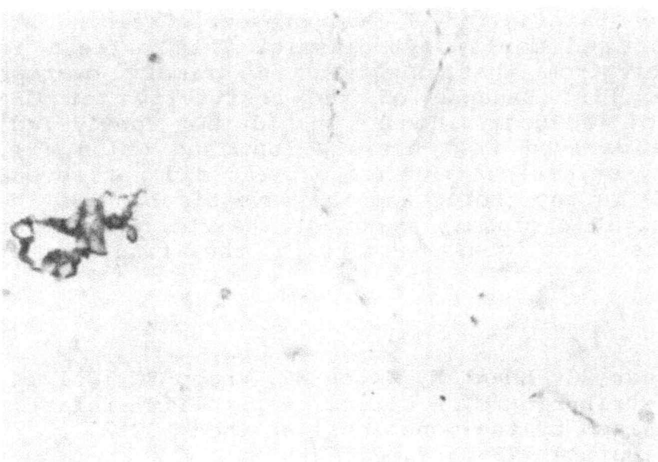

Fig.3 Mesothelial lining and groups of mesothelial cells show positive staining for CA 125, (Frozen section, x 400).

TREATMENT AND CLINICAL COURSE

Two weeks after surgery the patient presented with abdominal pain, vomiting and disturbed defaecation. One week later she developed an ileus. At operation the ileo-coecal area appeared completely obstructed by a tumor in the colon and peritoneal carcinomatosis was present. A palliative surgical procedure i.e. a bypass was performed.

DISCUSSION

The further classification ot adenocarcinoma of ostensibly unknown origin has been improved by the application of immunohistochemistry using (monoclonal) antibodies recognizing antigens specificy for certain tumor types. The contribution of immunohistochemistry is especially relevant if treatment is different for the different tumor types. This is the case in adenocarcinoma of the thyroid, the prostate or the ovary.

In the presented case, clinically metastatic ovarian carcinoma or colon carcinoma were the most likely possibilities. Several monoclonal antibodies with varying specificity are known to react with nonmucinous ovarian carcinoma. Although none of these antibodies is specific, a combination of antibodies seems to be adequate in most cases to discrimate primary ovarian cancers from metastases to the ovary. As discussed in chapter 13, OV632 and anti-CEA antibodies are very useful for this purpose. Also OC125 sometimes can be informative (1).

The data presented in this case presentation indicate that these antibodies are especially useful when a metastasis either from a tumor of the gastro-intestinal tract or of the ovary is a possibility. In the present case OV632 and OC125 did not react with the metastatic tumor tissue. On the other hand an extensive staining for CEA was present. Staining was diffusely present and merely cytoplasmic. This pattern is totally different from that observed in primary ovarian cancers (chapter 13). Because of the positivity for CEA several types of adenocarcinomas should be considered, especially those derived from breast, lung and colon (2). Because X-ray investigations in this patient did not reveal any abnormalities in the thorax and the investigation of the breast was negative, a primary tumor ot the colon was most likely. This was also consistent with the findings at laparotomy.

REFERENCES

1. Kabawat SE, Bast RC, Bhan AK, Welch WR, Knapp RC, Colvin RB. Tissue distribution of a coelomic-epithelium-related antigen recognized by the monoclonal antibody OC125. Int.J.Gynecol.Pathol. 1983; 2: 275-285.
2. Nap M, Keuning H, Burtin P, Oosterhuis JW, Fleuren GJ. CEA and NCA in benign and malignant breast tumors. Am.J.Clin.Pathol. 1984; 82:526-534.

CASE PRESENTATIONS

25. CASE 8: TYPE OF CARCINOMA IN THE LIVER?

M. NAP

CLINICAL FINDINGS

A 60 year old male was admitted to an outside hospital for surgery because of an atherosclerotic aneurysm of the abdominal aorta.

During operation inspection of the abdominal cavity revealed a 2.5 cm large nodule in the left liver lobe that was excised with a margin of surrounding liver tissue.

HISTOPATHOLOGICAL FINDINGS

Histological examination showed a relatively well circumscribed lesion, composed of gland-like structures which varied in size and shape. Locally the gland-like structures infiltrated into the adjacant liver parenchyma (Fig. 1).

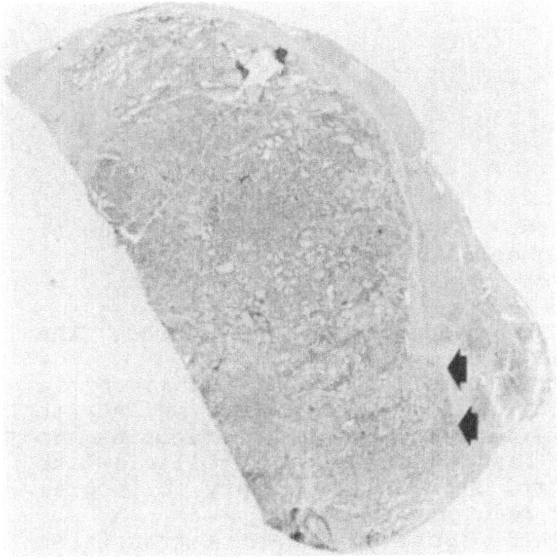

Fig.1 Low-power view section of the tumor illustrating the infiltrative growth (arrows) into the preexisting liver parenchyma.
(H and E stain, x 5)

The lumina of these structures contained an eosinophilic substance with a moth eaten aspect at the epithelial surface resembling thyroid follicles (Fig. 2).

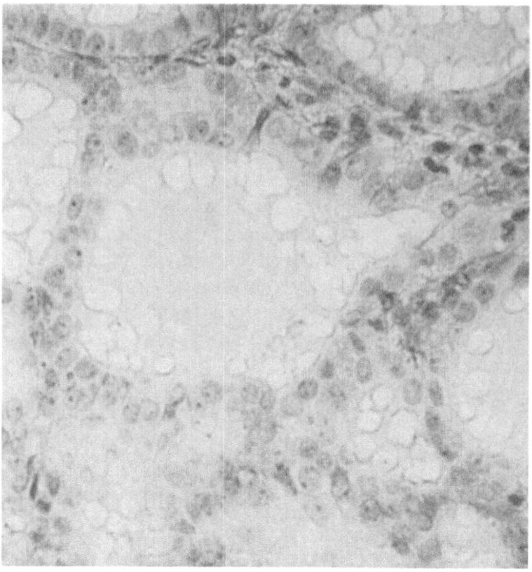

Fig.2 High-power view to illustrate the follicular structures containing colloid-like material (H and E stain, x 400)

Mitotic figures were rare; no necrosis was found. The resection margins were free of tumor.
Sections and blocks were then referred to our laboratory in order to confirm the histological diagnosis: metastatic thyroid carcinoma in the liver. However, antibodies to thyroglobulin did not react with the follicle-like structures, whereas a control section of primary follicular thyroid carcinoma strongly reacted positive.
Careful examination of H.& E. sections showed a transition between the cuboid tumor cells lining the follicular structures and tumor cells in a more trabecular arrangment, suggestive of hepatocellular differentiation (Fig. 3).

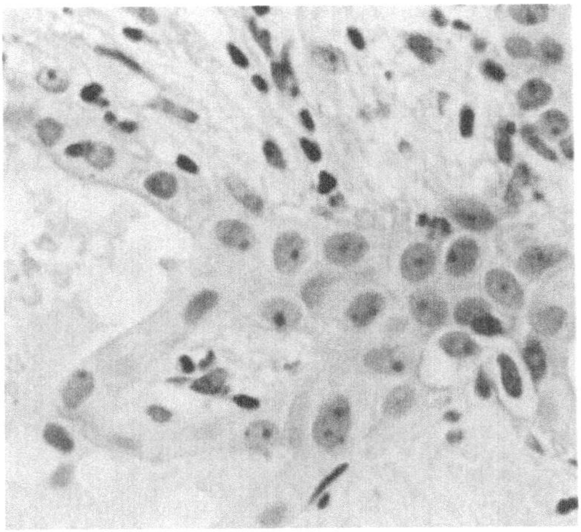

Fig.3 Trabecular growth pattern suggestive of hepatocellular differentiation. (H and E stain x 400)

Therefore, hepatocellular carcinoma resembling follicular thyroid cancer (1) was then considered as one of the differential diagnostic possibilities. In support of this diagnosis extensive clinical examination did not give evidence for a primary thyroid carcinoma or any other tumor.

FURTHER IMMUNOHISTOCHEMICAL STUDIES

In order to verify this diagnosis and to exclude others, like metastatic carcinoid, metastatic adenocarcinoma from the gastro-intestinal tract, or prostate further immunohistochemical examination was done. Staining of paraffin sections with antibodies against alphafetoprotein (AFP), carcino embryonic antigen (CEA), and prostate specific antigen (PSA) was negative. No argyrophylic granules could be demonstrated using the Grimelius reaction. In a recently completed study concerning the immunohistological distribution of AFP, CEA, alpha-1-antitrypsin (AAT) and HBsAg, in primary hepatocellular tumors, we have demonstrated a peculiar staining reaction of bile canalicular structures of some anti-CEA antibodies (2), which was the result of "crossreaction" with the biliary glycoprotein 1 (BGP_I). This staining pattern was never observed using monospecific antibodies to CEA. In 80% of primary liver cell carcinomas such a bile canalicular staining pattern could be observed whereas in tumors of non hepatocellular origin this characteristic staining pattern was never observed. Incubation of sections from the present tumor with polyclonal anti-CEA serum, containing amongst others antibodies cross reactive with BGP_I, resulted in this typical bile canalicular staining pattern (fig. 4a, b).

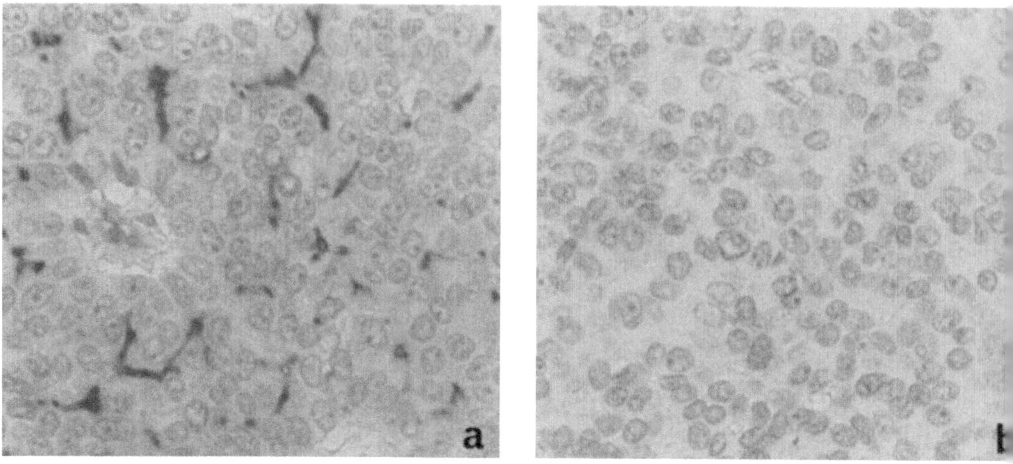

Fig.4a Bile canalicular staining pattern obtained after incubation with BGP_I-cross reactive anti CEA serum on pariffin section.
(immunoperoxidase, Haematoxylin counterstain, x 400)

Fig.4b Same area as 4a showing no reactivity with non cross reactive anti CEA antibodies.
(Immunoperoxidase, Haematoxylin counterstain, x 400)

Therefore, a definite diagnosis of primary hepatocellular carcinoma could be made.

CLINICAL COURSE

Two years after the initial operation because of an aortic aneurysm the patient died. At autopsy (Dr. H.B. Oey, Department of Pathology, Hoogeveen) a rupture of one of the sutures of the artificial aortic graft was found, with consequent intraabdominal bleeding. This was interpreted as the cause of death. No tumor could be found in the liver or any other organ including thyroid, stomach, intestine, lungs, pancreas or prostate.

DISCUSSION

In a immunohistochemical study on 125 primary thyroid carcinomas and their metastasis all follicular structures were positive for thyroglobulin (4). Absence of reactivity with such antibodies in the presence of a good positive control therefore excluded the possibility of metastatic follicular thyroid cancer in our patient. The absence of CEA (with mono specific antibodies) in this liver tumor made a metastatic gastro-intestinal carcinoma highly unlikely. Similarly, the absence of PSA reactivity excluded a metastasis from a prostatic adenocarcinoma. Although AFP is often advocated as an excellent marker of primary hepatocellular carcinoma, its absence in this particular case illustrates its limited sensitivity, as indicated by the literature (5) and our own study (2) in which only in 12% of primary liver cancers AFP could be demonstrated. On the contrary using anti-BGP_I in over 80% of primary liver tumors a bile canalicular staining pattern can be demonstrated, as mentioned earlier (2).

The bile canalicular staining pattern has a higher sensitivity for hepatocellular differentiation than the presence of bile pigment in tumor cells, because bile pigment is seen in only 60% of primary hepatocellular carcinomas (6). Therefore the use of anti-BGP_I antibodies has significance for the diagnosis of hepatocellular carcinoma. The application of immunohistology using antibodies recognizing more or less organ specific antigens in this particular case was clinically relevant, because in our patient no additional invasive diagnostic procedures in search for a possible primary had to be performed.

In conclusion, the major evidence for primary hepatocellular tumor in this case was:

1. Bile canacular staining pattern with anti-BGP_I antibody
2. Absence of tumor in any other organ at autopsy
3. Presence of invasive growth. Therefore our final diagnosis is hepatocellular carcinoma with follicular aspect.

REFERENCES

1. Edmundson H., Tumors of the liver and intrahepatic bile ducts. AFIP fasc. 25, 1958 (Fig. 38).
2. Koelma I.A., Nap M., Huitema S., Krom R.A.F., Houthoff H.J. Hepatocellular Carcinoma, Adenoma and Focal Nodular hyperplasia. A comparative histoplastic study with immunohistochemical parameters. Arch. Path. Lab. Med., 1986 in press.
3. Sijperda A., Thyreoglubine bij hyperthyreoidie en schildkliercarcinoom. Academic Thesis, Groningen, 1984.
4. Mensink H.J.A., Prostaatcarcinoom. gradering en zure fosfatase. Academic Thesis, Groningen, 1984.
5. Thung S.N., Gerber M.A., Saruo E. et al., Distribution of five antigens in hepatocellular carcinoma. Lab. Invest. 1979; 41: 101-105.
6. Anthony P.P. Hepatic neoplasms. In: pathology of the liver. R.N.M. MacSween, P.P. Anthony, P.J. Scheuder (eds), Edinburgh. London, New York, Churchill Livingstone 1979, pp. 387-413.

CASE PRESENTATIONS.

26. CASE 9: METASTATIC MENINGIOMA:A RARE CAUSE OF DIFFUSE NODULAR LUNG DISEASE.

J.R.J. ELBERS, SJ.SC. WAGENAAR, J.K.TH.M. AUMANN, J.M.N. VAN DEN BOSCH

INTRODUCTION

It is reported that primary extracranial and extraspinal meningiomas occur in the vertebral and paravertebral regions, the paranasal sinuses, the orbita and the skin but are rarely found in the lungs (1, 4). Such an extracranial dissemination of an intracranial "benign appearing" meningioma is sporadically mentioned (3, 6) A high percentage of these metastasizing meningiomas was reported to be of the angioblastic subtype (3, 6)
The diagnosis of "meningioma-like" lesions in both lungs is very difficult (2), even with the use of various additional techniques.
In this brief report we describe a patient suffering from a nodular lung disease, preceded by a craniotomy for a meningioma of the transitional type 5 years earlier.

CLINICAL DATA

A 45 year old woman with a long history of asthma bronchiale was admitted because of multiple pulmonary nodules which had increased in size on sequential chest roentgenograms (Fig. 1).

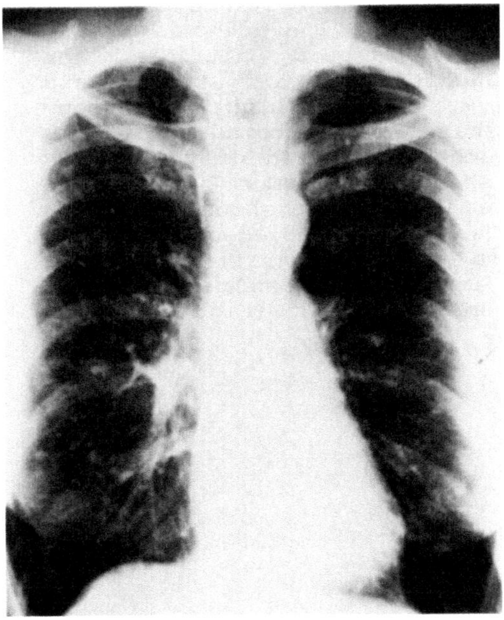

Fig. 1. Multiple nodular densities in middle and lower lung fields.

Five years earlier she had been admitted to our hospital with a frontal headache. At clinical examination a bilateral papilledema was found. An EEG revealed a left frontal hypofunctional area; the left carotid angiogram showed a frontal parasagittal mass. A CT scan demonstrated a large mass extending from the frontal bone with complete compression of the anterior horns and displacement to the right. A left frontal temporal craniotomy was performed and a meningioma of the transitional type, that had invaded the falx, was removed. There were no postoperative complications.

Until now no neurologic symptoms suggesting a cerebral relapse have occured.

On admission to the pulmonary clinic the patient was in good health and asymptomatic. Physical examination revealed no abnormalities, especially no neurologic dysfunction. Routine laboratory data were normal. No acid fast bacilli, pathogenic bacteria or fungi were found both in sputum or bronchial secretions. The PPD was positive.

The chest roentgenogram and tomograms showed multiple nodular, well demarcated densities, especially in the middle and lower lung fields, varying in size up to 1 cm, but uniform in density.

There were no calcifications or excavations. Pleura, mediastinum and heart showed no abnormalities. Intravenous pyelography, mammography and echography of the breast and thyroid revealed no tumor. Bronchoscopy and broncho-alveolar lavage were normal, as was the morphology of bronchial secretions and bronchial biopsies. Finally a left thoracotomy with open lung biopsy was performed.

PATHOLOGICAL DATA

The open lung biopsy specimens showed multiple whitish, glassy nodules of varying dimensions (0.1 - 0.8 cm). Tissue samples were snap frozen in liquid nitrogen for enzymehistochemical and immunohistochemical studies and fixed in glutaraldehyde for E.M. studies. Light microscopy showed deposits of tumor sharply demarcated from the surrounding parenchyma. The tumors consisted of cell nests located in the interstitial space. The tumor cells often surrounded small veins, but a relation to bronchioles or arteries could not be shown. They were spindled or elongated with an eosinophilic cytoplasm and indistinct cytoplasmic borders, and were arranged in whorls, bands and small clusters with oval nuclei and small nucleoli (Fig. 2).

Fig. 2. Arrangement of tumor cells in whorls. (H and E x 200).

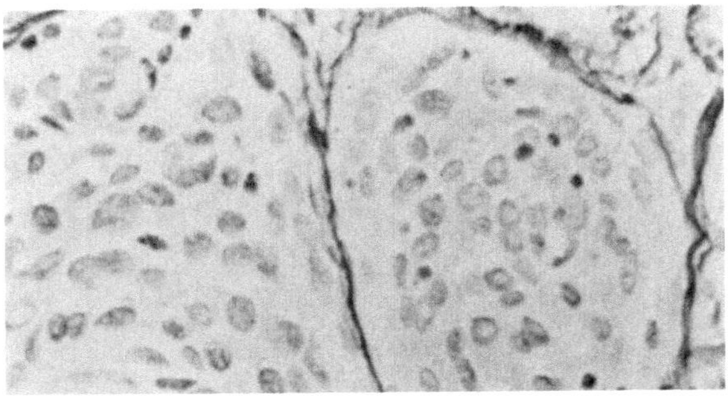

In some nests a psammoma body was seen (Fig. 3).

Fig. 3. Nests of tumor cells with psammoma body. (H and E x 400).

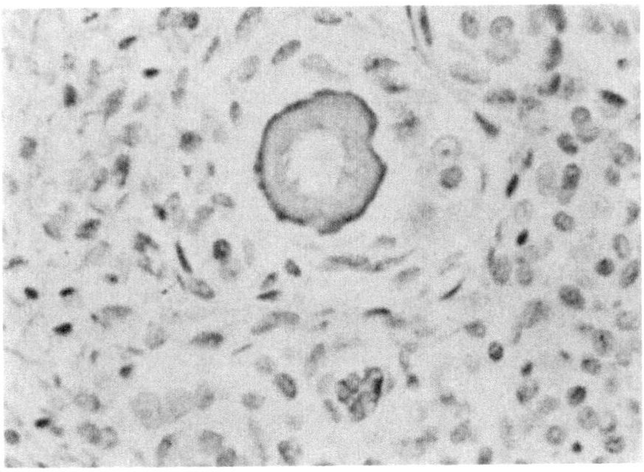

The Grimelius stain was negative. By electronmicroscopical examination the most important features were the presence of interdigitating cell processes, numerous typical desmosomes and absence of basement membranes (Fig. 4).

Fig. 4. Electron micrograph showing typical desmoses, cell processes and absence of basement membranes (x 10.000).

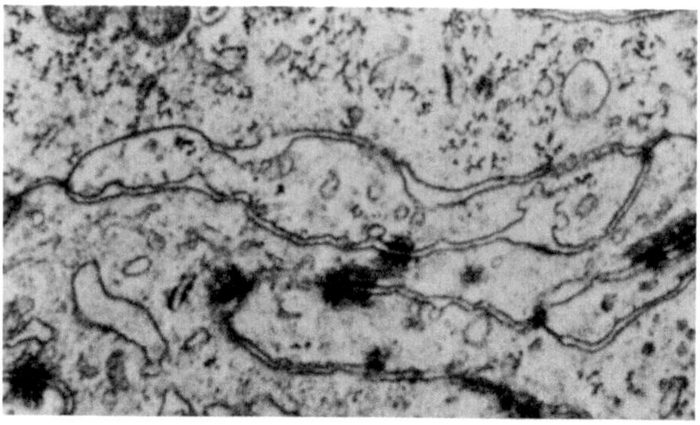

The results of enzyme- and immunohistochemical examination are summarized in table 1.

Table 1. Results of enzym- and immunohistochemical examination of the pulmonary lesions in the patient.

Enzym-histochemistry		Immuno-histochemistry	
Acid Ph.	+	Factor VIII R-ag.	-
Alk. Ph.	+	Vimentin	+
B-Gluc.	+	Keratin	-
Non-Spec. Est.	+	123-C3*	+
ATP-ase	+	Neurofil.	-
5-Nucl.	+	S100	-

*123-C3 = Monoclonal antibody recognizing a neuroendocrine related antigen.

The light- and electron-microscopic, the immuno- and enzymehistochemical findings were consistent with metastatic meningioma. Comparison with the craniotomy specimen showed an identical histological appearance.

DISCUSSION

Tumors in the lung with the histologic appearance of meningiomas are extremely rare.

Primary meningioma of the lung is an extremely rare solitary tumor whose light microscopical and ultrastructural features are identical to intracranial and spinal meningiomas.

Pulmonary lesions originally described by Korn et al. (5) as multiple minute pulmonary chemodectomas have similarities with our case. Light microscopical examination of these lesions reveals interstitial nests of tumor cells with ill-defined cytoplasmic borders often showing a close relation to small veins. The tumor cells are spindled or elongated with sometimes indented vesicular nuclei with finely divided chromatin and small nucleoli. However, most of these cases reported are incidental findings at autopsy in female patients ranging in age from 16-85 years (average 58 years). Over 50% of the cases published show a diffuse distribution over both lungs. Furthermore, minute pulmonary tumors have a maximal diameter of 2 mm.

It is remarkable that Kuhn and Askin (6) and Churg and Warnock (2) have shown, by means of electron microscopical examination, that these lesions have no features of chemodectomas, but resemble meningeoma. The electronmicroscopical features of the both lesions in comparison of those of classical chemodectoma (of the carotid body) are listed in Table 2.

Table 2. Ultrastructural features of minute pulmonary chemodectoma and meningioma and chemodectoma (carotid body).

	Minute pulmonary chemodectoma and meningioma	Classic chemodectoma
Basal lamina	None	Complete
Capillaries	Non-fenestrated	Fenestrated
Cyt. Processes	Long, complex inter-digitating	Long, straight
Cell junctions	Typical desmosomes	Atypical junctional structures
Mitochondria	Few	Many
Dense core granules	Absent	Present

In our case the ultrastructural features were identical to those found in meningioma and so-called minute pulmonary chemodectoma.

Furthermore, enzymehistochemical and immunohistochemical studies were performed on a classical case of (transitional) meningioma and a typical case of chemodectoma (carotid body) and the results were compared with the findings in our patient (Tables 3 and 4).

Table 3. Results of enzymehistochemical examination in our patient and in cases of transitional meningioma and classical chemodectoma.

	Results of this case	Meningioma (transitional)	Classic chemodectoma
Ac. Phosph.	+	+	+
Al. Phosph.	+	+	-
B-Gluc.	+	+	+
N-spec. Esterase	+	+	+
ATP-ase	+	+	-

Table 4. Features of immunohistochemical examination in our patient and in cases of transitional meningioma and classical chemodectoma.

	Results of this case	Meningioma (transitional)	Classic chemodectoma
Vimentin	+	+	+
Keratin	-	-	-
Neurofil.	-	-	+
S100	-	-	-
123-C3*	+	+	+

*see Table 1 for further specification.

The results of immunohistochemical staining were identical in all 3 cases except for staining with anti-neurofilament. The enzymehistochemical results of our case were similar to those of the case of transitional meningioma and deviated of those seen in classical chemodectoma.
Unfortunately, results of enzyme and immunohistochemical studies in so-called minute pulmonary chemodectoma have not been reported in the literature. Perhaps the techniques mentioned could be of further help in differentiating these pulmonary lesions.
Only a few cases concerning extra-cranial metastasis of benign appearing meningiomas in the lungs have been reported (3, 7). It is noteworthy that in these cases intracranial surgery was usually performed.

Review of the slides of the primary tumor in our case, surgically removed 5 years before, revealed no histologic signs of malignancy. We believe that the pulmonary lesions are metastases of meningioma, because of the multiplicity and the relatively large size of the pulmonary lesions and the histological similarity of the pulmonary nodules with the craniotomy specimen.
The results of light microscopic examination, immuno- and enzymehistochemical study and electronmicroscopy of the pulmonary nodules of our patient were identical with the results obtained in another case of transitional meningioma.
In conclusion, it is our opinion that we are dealing with an extremely rare case of pulmonary metastases of a benign-appearing intracranial meningioma.

ACKNOWLEDGEMENT
The authors thank Dr. K.P. Dingemans, Department of Pathology, University of Amsterdam, for performing the electronmicroscopical examination, Felie Schmitz du Moulin and Ella Vaarkamp for their excellent technical assistance, Loes Marijnen for skilfully typing this manuscript and M. Blinde and G. Kropheller for the photography.

REFERENCES
1. Chumas JC, Lorell CA. Pulmonary meningioma: A light and electron microscopic study. Am. J. Surg. Path.1982; 6: 795-801.
2. Churg AM, Warnock ML. So-called "minute pulmonary chemodectoma". Cancer 1976; 37: 1759-69.
3. Glasauer FE, Yuan RH. Intracranial tumors with extracranial metastasis: a case report and review of the litterature. J. Neurosurg. 1963; 20: 474-93.
4. Kemnitz P, Spormann H, Heinrich P. Meningioma of lung: first report with light- and electronmicroscopic findings. Ultrastruct. Pathol.: 1982; 3: 359-65.
5. Korn D, Bensch K, Liebow AA, Castleman B. Multiple minute pulmonary tumors resembling chemodectomas. Am. J. Pathol. 1960; 37: 641-672.
6. Kuhn C, Askin FB. The fine structure of so-called minute pulmonary chemodectomas. Hum. Pathol. 1976; 6: 681-691.
7. Shuangshoti, S., Hongsaprabhas C, Netsky MG. Metastasizing meningioma. Cancer 1970; 26: 832-841.

APPENDIX

I. LIST OF MONOCLONAL ANTIBODIES USEFUL IN HISTOPATHOLOGY.

Over the years a growing number of firms have become distributors of monoclonal antibodies. Although very few antibodies are of poor quality there often is some difference in titers, unexpected crossreactions and in amount of unwanted background staining, especially at high concentrations of primary antibody.
In this appendix a list is presented of antibodies that have been found satisfactory by authors of this book. For the staining characteristics of the antibodies in this list the reader should consult the information provided by the distributors.
Additional information can be found in various chapters of this book.

Antibodies recommended by authors of this book.

a. Anti cytoskeletal antibodies:

anti vimentin: MV1 (Eur), MonF 3005 (San)
anti GFAP : PGF (Eur), MonF 3002 (San)
anti desmin : PDE (Eur), MonF 3001 (San)
anti neurofilament: MNF (Eur), MonF 3004 (San)
anti cytokeratin
(broad spectrum): MonF 3003 (San)
anti cytokeratin 10: RKSE60 (Eur)
anti cytokeratin 18: RGE53 (Eur)

b. anti T cell markers:

CD1: Leu6 (B/D), OKT6 (Ortho) (+ Langerhans cells)
66 IL C7 (San)

CD2: Leu5 (B/D) T11 (CC)

CD3: Leu4 (B/D) OKT3 (Ortho)

CD4: Leu3 (B/D)

CD5: Leu1 (B/D), T1 (CC) (+ fraction of B cells)

CD6: Tu 33 (Clon)

CD7: Leu9 (B/D), WT1 (ATCC, SAN)

CD8: Leu2 (B/D), T3 (CC)

c. B cell markers:

CD9: BA2 (Hy)
CD10: BA3 (Hy)
CD19: Leu12 (B/D)
CD20: B1 (CC)

CD21:	10B/a (S.T)
	B2 (C.C.)
CD22:	Leu14 (B/D) M708 (Dako)
CD24:	BA1 (Hy)
anti IGM:	M702 (Dako)
anti IGD:	M703 (Dako)
anti λ :	MonP 5002 (San)

d. myeloid/monocyt markers:

CD11:	OKM1 (Ortho)
CDW13:	My7 (CC)
CDw14:	FMC17 (SL)
	Leu M1 (B/D) (+ fraction of B cells)
-	Leu M5 (+ hairy cells)
-	Mon1 (BRL)

Other antibodies:

I Generally occurring:

HLA-ABC:	W6/32 (SL)
	34/28 HLK (SL)
HLA-DR:	OKIa (Ortho)
	L243 (B/D)
Transferrin receptor	MonCS 1009 (San)
	B3/25 (Hy)

II Partially restricted.

epithelial cells:	HMFG2 (Unip)
	HMFG1 (Unip)
	EMA115 D8 (Euro)
	CEA F6 (CIS)
melanoma	NK1 C3 (EORTC)
	MA 7001(San) Ma 7002 (San)
hemato-/ lymphopoietic	Common leucocyte antigen:
	DAKO-LC, MAL (Clonab)
	C3b receptor: DAKO C3br.
	Interleukin 2 receptor: a IL2r (B/D, Clonab).

III Restricted

Thrombocytic/megakaryocytic :	C8.13 (CLB)
	C17.27 (CLB)
Dendritic cells:	DRC1 (Dako)
K/ NK cells :	Leu7 (B/D)
Endothelial cells :	Mon HA 6001 (San)

II. SUPPLIERS/DISTRIBUTORS

Dako=Dakopatts a/s Produktionsvej 42. P.O.Box 1359
DK 2600 Glostrup Denmark

San= Sanbio b.v. P.O.Box 540, 5400 AM Uden, the Netherlands

Euro= Eurodiagnostics b.v. P.O. Box 2820
7303 GC Apeldoorn, the Netherlands

C.L.B.= Central Laboratory for Blood Transfusion Service Amsterdam, The Netherlands.
Distributor: Amstelstad B.V. Dennenlaan 34 1161CR Zwanenburg, P.O.Box 9100 AC Amsterdam

B.D. = Becton Dickinson Monoclonal Center Inc. 2375 Garcia Avenue, Mountain View California 94043, USA

BRL = Bethesda Research Laboratories Life Technologies Inc. Gaithersburg Maryland 20877, USA

Unip = Unipath, distributor Bio Trading P.O. Box 32, 3648 ZG Wilnis, The Netherlands

CC = Coulter Clone: Coulter Electronics Limited, Northwell Drive Luton, Bedfordshire LU 33RH, England

Clonab: Biotest Serum Institute GmbH, D6072 Dreieich, W. Germany

C.I.S.: Compagnie Oris Industrie
CIS, France BP 21 91190 Gif sur Yvette, France

Hy = Hybritech Inc. 11085 Torreyana Road, San Diego, California 92121, USA

SL= Seralab Ltd. Crawley Down RH10 4FF, Sussex, England

ST = Serotec. Distributor: Instruchemie b.v., P.O.Box 1585, 1200 BN Hilversum, The Netherlands

EORTC: EORTC Melanoma Mabs Research and Development project: Dr. F.J. Lejeune. Institut Jules Bordet, Rue Héger-Bordet, 1000 Brussels, Belgium

ATCC: American Type Culture Collection, 12301 Park Lawn Drive, Rockville, Maryland 20852, USA

INDEX OF SUBJECTS

GPSR Compliance

The European Union's (EU) General Product Safety Regulation (GPSR) is a set of rules that requires consumer products to be safe and our obligations to ensure this.

If you have any concerns about our products, you can contact us on ProductSafety@springernature.com

In case Publisher is established outside the EU, the EU authorized representative is:

Springer Nature Customer Service Center GmbH
Europaplatz 3
69115 Heidelberg, Germany

Batch number: 10583998

Printed by Printforce, the Netherlands